Implementation Science

This core textbook introduces the key concepts, theories, models and frameworks used in implementation science, and supports readers applying them in research projects.

The first part of the book focuses on the theory of implementation science, providing a discussion of its emergence from the evidence-based practice movement and its connections to related topics such as innovation research. It includes chapters looking at a wide range of theories, methods and frameworks currently used in implementation science, and a chapter focusing on suitable theories that could be imported from other fields. The first part also addresses strategies and outcomes of implementation and discusses how researchers can build causal pathways adapted to their study. The second part of the book focuses squarely on putting the theory of implementation science to work in practice, with chapters discussing research methods used in the field and how to select the most appropriate approach. This section also features several chapters presenting in-depth case studies of specific applications.

This multidisciplinary text is an essential resource for graduate students from a range of healthcare backgrounds taking courses on implementation science, as well as researchers from medicine, nursing, public health, allied health, economics, political science, sociology and engineering.

Per Nilsen is a professor of social medicine and public health at Linköping University and a professor of implementation science at Halmstad University, Sweden.

Professor Nilsen has been providing thought leadership to the field of implementation science for many years. This new book provides a positive feast for those interested in learning more about implementation science. It tells the story of how we got to where we are and pulls together a compendium of key content ranging from theory to tools and techniques. This is definitely a book I will be recommending to students and colleagues to both dip into for information about key concepts and also to read from cover to cover.

Professor Annette Boaz, King's College London, UK

Professor Nilsen has been "making sense" of complex issues in implementation science for a long time. Indeed, he has been an international field leader, teacher and ambassador for implementation science since its early days. This book is the culmination of his efforts to communicate with clarity and guide by example. Packed with practical applications, it also provides a history of the field and guidance on where it needs to go (and not go). It will immediately become a core resource for my own teaching and mentoring.

Professor Geoffrey M. Curran, University of Arkansas
for Medical Sciences and University of Limerick, Ireland

The proliferation of specialist methods, models, frameworks and theories in implementation science makes for an increasingly complex and sometimes confusing field. This book identifies the core ideas and methods in implementation science, presents them in an accessible way and shows how they can be applied in practice. A book that does this is long overdue. It will be invaluable for students, early career researchers, health professionals, health system managers and policy makers.

Professor Carl May, London School of Hygiene
and Tropical Medicine, UK

I first met Professor Nilsen when he stayed in Hong Kong in 2017 as a Visiting Professor at the Chinese University of Hong Kong. There was burgeoning interest in implementation science at that time, but its importance has grown rapidly in Asia and I believe this book is very timely in Asia now. The insightful book provides a comprehensive understanding of the unique challenges and opportunities faced in implementing evidence-based interventions in diverse settings. It is an indispensable resource for anyone interested in implementation science and its application to solving real-world problems in Asia and beyond.

Associate Professor Vincent Chung, Jockey
Club School of Public Health and
Primary Care, Chinese University of Hong Kong

This book is a gift in providing an overview and multiple applications of commonly used theories and frameworks in implementation science. Importantly, it signals the importance of drawing deeply from theories and concepts from other fields and of the discipline of theorizing in implementation science. The authors, international experts, adeptly balance the need to provide a thorough overview of implementation science while maintaining a constructively critical stance that will advance the field in the years to come.

Associate Professor Byron J. Powell,
Washington University in St. Louis

Implementation Science
Theory and Application

Edited by Per Nilsen

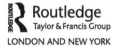

Routledge
Taylor & Francis Group

LONDON AND NEW YORK

Designed cover image: © Getty Images

First published 2024
by Routledge
4 Park Square, Milton Park, Abingdon, Oxon OX14 4RN

and by Routledge
605 Third Avenue, New York, NY 10158

Routledge is an imprint of the Taylor & Francis Group, an informa business

British Library Cataloguing-in-Publication Data
A catalogue record for this book is available from the British Library

Library of Congress Cataloging-in-Publication Data
Names: Nilsen, Per (Professor of social medicine and public health), editor.
Title: Implementing science : theory and application / edited by Per Nilsen.
Description: 1 edition. | New York, NY : Routledge, 2024. | Includes bibliographical
    references and index.
Identifiers: LCCN 2023050497 (print) | LCCN 2023050498 (ebook) |
    ISBN 9781032330853 (hardback) | ISBN 9781032330846 (paperback) |
    ISBN 9781003318125 (ebook)
Subjects: LCSH: Research. | Evidence. | Evidence-based medicine.
Classification: LCC Q180.A1 .I587 2024 (print) | LCC Q180.A1 (ebook) |
    DDC 507.2—dc23/eng/20240131
LC record available at https://lccn.loc.gov/2023050497
LC ebook record available at https://lccn.loc.gov/2023050498

ISBN: 978-1-032-33085-3 (hbk)
ISBN: 978-1-032-33084-6 (pbk)
ISBN: 978-1-003-31812-5 (ebk)

DOI: 10.4324/9781003318125

Typeset in Sabon LT Pro
by Apex CoVantage, LLC

Contents

List of figures and tables

Figures

List of tables

List of contributors

Gregory A. Aarons, PhD is a clinical and organizational psychologist, Professor of Psychiatry at University of California Diego (UCSD), Director of the Child and Adolescent Services Research Center and Co-Director of the UCSD ACTRI Dissemination and Implementation Science Center and IN-STEP Team Effectiveness Center, USA. His research, funded by the US National Institutes of Health, Centers for Disease Control and William T. Grant Foundation, focuses on identifying and improving system, organizational and individual factors that support implementation and sustainment of evidence-based practices in health and allied health care settings, involving multi-level leadership alignment. He co-developed the Exploration, Preparation, Implementation, Sustainment (EPIS) framework. Dr Aarons's recent projects seek to align policies with payment and quality metrics for public sector behavioural health treatment agencies, HIV prevention and implementation of cancer control, with work in the USA, Mexico, Norway and sub-Saharan Africa.

Hanna Augustsson is a Research specialist at the Medical Management Centre, Karolinska Institute and an implementation specialist at the Center for Epidemiology and Community Medicine, Region Stockholm, Sweden. Dr Augustsson's research interests include implementation and evaluation of evidence-based practices, interventions and organizational changes, particularly in the context of health and social care. Her research also addresses equity issues in relation to implementation and she has a focus on the de-implementation of low-value care from the perspectives of healthcare professionals' and from a governance perspective.

Mark S. Bauer is Professor of Psychiatry, Emeritus, at Harvard Medical School, USA. Dr Bauer's career-long passion has been improving care for those with serious mental health conditions. His focus has been in particular on how to organize systems of care using the Collaborative Chronic Care Model (CCM) to improve care quality, clinical outcomes and quality of life. The challenge of moving evidence-based models like the CCM off the shelf and into widespread practice galvanized his interest in implementation science. His dual expertise in clinical trials and implementation science bridges the gap between these two critically important areas of healthcare research.

Theresa S. Betancourt is the inaugural Salem Professor in Global Practice at the Boston College School of Social Work and Director of the Research Program on Children and Adversity, USA. Her primary research interests are understanding risk and protective processes shaping risky and resilient mental health and child development outcomes. Dr Betancourt has led initiatives to adapt and test evidence-based behavioural and parenting interventions and strategies for scaling out these interventions. She is Principal Investigator of a National Institute of Mental Health-funded intergenerational study of war/prospective longitudinal study of war-affected youth in Sierra Leone, research on scaling a home-visiting intervention to promote early childhood development and prevent violence among families in poverty with a child (0–3 years) in Rwanda and participatory research to adapt and test family-based prevention programmes among Somali Bantu, Bhutanese and Afghan resettled families in the USA.

Sarah A. Birken is an Associate Professor in the Department of Implementation Science in the School of Medicine at Wake Forest University School of Medicine and a member of the Comprehensive Cancer Center, USA. Dr Birken's research focuses on translating evidence into practice. Specifically, Dr Birken studies middle managers' role in implementing evidence-based practices, the implementation of innovations in cancer care, improving care coordination and the selection and application of implementation theories.

Ingemar Bohlin is a Senior Lecturer in Theory of Science at the Department of Philosophy, Linguistics and Theory of Science, University of Gothenburg, Sweden. His research covers a range of topics, always relying on analytical tools from the area of Science and Technology Studies. In recent years his research has addressed formats in which primary research is being synthesized in order to make relevant evidence available to policymakers and professional practitioners in different areas, including medicine, education and climate policy. A central theme in Bohlin's analyses of formats employed for this purpose is the type and degree of standardization adopted and the concomitant tension between formalized procedures and informal, professional competence.

Matthew Chinman, PhD, is a Senior Behavioral Scientist at the RAND Corporation and a Research Career Scientist at Veterans Affairs Pittsburgh Healthcare System, USA. Dr Chinman is a psychologist who has focused on developing and conducting randomized trials on implementation strategies, most notably Getting To Outcomes, and developing frameworks to support implementation science including the Expert Recommendations for Implementing Change (ERIC) and the Implementation Replication Framework (IRF).

Erika L. Crable, PhD, MPH is an Assistant Professor and health services researcher at the University of California San Diego (UCSD), an Investigator with the UCSD ACTRI Dissemination and Implementation Science Center and an alumna of the Implementation Research Institute, USA. Dr Crable's research focuses on developing and testing dissemination and implementation strategies aimed at improving evidence-informed policymaking related to substance use treatment services. Her research addresses government and organizational policies that influence access to and the quality of services delivered in publicly funded settings. Her research employs dissemination and implementation science strategies to mitigate structural barriers to behavioural health services for low-income and criminal-legal involved populations. She is currently conducting research studies at national scale across the USA and in Norway.

Danielle D'Lima is the Teaching Lead for the UCL Centre for Behaviour Change, UK. Her role includes designing and delivering teaching and training in Behaviour Change, as well as overseeing research projects on Implementation Science. She has an evolving interest in capacity building in Behaviour Change Science and Implementation Science as well as the application of these to the education setting. Danielle has a PhD from Imperial College London on the influence of feedback on professional behaviour change in healthcare. She has been involved in research projects on patient safety in the mental health setting, the use of routinely collected information for quality improvement in the NHS and process evaluation methodology.

Signe Flottorp is a senior researcher at the Division for Health Services at the Norwegian Institute of Public Health and professor at the Department of Health Management and Health Economics, Institute of Health and Society at the University of Oslo, Norway. Signe is a general practitioner and has worked in primary care for more than 30 years, though she left clinical practice in 2013. Since 1994, she has mainly focused on health services research exploring how to support informed decisions in health care. She has been involved in several projects both to conduct and improve methods for systematic reviews, guideline development and implementation research. She is among the founding members of the GRADE working group and a member of the editorial team of the Effective Practice and Organisation of Care (EPOC) Group in Cochrane.

Russell E. Glasgow is the Director of the Dissemination and Implementation Science Program of ACCORDS (https://bit.ly/2BnJzuk) and research professor in the Department of Family Medicine at the University of Colorado School of Medicine, USA. Dr Glasgow is one of the original developers of the RE-AIM (www.re-aim.org), PRISM and Dynamic Sustainability frameworks and currently directs an NIH-funded implementation science centre in cancer control. He is an implementation scientist whose work focuses on public health issues of studying and enhancing the reach and adoption of evidence-based programmes; assessing and guiding contextually based adaptations; and pragmatic research methods and measures to enhance health equity and sustainment.

Rebecca J. Guerin is a behavioural scientist and chief of the Social Science and Translation Research Branch, National Institute for Occupational Safety and Health, US Centers for Disease Control and Prevention, USA. Her research focuses on improving public health outcomes in community settings by designing and delivering evidence-based interventions to reduce job-related injuries and enhance well-being among worker populations at increased risk. Dr Guerin uses dissemination and implementation (D&I) science models, methods, and measures to expand the equitable reach, adoption, implementation, and sustained use of these interventions and to build partnerships and D&I capacity in the occupational safety and health community.

Gillian Harvey is a Matthew Flinders Professor of Health Services and Implementation Research in the College of Nursing and Health Sciences at Flinders University, Adelaide, Australia. She is a Deputy Director (Knowledge Translation) in the College's Caring Futures Institute and a Co-Director in Aged Care Research and Industry Innovation Australia (ARIIA). Her research interests are in implementation science, knowledge translation and quality improvement, spanning theory development and the development and testing of implementation interventions.

Rene Hawkes is a Research Project Manager at the Kaiser Permanente Washington Health Research Institute, Seattle, Washington, USA. She has 24 years' experience managing public health research studies, including Clinical Trials, Pragmatic Trials and studies embedded within healthcare delivery systems and community hospitals. Her research portfolio has included Complementary and Integrative Health modalities for Chronic Low Back Pain, Neck Pain and Generalized Anxiety Disorder, Animal Assisted Activities for Pediatric Cancer Patients and improving alignment with evidence based treatments for Pediatric Acute Respiratory Tract Infections. She has experience with mixed methods and draws on her research experience to help research teams embed implementation science methods within their studies.

Alyson Hillis is a Research Fellow in the Health Services Research and Policy (HSRP) department of the Public Health and Policy (PHP) faculty at the London School of Hygiene and Tropical Medicine (LSHTM), UK. Dr Hillis's research largely encompasses qualitative methodologies and systematic reviews or evidence syntheses, with interests in incorporating equity, power and justice into the implementation science field, particularly relating to service delivery; sexual health and HIV; travel medicine; prisoner health; and women's health and rights (reproduction and menstruation practices).

Jodi Summers Holtrop is the Associate Director of the Dissemination and Implementation Science Program of ACCORDS (https://bit.ly/2BnJzuk) and Professor and Vice Chair for Research in the Department of Family Medicine at the University of Colorado School of Medicine, USA. Dr Holtrop is an implementation scientist whose work focuses on study designs and methods, particularly qualitative and mixed methods. As a master certified health education specialist with 25 years in Family Medicine, her research centres on improving health promotion and preventive care in primary care. She has lead research in smoking cessation, chronic disease management, diabetes prevention, and obesity treatment in primary care.

Amy G. Huebschmann is a primary care physician and Associate Professor at the University of Colorado School of Medicine in the Division of General Internal Medicine. Dr Huebschmann's independent line of research inquiry seeks to advance the dissemination and implementation (D&I) science methods available to translate evidence-based interventions into real-world practice settings with attention to health equity concerns. Huebschmann currently serves as MPI and lead D&I investigator for one of only seven NHLBI-funded UG3/UH3 dissemination trials to improve cardiopulmonary disparities and is the lead D&I co-investigator or consultant on several other NIH-funded studies.

Sarah C. Hunter is a Research Fellow in a Joint Position between Flinders University and Wellbeing SA. Dr Hunter is a social psychologist and implementation scientist, and she applies her knowledge translation and implementation skills to shape an evidence-informed Early Years System in Australia that engages and supports parents and caregivers. Her research focuses on understanding the complex and diverse ways in which caregivers enact child rearing and how they navigate services and support. This programme of research intersects with implementation science as it explores facilitating and implementing evidence into complex multi-sector systems, with a focus on the contextual and recipient factors that influence success.

Soohyun Hwang is a Research Scientist Intern at VivoSense. Dr Hwang's research focuses on improving the quality of cancer care across the cancer care continuum by engaging various stakeholders and using mixed methods. Currently, Dr Hwang's research focuses on improving patient experiences in clinical trials and ensuring patient-centred approaches in clinical trials with wearable technology.

Ryan G. Kenneally received her Bachelor of Arts degree with honours from Emory University in 2022, majoring in Psychology and Sociology. Ryan currently works as an Organizational Research Assistant at the Child and Adolescent Services Research Center within the University of California San Diego Department of Psychiatry, assessing the impact of organizational- and system-level factors that influence the delivery of behavioural healthcare. Her research interests include the implementation, dissemination and sustainment of evidence-based practices in mental health and substance use treatment and the use of research evidence in multi-level outer- and inner-context service settings.

Sobia Khan is the Director of Implementation at the Center for Implementation based in Canada. She is an award-winning expert on how to practically implement complex interventions in complex systems. Globally, she has supported and advised both researchers and practitioners on over one hundred change initiatives across five continents, integrating multiple fields such as implementation science, systems thinking and social network theory to achieve meaningful and large-scale change. She emphasizes pragmatic and equity-driven approaches, with a particular focus on the need for relationship building, advocacy and collective action to create change at all levels of the system.

JoAnn E. Kirchner, MD, is Professor, Department of Psychiatry, at the University of Arkansas for Medical Sciences and an implementation science leader in the US Department of Veterans Affairs. The primary focus of her research has been developing, evaluating and spreading strategies that support the implementation of clinical innovations in settings unable to implement programmes without assistance. Her most recent work supports the transfer of evidence-based implementation strategies to implementation practitioners.

Alison L. Kitson is the Vice President and Executive Dean of the College of Nursing and Health Sciences at Flinders University in South Australia. Professor Kitson is recognized internationally as a leading research translation scientist, nurse leader and champion of improving fundamentals of care research and practice. In 2019, she established the Caring Futures Institute, the first research institute in Australia fully dedicated to the study of self-care and caring solutions as an answer to rising complex health challenges. Professor Kitson has published over 300 peer reviewed articles and has received many honours in recognition of her work in knowledge translation, fundamentals of care and nursing leadership.

Predrag "Pedja" Klasnja, PhD, is an Associate Professor in the School of Information at the University of Michigan. He focuses on the design and optimization of novel mHealth technologies for health behaviour change. He is particularly interested in the design and evaluation of just-in-time adaptive interventions (JITAIs), interventions that continuously adapt their functioning to provide optimal support to individuals as their needs and circumstances change. In addition to his intervention development work, Dr Klasnja develops optimization methods for implementation science, with an emphasis on causal modelling of processes hypothesized to underlie the functioning of implementation strategies.

Bethany M. Kwan, PhD, MSPH is an Associate Professor and Associate Vice Chair for Research in the Department of Emergency Medicine at the University of Colorado School of Medicine, Anschutz Medical Campus, USA. She is a dissemination and implementation (D&I) scientist with the University of Colorado's Adult & Child Center for Outcomes Research and Delivery Science (ACCORDS). She is the Director of D&I for the Colorado Clinical & Translational Sciences Institute (CCTSI). Her research addresses community and partner engagement and methods for designing for dissemination and pragmatic trials, chronic disease self-management, and enhancing quality of life for patients and care partners.

Cara C. Lewis, PhD, is the Deputy Director of the Center for Translation Research and Implementation Science at the National Heart, Lung and Blood Institute within the National Institutes of Health in Bethseda, Maryland, USA. Dr Lewis has a Ph.D. in clinical psychology with research expertise focused on advancing pragmatic and rigorous measures and methods for implementation science and practice.

Fabiana Lorencatto is the Research Lead at the Centre for Behaviour Change, University College London, UK. Dr Lorencatto is a psychologist by background with expertise in behavioural and implementation science. Her research focuses on the application of behavioural science theories, frameworks and methods to identify the individual, socio-cultural and environmental influences on behaviour, as a basis for the designing theory- and evidence-based interventions. Her research has primarily focused on healthcare provider behaviour change and healthcare quality improvement across a range of areas, such as antimicrobial resistance and maternal health. She is an Associate Editor of Implementation Science Communications and has a particular methodological interest in process evaluations and evidence synthesis of healthcare quality improvement interventions.

Kayne D. Mettert is a research specialist at Kaiser Permanente Washington Health Research Institute (KPWHRI) in Seattle, Washington, USA, and a graduate student pursuing a PhD in clinical psychology at the University of Washington, Seattle. Kayne's research focuses on the convergence of evidence-based interventions for substance and alcohol use disorders with implementation and dissemination methodology and measurement. He is particularly interested in bridging the gap between research and practice, ultimately striving to improve the lives of individuals struggling with addiction.

Rosemary D. Meza, PhD, is a Collaborative Scientist and Clinical Psychologist at Kaiser Permanente Washington Health Research Institute (KPWHRI) in Seattle, Washington, USA. Her work focuses improving pragmatic models of mental health care delivery, designing interventions to leverage leaders and supervisors in improving innovation implementation and advancing methods to improve the rigor of implementation science.

Julia E. Moore is the Executive Director of the Center for Implementation, a social enterprise based in Canada that trains, supports and empowers individuals and organizations in applying theory and evidence-informed change methods to improve outcomes.

She is known internationally for her ability to communicate complex implementation science concepts in clear and actionable ways. As an expert on the practical applications of implementation science, her work focuses on the spread and scale of accessible training and supporting hundreds of change initiatives around the world. She has designed and taught courses and workshops taken by over 10,000 professionals from a wide range of fields.

Margit Neher is a Senior Lecturer in Implementation Science at Halmstad University, Sweden. Dr Neher' s research has included implementation of diverse clinical interventions within cardiology, cancer rehabilitation and family health promotion. Her current research addresses challenges related to the complexity of implementing information-driven healthcare solutions, including artificial intelligence systems and applications. Dr Neher has a research focus on the learning processes related to change in individuals, groups and organizations.

Andrea Nevedal, PhD, is an Investigator and Senior Qualitative Methodologist with the VA Center for Clinical Management Research in Ann Arbor, Michigan, USA. Dr Nevedal is a medical anthropologist whose research focuses on understanding the socio-cultural dimensions of health/illness and health care delivery. She also focuses on understanding long-term sustainment of evidence-based innovations and advancing the field of rapid qualitative methods, especially in using the Consolidated Framework for Implementation.

Per Nilsen is a Professor of Social Medicine and Public Health at Linköping University and a Professor of Implementation Science at Halmstad University, Sweden. An economist by training at Stockholm School of Economics, Sweden, Nilsen was responsible for building a research and educational programme on implementation science at Linköping University, including a PhD course which is running annually since 2011. He takes particular interest in applying concepts and theories from beyond implementation science for improved understanding of the challenges involved in achieving practice change. Nilsen has broad interests and has also authored books on rock artists like Prince, David Bowie and Iggy & the Stooges.

Lorella Palazzo, PhD, is a Collaborative Scientist and Sociologist at Kaiser Permanente Washington Health Research Institute (KPWHRI) in Seattle, Washington, USA, who specializes in optimizing care delivery and improving access to health services. She has extensive experience in evaluating health care improvement efforts using implementation science and mixed methods. Dr Palazzo has used this expertise to assess the progress and results of projects from pilots to pragmatic clinical trials. She has supported research at KPWHRI on aging and dementia, cancer, paediatrics, mental health, substance use disorders and safe medication use.

Mónica Pérez Jolles, PhD, MA, is an Associate Professor in the Department of Pediatrics at the University of Colorado School of Medicine, USA. Dr Pérez Jolles is also a Faculty and co-leads the Equity and Engagement workgroup at the Dissemination and Implementation Science Program at ACCORDS. She is a health services and implementation scientist seeking to close the health gap through team-based science and co-creation partner engagement. Her focus is on supporting Federally Qualified Health Centers in their efforts to implement complex interventions; particularly family-centred and trauma-informed care, and the implementation of psychosocial screenings to address social determinants of health.

James Pittman, PhD, LCSW is an Associate Professor at the University of California, San Diego, School of Medicine, Department of Psychiatry and a consultant with the UC San Diego Dissemination and Implementation Science Center, USA. Dr Pittman oversees Integrative Mental Health Services and Mental Health Social Work at the VA San Diego Healthcare System. His research focuses the development and implementation of technology to improve healthcare and the use of multicomponent implementation strategies to support adoption of complex interventions.

Michael D. Pullmann, PhD, is a methodologist and biostatistician at the University of Washington in Seattle, USA. His research focuses on digital mental health, the possible unforeseen consequences and outcomes associated with implementation strategies and community-based and participatory approaches in cross-system collaborative efforts to serve youth and families with complex needs. He provides research and methodological leadership across multiple research centres, including the UW School Mental Health Assessment, Research and Training (SMART) Center, the UW ALACRITY Center and the UW Impact Center.

Borsika A. Rabin is an Associate Professor at the UC San Diego Herbert Wertheim School of Public Health and Human Longevity Science and the Co-Director of the University of California San Diego Dissemination and Implementation Science Center (http://disc.ucsd.edu). Dr Rabin's research focuses on improving population health outcomes in clinical and public health settings through co-creation with partners with the intent to increase the equitable reach, adoption, implementation, and sustained use of evidence-based interventions. Dr Rabin has developed and implemented novel capacity building approaches for implementation science including the D&I Models in Health webtool and serves as the Co-Director for the ACCORDS D&I Science Certificate Program at the University of Colorado, USA.

Caitlin Reardon, MPH, studied Health Behavior and Health Education at the University of Michigan School of Public Health in Ann Arbor, Michigan, USA. She is a qualitative methodologist and a developer of both the Updated CFIR and the CFIR Outcomes Addendum. Ms. Reardon was trained and mentored by Ms. Laura Damschroder, the lead developer of the original CFIR, and has over 10 years of experience using the framework to plan and evaluate the implementation of diverse evidence-informed practices within and outside of healthcare settings; she has conducted and analysed hundreds of CFIR-based interviews. In addition, she has worked with and/or trained over one hundred investigators and analysts in the USA and abroad on using the CFIR.

Shari Rogal, MD, MPH, is an Associate Professor of Medicine, Surgery and Clinical and Translational Science at the University of Pittsburgh, USA, and the Co-Director of the Dissemination and Implementation Science Core of the Center for Health Equity Research and Promotion. As a gastroenterologist, transplant hepatologist and implementation scientist. Dr Rogal's research focuses on developing empirical approaches to select implementation strategies to improve the equity and quality of healthcare delivery.

Rachel Rosenblum, MD, is an Assistant Attending Physician at Memorial Sloan Kettering Cancer Center, New York, USA. Dr Rosenblum is a thoracic oncologist whose research focuses on the integration of palliative care with oncology care in patients with advanced cancer. She has used implementation science frameworks and quality improvement methodologies to inform the development of targeted strategies for early specialty palliative care implementation in various practice settings and patient populations.

Anne Sales is a nurse and Professor in the Sinclair School of Nursing and the Department of Family and Community Medicine in the School of Medicine at the University of Missouri in Columbia, USA, and she is the Associate Dean for Implementation Research and Health Delivery Effectiveness in the School of Medicine. She is also a Research Scientist at the Center for Clinical Management Research at the VA Ann Arbor Healthcare System. Her training is in nursing, sociology, health economics, econometrics and general health services research. She is a founding co-Editor-in-Chief of *Implementation Science Communications*. Her work involves theory-based design of implementation interventions, including understanding how feedback reports affect provider behaviour and impacts on patient outcomes, the role of social networks in implementation interventions and effective implementation methods using electronic health records and digital interventions. She has completed over 40 funded research projects, many focused on implementation research.

Christina R. Studts, PhD, MSW, MSPH is an Associate Professor in the Department of Pediatrics at the University of Colorado Anschutz Medical Campus, USA. She is an implementation scientist in the Dissemination & Implementation Science Program at ACCORDS and directs and co-teaches in the Dissemination & Implementation Science Graduate Certificate Program. Her research focuses on increasing the accessibility and acceptability of evidence-based behavioural parent training interventions with marginalized communities and populations. In this programme of research and in other projects she supports methodologically, Dr Studts focuses on assessment of context, engaging partners in adaptations, and implementation mapping to improve implementation outcomes.

Kristin Thomas is an Associate Professor in Public Health at the Department of Health, Medicine and Caring Sciences at Linköping University, Sweden. Her research interests are to understand the implementation processes in health promotion and disease prevention such as the use of new patient pathways, practice models and digital tools in healthcare. Her current research focuses on the implementation of interventions promoting mental health and wellbeing in childcare and school health care. She is also active in teaching and supervision of implementation science students at master and doctoral levels at Linköping University.

Katy E. Trinkley is an Associate Professor and implementation scientist at the University of Colorado in the Department of Family Medicine with secondary appointments in the Department of Biomedical Informatics and the Colorado Center for Personalized Medicine, USA. She is also a primary care clinical pharmacist and clinical informaticist at UCHealth. Dr Trinkley's research focuses on advancing the visionary goals of learning health systems and leveraging data and implementation science to create innovative health information technologies to optimize safe and effective medication use. Much of her research focuses on clinical decision support tools within the electronic health record to optimize therapies for chronic cardiovascular disease.

Bryan J. Weiner, PhD, is Professor, Department of Global Health and Department of Health Services, at the University of Washington, Seattle, USA. Dr Weiner's research focuses on the adoption, implementation and sustainability of innovations and evidence-based practices in health care delivery and other organizational settings. He has studied a wide range of innovations including quality improvement practices, care management practices, patient safety practices, clinical information systems, collaborative service delivery models, cancer prevention and control in communities and evidence-based diabetes practices. His research has advanced implementation science by creating new knowledge about the organizational determinants of effective implementation, introducing and developing new theories and improving the state of measurement in the field.

Michel Wensing is professor and head of the Master of Science programme for health services research and implementation science at Heidelberg University, Germany. He is a social scientist with an interest in healthcare practice, particularly primary care. His work focuses on the organization and delivery of healthcare, concepts and strategies of implementation and patients' perspectives. He is also deputy head of the Department of General Practice and Health Services Research at Heidelberg University Hospital. After receiving degrees in sociology and the medical sciences, he conducted research on the implementation of clinical guidelines, the organization of ambulatory healthcare and patients' perspectives on healthcare. He has been a member of the *Implementation Science* editorial team since the journal started in 2006. From 2012 until 2022, he was co-Editor-in-Chief.

Preface

Per Nilsen

Research is often depicted as a pipeline or process that begins with basic research, followed by increasingly applied research, ultimately leading to the adoption of research findings that benefit the health and welfare of individuals and societies. However, there are countless examples that indicate that the progression from discovery to application is not as straightforward or unproblematic as is implied in linear models like this. History has shown that the proof of the beneficial effect of an intervention is not sufficient in itself to guarantee adoption. A classic example of this is the fight against scurvy. It took almost 200 years from the discovery that lemon juice could save the lives of sailors to the introduction of daily intake of vitamin C into the diet of the fleet. Other more recent examples include dialysis treatment, which did not come into widespread use until the 1960s, despite the availability of a fully usable method of haemodialysis already around 1940. Penicillin also took two decades to become more widely accessible after Fleming's discovery in 1928. These examples are consistent with the frequently quoted statement that it takes 17 years to turn 14% of original research to real benefit in patient care.

However, there is not always a long lapse between scientific discovery and routine practice. Two notable examples of shorter routes from research to practice are antiretroviral medicines to stop HIV replicating in the body, and drug-eluting stents to reopen and maintain coronary arteries narrowed by arteriosclerosis. A recent success story is that of COVID-19 vaccines, which were developed and made available faster than any other vaccine against a new disease in history. Before COVID-19, it often took a decade or longer to develop and make a vaccine widely available to the public. The COVID-19 vaccine was developed and approved for use in less than a year, showing what can be achieved when a large-scale and coordinated effort is in place.

The fact that research-to-practice diffusion processes take very varied amounts of time in different instances raises obvious questions about the reasons or explanations for these differences. What factors influence the implementation of research findings? Why are some research results quickly translated into practice and policy, whereas other findings may take decades to achieve impact? What strategies might be used to speed up the process from research to practice? Why do some practices spread widely despite a lack of convincing evidence? Questions like these have become increasingly important in times of high expectations of the benefit of the results of research for individuals and society.

Implementation science has emerged in response to the challenges of getting evidence into practice and achieving an evidence-based practice. If an intervention is poorly implemented, or not implemented at all, then it is unlikely to produce its expected benefits.

Many studies have shown positive relationships between the level of implementation of a given intervention and quality of outcomes for the end-users, highlighting the importance of implementation. The need for practice to be informed by the most up-to-date, valid and reliable research findings has become a self-evident truth, a mantra expressed by a vast range of societal actors, including government agencies, professional organizations, policy makers, managers, practitioners and researchers.

The focus of implementation science is usually the study of factors, including contextual influences, that impact on the implementation of evidence-based practices (interventions, programmes, services, etc.) in healthcare and other areas of society. It is also the study of strategies to support the implementation based on the recognition that this evidence does not spread automatically. However, implementation science can also be much more; for example, studies presenting economic evaluations of implementation endeavours, matching determinants and strategies, investigating how adaptations influence implementation outcomes, identifying determinants of sustainability of evidence-based practices and evaluating strategies to support de-implementation of low-value care.

The origins of implementation science lie in numerous disciplines, and the field emerged in the 2000s under considerable expectations to accelerate the translation of scientific discovery into routine practice. The term implementation science came into being when the journal *Implementation Science* was launched in 2006. This journal quickly became a focal point for researchers involved in research on implementation. The field has seen a rapid expansion in recent years, with an almost doubling of the number of scientific publications every second year. Significant investments are being made in research funding, conferences, training and courses in implementation science.

My involvement in implementation science began in 2008 at Linköping University where I had defended my PhD thesis two years earlier. As it happened, I was co-supervising a PhD student who had read up on Rogers's Theory of Diffusion and was eager to apply some aspects of the theory in her PhD project which concerned provision of lifestyle advice in healthcare. She felt it would be more relevant to study why a particular intervention was adopted, or not, since evidence of effectiveness had already been demonstrated. The next year I was invited to head up a group of more junior researchers to lead research on implementation issues at Linköping University. The county council had decided to fund research to support more rapid implementation of new research-based knowledge. County councils are responsible for provision healthcare in Sweden, but they also invest in research and development to learn and improve healthcare. The local county council provided multi-year funding for research on the implementation of research in healthcare.

Thus, "implementation and learning" was appointed a strategic research area in 2009, with shared funding from the county council and Linköping University (its medical faculty). I felt, and still feel, learning is an integral but somewhat overlooked aspect of implementation since learning can be understood of changes in behaviours, attitudes, beliefs, etc., and implementation is essentially about changes. The concept of learning health systems also acknowledges the importance of learning to effect change and seek mechanisms to link learning with change. "Learning" also applied to what we did ourselves; it was a steep learning curve for all of us, researchers, teachers and students alike.

I immediately felt at home in implementation science, with its interdisciplinary and multi-professional approach. This research was a good fit with my background as an economist with an organizational perspective and several years of consultancy work for private and public organizations. Like many researchers who became involved in implementation science, I had previously done research with a focus on patients and populations, but I felt the new focus on the providers, both practitioners and organizations, was a better match with my background. My preceding research had also familiarized me with issues of implementation as my PhD thesis concerned injury prevention and my postdoctoral focus was on alcohol prevention, two fields where many interventions and programmes failed to spread or scale up despite convincing evidence.

Our implementation science programme launched several implementation science PhD projects, we developed a PhD course in implementation science (still running and attracting a highly international audience and with many guest lectures by prominent researchers in the field) and I assembled and edited a book (in Swedish) with contributions from researchers at the faculty that had expressed an interest in becoming involved. We invited several leading implementation science researchers for presentations and discussions. The PhD course generated many questions from participants, which prompted me to write a paper, "Making sense of implementation theories, models and frameworks". The paper has been a sort of "one-hit wonder" in terms of the number of citations, proving the need for an attempt to provide a structure of a large and growing number of theories, models and frameworks in the field.

Implementation science has developed into a thriving and close-knit community of researchers who are actively engaged in this field. Research in implementation science has become a collective and social endeavour that involves researchers across the globe with diverse perspectives, backgrounds and interests. For me, the opportunity to discuss, reflect and collaborate with numerous international and national researchers in the field has enriched my understanding of many implementation issues and the challenges of translating scientific discovery into routine practice. Many of these researchers have contributed to this book, for which I'm very grateful. It is my hope that this book will offer the reader insights into the topic of implementation science through the perspectives of chapter authors with a long experience and deep knowledge of different research and practice-related implementation issues.

The book is divided into two sections: the theory of implementation science and the practice of conducting implementation science research. The first section describes the historical roots of implementation science. It is important to provide a context for today's research in the field because this research did not appear in a vacuum. The book accounts for the fact that implementation science is an interdisciplinary endeavour; implementation problems and solutions are often multifaceted and need to be understood from multiple perspectives. Implementation science has drawn upon, and continues to be influenced by, an array of academic and scientific disciplines.

The first section of the book discusses several key concepts, theories, models and frameworks that can help scholars in the field to analyse and understand the challenges of implementation, including the changes required to achieve an evidence-based practice. This section also features a chapter on how to build causal pathways as an alternative to applying an existing approach.

The book also aims to facilitate hands-on research on implementation issues. Therefore, the second section of the book addresses numerous approaches for conducting implementation science research. This section features descriptions of research methods and study designs for use in this research and presents tools to select appropriate theories, models and frameworks. Several chapters are devoted to the application of theories, models and frameworks in studies of implementation issues. Although the "implementation" of implementation science as an academic endeavour has been successful, its impact on practice has been more limited. The final chapter of the book therefore explores some challenges that need to be addressed to maximize the impact of implementation science.

I am joined by the chapter authors in the hope that the book, with its collection of different concepts, theories, models, frameworks and tools of relevance in implementation science, will contribute not only to a wider knowledge about implementation science as a field, but also guide the reader in his or her own implementation project, be it academic or practice-based. Ultimately, the book hopes to inspire the readers to engage with the science of implementation and contribute to the development of the field. Improved understanding and explanation of implementation issues combined with the application of this knowledge can contribute to increased use of research findings to benefit the health and welfare of individuals and societies.

Part I

Theory

1 Origins of the evidence movement

Ingemar Bohlin

Introduction

In the early 1990s, Evidence-Based Medicine (EBM) was launched as a new medical training and practice paradigm. Ensuring that clinical practice is based on robust scientific evidence, the proponents of this concept argued, requires a new set of basic principles. Those principles were derived from areas that to a large extent had developed independently. This chapter outlines four separate lines of inquiry that converged in the emergence of EBM: the outcomes movement, clinical epidemiology, randomized clinical trials, and the methodology of research synthesis. The chapter provides a summary of these lines of development and their relevance for the birth of EBM. The final section addresses tensions between some of the developments.

The outcomes movement

In a series of publications appearing from the early 1970s on, epidemiologist John Wennberg demonstrated considerable variation in healthcare practices across regions in the United States. Drawing on local hospital discharge records as well as large national databases of health insurance claims such as Medicare and Medicaid, Wennberg found, for instance, that in Maine, the proportion of women aged 70 years who had undergone a hysterectomy was 20% in one hospital market and 70% in another, and that the proportion of children in Vermont who had a tonsillectomy ranged from 8% in one hospital market to almost 70% in another (Wennberg, 1984). Wennberg ascribed variations like these to "the practice style factor", that is, different approaches adopted locally within the medical profession. Alternative explanations have been proposed, such as that many medical conditions are unevenly distributed geographically, and that the pace at which new treatment methods are adopted across regions varies (Smits, 1986). These reservations notwithstanding, Wennberg's findings were received as clear evidence that at least in the United States, clinical decisions were not based on universally valid scientific knowledge to the extent one would expect.

In 1989, the Agency for Health Care Policy and Research (AHCPR) was set up in the United States. The responsibilities of the new agency included supporting research documenting the outcomes of medical interventions. This type of research, a recent development at the time, was sometimes referred to as medical treatment effectiveness research, but a more common term was patient outcomes research, or outcomes research, for short. The data included information about individual patients' interventions, complications and mortality, collected from databases of the kind on which Wennberg, who led

DOI: 10.4324/9781003318125-2

one of the agency's projects, had long been relying. The aim of the research funded by AHCPR was to document the outcomes of interventions within specific patient categories to build a knowledge base on the effectiveness and costs of various medical treatments. On the basis of this knowledge, guidelines supporting clinical decision-making were developed (Raskin and Maklan, 1991). In 1999, AHCPR was renamed the Agency for Healthcare Research and Quality, with a partly new mandate (Gray et al., 2003).

Guidelines for clinical practice had been issued by professional medical associations since the early 1930s. From the mid-1970s on, the number of published practice guidelines increased steadily, and in the early 1990s, their volume prompted the National Library of Medicine (responsible for Medline, the world's largest bibliographic database for biomedical literature) to define practice guidelines as a separate publication type (Weisz et al., 2007). By the late 1980s, the practice variations identified by Wennberg and colleagues of his were widely recognized among US policy makers responsible for healthcare, and guidelines for clinical practice offered a potential solution (Woolf, 1990). The foundation of AHCPR represented a significant step; a key part of its mandate was to regulate physicians' clinical decisions by means of guidelines. The act that established the new agency, signed by President Bush in December 1989, required the AHCPR to issue guidelines for the treatment of three medical conditions just 1 year later, in January 1991, and report to Congress on their effects on the quality and cost of medical care 2 years later (Woolf, 1990; Gray et al., 2003).

Outcomes research produces knowledge about the effects of specific interventions on large populations. The evidence generated is probabilistic. The rise of outcomes research represented a new phase in a long-standing conflict over whether laboratory science or statistics ought to provide the scientific foundation of medicine. Rosser Matthews (1995) documents successive phases in this conflict, covering debates in France, Germany and the United Kingdom from the early 19th to the mid-20th century. In the second half of the 19th century, Claude Bernard was a leading advocate of the view that medicine ought to become an experimental laboratory-based science, and a few decades later, the biometrical approach pioneered by Karl Pearson gave rise to the discipline of medical statistics. The link between medicine and mathematical statistics forged in this period subsequently became very strong, but before that, physiology, pathology and allied disciplines dominated medical training for several decades. This was partly due to the publication in 1910 of an influential report on medical education in the United States and Canada, in which the need for physicians to understand the basic mechanisms of disease was stressed (Bluhm and Borgerson, 2011; Newton, 2001). Biomedical science remained the fundament of medicine on both sides of the Atlantic in the post-World War II era.

Guidelines aimed at governing the practice of professional communities are typically perceived as a threat to their members' professional judgement. Given the medical profession's long-standing reliance on pathophysiology, practice guidelines based on population-based, probabilistic data could potentially conflict sharply with the professional discretion of physicians. To forestall resistance on the part of clinicians, some staff at AHCPR stressed that the practice guidelines issued by the agency were "meant to supplement, not supplant, what health care providers already know". The guidelines did not instantiate "a rigid form of 'cookbook medicine'", two AHCPR representatives asserted (Raskin and Maklan, 1991).

The approach of outcomes research grew strong in the course of the 1980s, particularly in the United States and the United Kingdom, and by the end of the decade the term "the outcomes movement" was introduced (Epstein, 1990). Apart from the clinical relevance of the data collected, this movement was driven by economic considerations. After World War II, healthcare expanded rapidly in the United States and expenses spiralled, and in the 1960s, serious efforts at containing expenditures began. The techniques by which data from large registries were gathered and analysed in outcomes research opened a new avenue for cost control, previous attempts at which had not been successful. Provided the costs of specific interventions are estimated, not only clinical decisions, but also policy decisions on which pharmaceuticals or surgical procedures to prioritize, too, may be based on information about the outcomes of interventions in large populations. In 1988, Arnold Relman, editor-in-chief of the *New England Journal of Medicine*, designated the emergence of outcomes research the third revolution in US healthcare; after the Eras of Expansion and Cost Containment, the US healthcare system was now about to enter "the Era of Assessment and Accountability" (Relman, 1988).

Clinical epidemiology and randomized clinical trials

At the time the outcomes movement was emerging, it had already been suggested that methods long used in public health might be useful in clinical practice. In the 1960s and 1970s, the term "clinical epidemiology" gradually came into use in the United States and Canada to designate a new approach to medical training and practice. The core idea was that clinical decisions about individual patients should be informed by epidemiological evidence, that is, findings from quantitative, population-based studies. Laboratory-based evidence on biological processes, to which medical training had long given priority, was increasingly regarded as an inadequate basis for clinical practice, and a new scientific foundation was deemed necessary (Daly, 2005). Clinical epidemiology, in other words, was part of the same shift that the outcomes movement helped bring about in the last few decades of the 20th century, from pathophysiology and allied disciplines to probabilistic, population-based evidence as the basis for medical practice.

The term clinical epidemiology was introduced in 1938 by John Paul, president of the American Society for Clinical Investigation, who went on to publish a book on the subject 20 years later (Paul, 1938, 1958). The principle that clinical decision-making needed to be based on epidemiological data was not widely accepted at the time, but in the first half of the 1980s, three separate volumes appeared bearing the same title as Paul's book published a quarter of a century previously, *Clinical Epidemiology* (Fletcher et al., 1982; Feinstein, 1985; Sackett et al., 1985).

Sackett et al. (1985) was a textbook whose three authors were all based at McMaster University outside Toronto. At the McMaster Medical School, the skill chiefly fostered in soon-to-be doctors was proficiency in identifying and assessing studies of potential relevance to any given clinical problem. Specifying procedures for doing this was at the core not only of clinical epidemiology as set out in the 1985 textbook by Sackett et al. but also of many later publications by the McMaster group. The significance they attributed to these procedures, referred to as comprising "critical appraisal", was such that that term was often used synonymously with clinical epidemiology. This emphasis on critical appraisal was consistent with a strongly sceptical attitude towards physicians' clinical experience and, in particular, recommendations issued by recognized experts. The McMaster group have consistently stressed the importance of randomized clinical trials (RCTs).

The use of control groups is a key step in the development of experimental methods. Randomized allocation to experiment and control groups is another. Each step has been taken at different points in different disciplines, often independently of developments in other areas. In American psychology and social science, for example, controlled experiments were common in the first decades of the 20th century (Oakley, 2000). A famous, much earlier example is the scurvy experiment conducted by James Lind, a Scottish naval surgeon, in the mid-18th century (Carpenter, 1986). Procedures of randomization were applied in experimental psychology in the mid-1880s (Stigler, 1978, 1999) and in educational research in the early 1920s (Oakley, 2000), in both cases in the United States. However, it was through the work of Ronald A. Fisher in the United Kingdom that randomization became an established statistical technique. Fisher's book *The Design of Experiments* has been particularly influential (Fisher, 1935).

Fisher's ideas, which were developed in the context of agricultural experimentation, were implemented rigorously in a clinical trial reported in 1948. In this trial, designed by Austin Bradford Hill, professor of medical statistics at the University of London, patients were randomly assigned either to the treatment group, receiving the substance whose effects were to be determined, or to the control group. Hill's 1948 study has widely been hailed as ground-breaking, opening a new era in medical research (Gehan and Lemak, 1994; Rosser Matthews, 1995). The standard for modern clinical trials, however, was not set by the medical profession or by the community of clinical researchers. It was through decisions made by regulatory bodies that the double-blind RCT was established as the required study design in medical research; double-blind means that neither patients nor investigators are aware of who receives the treatment tested. After a series of legal proceedings, the US Food and Drug Administration imposed this standard on the pharmaceutical industry in 1970, and by the late 1970s, the same standard had been adopted by government agencies in most western countries (Bodewitz et al., 1987; Rosser Matthews, 1995; Marks, 1997).

The textbook by Sackett et al. (1985) encouraged practising physicians to find answers to clinical problems themselves rather than rely on the judgement of some senior colleague. The book offered physicians hands-on guidance on how to appraise evidence of causation relevant to problems they were facing in their clinical practice. The guidance included "rules of evidence" by which the relative strength of methods used in clinical research can be determined. The advantages of randomized trials over other study designs were stressed again and again, and a simple scale placing RCTs at the top level, followed by cohort studies, case-control studies and case series was offered (Sacket et al., 1985, pp. 225, 297). In the revised and expanded second edition of the book, the term "study hierarchy" was introduced (Sackett et al., 1991). Dubbed the "hierarchy of evidence", an expanded version of the scale later became a central feature of evidence-based medicine (EBM) (e.g. Rinchuse et al., 2008; Greenhalgh, 2019). The latter term appeared twice in the 1991 edition of the McMaster textbook. It is mentioned in passing in the preface, and then in this remark, inserted under an asterisk in the concluding chapter: "Around our town, the incorporation of critical appraisal into clinical practice often is called 'evidence-based medicine'" (Sackett et al., 1991, pp. xii, 398). In an editorial appearing in a supplement to one of the main medical journals that same year, Gordon Guyatt, who had entered the author team for the book's second edition, outlined the new concept more fully (Guyatt, 1991).

It was in a programmatic article in the *Journal of the American Medical Association* the following year, however, that EBM was launched in a manner that drew wide attention. In this article, authored by a large collective chaired by Guyatt, the concept was presented as a new paradigm in medical practice (Evidence-Based Medicine Working Group, 1992). The new paradigm emphasized practitioners' skills in critical appraisal relying on rules of evidence, and de-emphasized clinical experience and the understanding of pathophysiological processes. The paradigm shift was a result, it was suggested, of recent advances in clinical research. Two methods were described as particularly important. One was the RCT, the other was meta-analysis, a technique that "may have as profound an effect on setting treatment policy as have randomized trials themselves" (Evidence-Based Medicine Working Group, 1992, p. 2420).

Meta-analysis and systematic reviews

By the early 1970s, the volume of research published in the social sciences had reached such a level that the adequacy of established routines for summarizing results was questioned. Hence, a new method proposed by Gene Glass, professor of educational psychology at Colorado University, as an alternative to reviews authored by experts not relying on any explicit method, was mostly received very favourably. Meta-analysis, as Glass (1976) called his innovation, was a technique for aggregating quantitative data from individual studies addressing similar topics. Glass and a colleague developed the method when compiling findings from almost 400 studies on the effects of psychotherapy (Smith and Glass, 1977), and they went on to summarize 80 studies on the effects of class size on pupils' achievements (Glass and Smith, 1979). Independently of Glass and his team, two other groups of social researchers developed similar statistical techniques in this period, but the term meta-analysis was quickly adopted. By the mid-1980s, a handful of textbooks on meta-analysis had appeared, including Glass et al. (1981), Light and Pillemer (1984) and Cooper (1984), and the method was fairly well established in the quantitative social sciences.

Although clinical trials of any given treatment tended to be much fewer at this point than the number of social science studies cited above, the need to resolve the uncertainty generated by studies yielding very different results was by no means less pressing. Some early attempts were made to collate quantitative data from separate clinical studies, and several articles with this aim appeared in the 1970s, but it was in the early 1980s that statistical procedures for aggregating results from series of clinical trials were seriously launched as a new method in medical research. A group of researchers, mainly based in Oxford, were among the leading proponents.

The first meta-analysis published by this group addressed the effect of intravenous infusion of streptokinase in patients with acute myocardial infarction. Eight clinical trials were identified, all of them small. Five trials indicated that streptokinase reduced mortality and three suggested an increased risk of death, but only two of the results were statistically significant. Combining the results, however, the Oxford researchers found that they indicated that intravenous streptokinase therapy reduced mortality by 20%, and this finding was statistically significant (Stampfer et al., 1982). In a larger meta-analysis by the same team 3 years later, the same result was confirmed and strengthened (Yusuf et al., 1985).

These and similar assessments of the evidence available for various interventions were hailed as valuable contributions to clinical research, but strong objections were also raised to the methodology adopted. The main problem to which sceptics drew attention was that of deciding which studies to include in a meta-analysis. There were two aspects to this problem, concerning the heterogeneity and quality, respectively, of the studies available. On the one hand, because interventions vary with respect to diagnostic instruments, substances, dosages, the composition of patient groups, etc., comparisons may be misleading, critics argued. How can the level of homogeneity across trials be determined so that meta-analyses may yield meaningful results? On the other hand, critics found it unacceptable that results of carefully conducted clinical trials were sometimes pooled with data from trials with obvious methodological flaws. In 1986, a workshop was convened in Bethesda, Maryland, providing advocates and detractors of the new method an opportunity to discuss its merits and limitations. As is clear from the proceedings (Yusuf et al., 1987), little by way of consensus emerged at the workshop. Yet the standing of meta-analysis in clinical research was consolidated in the late 1980s and early 1990s.

Among the participants at the Bethesda workshop was Thomas Chalmers, who had held positions at Mount Sinai Medical Center and many other institutions in the United States. Assuming the role of leading champion of medical meta-analysis at a theoretical and programmatic level, Chalmers argued emphatically that meta-analysis ought to be established as a scientific discipline. The analyses should be held to the same rigorous standards as the clinical trials whose findings were being aggregated. To ensure the objectivity and replicability of medical meta-analyses, and hence the reliability of the results produced, Chalmers and his collaborators developed guidelines for this type of synthesis (e.g. Sacks et al., 1987). Leaving aside the question of how closely these guidelines were heeded, the number of meta-analyses appearing in the medical literature increased sharply in this period. In 1991, the year before the significance of meta-analytical techniques was signalled in the multi-author paper launching EBM as a new paradigm, 431 medical meta-analyses were reportedly published, up from 21, 5 years earlier (Dickersin and Berlin, 1992).

Starting in the late 1970s, under the leadership of British obstetrician Iain Chalmers (no relation of Thomas Chalmers), numerous teams of researchers conducted meta-analyses addressing research on various aspects of pregnancy and childbirth. After the publication of a massive two-volume work (Chalmers et al., 1989), Chalmers encouraged his author teams to continue combining findings from clinical trials. This was the seed of what was to become the leading international organization producing syntheses of research on all aspects of healthcare. In 1992, the Cochrane Centre was set up in Oxford, named in honour of Archie Cochrane, an epidemiologist who had been Chalmers's mentor, with financial support from the National Health Service. The following year, the Cochrane Collaboration, an international network, was founded.

In the late 1980s and early 1990s, it was recognized that the basic steps of guidelines for the conduct of meta-analyses were as relevant for literature reviews in which no attempts to aggregate quantitative data were made. This suggested the need for a more general term than meta-analysis. In publications around the time the Cochrane Collaboration was established, Iain Chalmers (e.g. Chalmers et al., 1992) started using the term "systematic review". The term was soon adopted to denote syntheses conducted in accordance with formalized guidelines, primarily of RCTs. Consequently, meta-analysis now mostly refers to the statistical computations that are usually part of systematic reviews (for a fuller account of the history of research synthesis, see Bohlin, 2012).

Tensions

The previous sections have outlined the emergence of four distinct approaches in the history of medical research in the 20th century: the outcomes movement, clinical epidemiology, RCTs, and research synthesis. Each of these approaches has been described by commentators as the central component of EBM. For example, it has been suggested that, by the early 1990s, "the outcomes movement had evolved into evidence-based medicine" (Tanenbaum, 2006). John Wennberg, whose documentation of geographical variation in medical practice provided impetus for outcomes research in the 1980s, has been portrayed as one of the founding fathers of EBM, along with Archie Cochrane and David Sackett

(Timmermans and Berg, 2003). Cochrane's being cited in this context is due to the importance of systematic reviews, which have been described as a cornerstone of EBM (e.g. Petticrew, 2001) or of the entire evidence movement (e.g. Dixon-Woods, 2006).

However, the manner in which EBM is related to the four distinct lines of inquiry considered in this chapter is more complex than is often assumed. Space does not allow a detailed discussion of parallels and disparities between the approaches addressed above, or between EBM and each of the others; a few remarks about discrepancies will have to suffice here concerning the relationship between randomized experiments and outcomes research, on the one hand, and between EBM and research synthesis methods, on the other.

From the early 1970s on, computerized databases containing information about individual patients' medical conditions, interventions they had undergone and outcomes of those interventions were proposed as a key resource for clinical practice (for an early example, see Rosati et al., 1973). From an early stage, the clinical significance of this type of data was questioned by researchers stressing the power of randomized trials (e.g. Byar, 1980). This dispute, in which the methodological rigour of well-conducted RCTs was set against the relevance of data gathered in actual healthcare practice, intensified in the early 1990s when the AHCPR started providing generous funding for outcomes research (Tanenbaum, 1995). Even though the evidence generated both by outcomes research and by RCTs is probabilistic and population-based, as opposed to evidence of physiological mechanisms, the issue of relevance versus rigour has been a constant source of tension between the two methods.

Another divide separates critical appraisal from research synthesis methods. In an editorial appearing some years after the launch of the concept of EBM, a team of McMaster clinical epidemiologists led by Gordon Guyatt distinguished between "evidence-based practitioners" and "evidence users". The former term refers to clinicians who have acquired the skills to identify, appraise and apply evidence from the primary medical literature, whereas the latter refers to those who rely, instead, on systematic reviews, clinical practice guidelines and other forms of "pre-appraised" evidence. The editorial was an admission that many clinicians – a majority, even – were not prepared to invest the time and effort needed to acquire the skills of critical appraisal, the teaching of which had been a top priority at McMaster from the outset (Guyatt et al., 2000). Interviewed a few years later, Guyatt affirmed that he had found it hard to abandon his view of the central task of EBM and that composing that brief editorial had cost him "a year of agonizing" (Daly, 2005).

In short, the four lines of inquiry traced in this chapter, providing building blocks for what would become evidence-based medicine and, subsequently, what is often referred to as the evidence movement, did not form a homogeneous entity. The constituents are interrelated in complex ways involving some deep tensions.

Acknowledgements

Two previous versions of this chapter have appeared in Swedish (Bohlin, 2011, 2014).

References

Bluhm, R., Borgerson, K. (2011) Evidence-based medicine. In: Gifford, F. (Ed.), *Philosophy of Medicine*. Amsterdam: Elsevier, pp. 203–238. https://doi.org/10.1016/B978-0-444-51787-6.50008-8

Bodewitz, H.J.H.W., Buurma, H., deVries, G.H. (1987) Regulatory science and the social management of trust in medicine. In: Bijker, W.E., Hughes, T.P., Pinch, T. (Eds.), *The Social Construction of Technological Systems*. Cambridge, MA: MIT Press, pp. 243–259.

Bohlin, I. (2011) Evidensbaserat beslutsfattande i ett vetenskapsbaserat samhälle: Om eviden-srörelsens ursprung, utbredning och gränser. In: Bohlin, I., Sager, M. (Eds.), *Evidensens många ansikten: Evidensbaserad praktik i praktiken*. Lund: Arkiv förlag, pp. 31–68.

Bohlin, I. (2012) Formalizing syntheses of medical knowledge: the rise of meta-analysis and systematic reviews. *Perspectives on Science* 20, 273–309. https://doi.org/10.1162/POSC_a_00075

Bohlin, I. (2014) Evidensrörelsens ursprung. In: Nilsen, P. (Ed.), *Implementering av evidensbaserad praktik*. Malmö: Gleerups, pp. 23–42.

Byar, D.P. (1980) Why data bases should not replace randomized clinical trials. *Biometrics* 36, 337–42. https://doi.org/10.2307/2529989

Carpenter, K.J. (1986) *The History of Scurvy and Vitamin C*. Cambridge: Cambridge University Press.

Chalmers, I., Enkin, M., Keirse, M.J.N.C. (Eds.) (1989) *Effective Care in Pregnancy and Child-birth*. Oxford: Oxford University Press.

Chalmers, I., Dickersin, K., Chalmers, T.C. (1992) Getting to grips with Archie Cochrane's agenda. *BMJ* 305, 786–788. https://doi.org/10.1136/bmj.305.6857.786

Cooper, H.M. (1984) *The Integrative Research Review: A Systematic Approach*. Beverly Hills, CA: Sage.

Daly, J. (2005) *Evidence-Based Medicine and the Search for a Science of Clinical Care*. Berkeley, CA: University of California Press; New York: Milbank Memorial Fund.

Dickersin, K., Berlin, J.A. (1992) Meta-analysis: state of the science. *Epidemiologic Reviews* 14, 154–176. https://doi.org/10.1093/oxfordjournals.epirev.a036084

Dixon-Woods, M. (2006) Evidence from qualitative and quantitative research. In: Killoran, A., Swann, C., Kelly, M.P. (Eds.), *Public Health Evidence: Tackling Health Inequalities*. Oxford: Oxford University Press, pp269–282.

Epstein, A.M. (1990) The outcomes movement – will it get us where we want to go? *New England Journal of Medicine* 323, 266–270. https://doi.org/10.1056/NEJM199007263230410

Evidence-Based Medicine Working Group (1992) Evidence-based medicine: a new approach to teaching the practice of medicine. *JAMA* 268, 2420–2425. https://doi.org/10.1001/jama.268.17.2420

Feinstein, A.R. (1985) *Clinical Epidemiology: The Architecture of Clinical Research*. Philadelphia, PA: Saunders.

Fisher, R.A. (1935) *The Design of Experiments*. Edinburgh: Oliver & Boyd.

Fletcher, R.H., Fletcher, S.W., Wagner, E.H. (1982) *Clinical Epidemiology: The Essentials*. Baltimore, MD: William & Wilkins.

Gehan, E.A., Lemak, N.A. (1994) *Statistics in Medical Research: Developments in Clinical Trials*. London: Plenum. https://doi.org/10.1007/978-1-4615-2518-9

Glass, G.V. (1976) Primary, secondary, and meta-analysis of research. *Educational Researcher* 5(10), 3–8. https://doi.org/10.3102/0013189X005010003

Glass, G.V., Smith, M.L. (1979) Meta-analysis of research on the relationship of class size and achievement. *Educational Evaluation and Policy Analysis* 1, 2–16. https://doi.org/10.3102/01623737001001002

Glass, G.V., McGaw, B., Smith, M.L. (1981) *Meta-Analysis in Social Research*. Beverly Hills, CA: Sage.

Gray, B.H., Gusmano, M.K., Collins, S. (2003) AHCPR and the changing politics of health services research. *Health Affairs* Supplement Web Exclusives, W3–283–307. https://doi.org/10.1377/hlthaff.W3.283

Greenhalgh, T. (2019) *How to Read a Paper: The Basics of Evidence Based Medicine and Health-care*. 6th edition. Chichester: Wiley Blackwell.

Guyatt, G.H. (1991) Evidence-based medicine. *ACP Journal Club* 114, A16A. https://doi.org/10.7326/ACPJC-1991-114-2-A16

Guyatt, G.H., Meade, M.O., Jaeschke, R.Z., Cook, D.J., Haynes, R.B. (2000) Practitioners of evidence based care. *BMJ* 320, 954–955. https://doi.org/10.1136/bmj.320.7240.954

Light, R.J., Pillemer, D.B. (1984) *Summing Up: The Science of Reviewing Research*. Cambridge, MA: Harvard University Press. https://doi.org/10.4159/9780674040243

Marks, H.M. (1997) *The Progress of Experiment: Science and Therapeutic Reform in the United States, 1900–1990*. Cambridge: Cambridge University Press.

Newton, W. (2001) Rationalism and empiricism in modern medicine. *Law and Contemporary Problems* 64, 299–316. https://doi.org/10.2307/1192299

Oakley, A. (2000) *Experiments in Knowing: Gender and Method in the Social Sciences*. Cambridge: Polity Press.

Paul, J.R. (1938) Clinical epidemiology. *Journal of Clinical Investigation* 17, 539–541. https://doi.org/10.1172/JCI100978

Paul, J.R. (1958) *Clinical Epidemiology*. Chicago, IL: University of Chicago Press.

Petticrew, M. (2001) Systematic reviews from astronomy to zoology: myths and misconceptions. *BMJ* 322, 98–101. https://doi.org/10.1136/bmj.322.7278.98

Raskin, I.E., Maklan, C.W. (1991) Medical treatment effectiveness research: a view from inside the Agency for Health Care Policy and Research. *Evaluation and the Health Professions* 14, 161–186. https://doi.org/10.1177/016327879101400203

Relman, A. (1988) Assessment and accountability: the third revolution in medical care. *New England Journal of Medicine* 319, 1220–1222. https://doi.org/10.1056/NEJM198811033191810

Rinchuse, D.J., Rinchuse, D.J., Kandasamy, S., Ackerman, M.B. (2008) Deconstructing evidence in orthodontics: making sense of systematic reviews, randomized clinical trials, and meta-analyses. *World Journal of Orthodontics* 9, 167–176.

Rosati, R.A., Wallace, A.G., Stead, E.A. (1973) The way of the future. *Archives of Internal Medicine* 131, 285–287. https://doi.org/10.1001/archinte.1973.00320080121017

Rosser Matthews, J. (1995) *Quantification and the Quest for Medical Certainty*. Princeton, NJ: Princeton University Press.

Sackett, D.L., Haynes, R.B., Tugwell, P. (1985) *Clinical Epidemiology: A Basic Science for Clinical Medicine*. Boston, MA: Little, Brown and Company.

Sackett, D.L., Haynes, R.B., Guyatt, G.H., Tugwell, P. (1991) *Clinical Epidemiology: A Basic Science for Clinical Medicine*. 2nd edition. Boston, MA: Little, Brown and Company.

Sacks, H.S., Berrier, J., Reitman, D., Ancona-Berk, V.A., Chalmers, T.C. (1987) Meta-analyses of randomized controlled trials. *New England Journal of Medicine* 316, 450–455. https://doi.org/10.1056/NEJM198702193160806

Smith, M.L., Glass, G.V. (1977) Meta-analysis of psychotherapy outcome studies. *American Psychologist* 32, 752–760. https://doi.org/10.1037/0003-066X.32.9.752

Smits, H.L. (1986) Medical practice variations revisited. *Health Affairs* 5(3), 91–96. https://doi.org/10.1377/hlthaff.5.3.91

Stampfer, M.J., Goldhaber, S.Z., Yusuf, S., Peto, R., Hennekens, C.H. (1982) Effect of intravenous streptokinase on acute myocardial infarction: pooled results from randomized trials. *New England Journal of Medicine* 307, 1180–1182. https://doi.org/10.1056/NEJM198211043071904

Stigler, S.M. (1978) Mathematical statistics in the early states. *Annals of Statistics* 6, 239–265. https://doi.org/10.1214/aos/1176344123

Stigler, S.M. (1999) *Statistics on the Table: The History of Statistical Concepts and Methods*. Boston, MA: Harvard University Press.

Tanenbaum, S.J. (1995) Getting there from here: evidentiary quandaries of the US outcomes movement. *Journal of Evaluation in Clinical Practice* 1, 97–103.

Tanenbaum, S.J. (2006) expanding the terms of the debate: evidence-based practice and public policy. In: Goodheart, C.D., Kazdin, A.E., Sternberg, R.J. (Eds.), *Evidence-Based Psychotherapy: Where Practice and Research Meet*. Washington, DC: American Psychological Association, pp. 238–259. https://doi.org/10.1111/j.1365-2753.1995.tb00014.x

Timmermans, S., Berg, M. (2003) *The Gold Standard: The Challenge of Evidence-Based Medicine and Standardization in Health Care*. Philadelphia, PA: Temple University Press.

Weisz, G., Cambrosio, A., Keating, P., Knaapen, L., Schlich, T., Tournay, V.J. (2007) The emergence of clinical practice guidelines. *Milbank Quarterly* 85, 691–727. https://doi.org/10.1111/j.1468-0009.2007.00505.x

Wennberg, J.E. (1984) Dealing with medical practice variations: a proposal for action. *Health Affairs* 3(2), 6–32. https://doi.org/10.1377/hlthaff.3.2.6

Woolf, S.H. (1990) Practice guidelines: a new reality in medicine. I. Recent developments. *Archives of Internal Medicine* 150, 1811–1818. https://doi.org/10.1001/archinte.1990.00390200025005

Yusuf, S., Collins, R., Peto, R., Furberg, C., Stampfer, M.J., Goldhaber, S.Z., et al. (1985) Intravenous and intracoronary fibrinolytic therapy in acute myocardial infarction: overview of results on mortality, reinfarction and side-effects from 33 randomized controlled trials. *European Heart Journal* 6, 556–585. https://doi.org/10.1093/oxfordjournals.eurheartj.a061905

Yusuf, S., Simon, R., Ellenberg, S.S. (Eds.) (1987) Proceedings of the workshop on methodologic issues in overviews of randomized clinical trials. *Statistics in Medicine* 6, 217–410. https://doi.org/10.1002/sim.4780060302

2 The historical background of implementation science

Per Nilsen

A new paradigm

The birth of the field of implementation science is usually linked to the emergence of the evidence-based movement in the 1990s. Evidence-based medicine (EBM) was introduced in 1992 in the *Journal of the American Medical Association* with a proclamation by the Evidence-Based Medicine Working Group (1992, p. 2420). It was launched as "a new paradigm of medical practice", which downplayed "the importance of intuition, unsystematic clinical experience, and pathophysiological explanations as sufficient grounds for clinical decision-making and emphasizes review of evidence from clinical research". Working in accordance with EBM would require "new abilities of the physician, including effective literature search and application of formal rules for the evaluation of evidence in clinical literature". EBM has been described as a disruptive innovation, meaning that it was "a new way of doing things that sought to overturn previous practices" (Wilson and Sheldon, 2019, p. 67).

In the ensuing years, EBM spread widely as evidence-based practice (EBP), not only to areas that are relatively close to those of medicine, such as nursing, mental health, physiotherapy and occupational therapy, but also to areas further from EBM's medical origins, for example, public health, social work, education and management. At the same time, a vertical spread occurred, from an early focus on various forms of treatments and interventions to also include the policy process concerning the use of evidence for identifying and prioritizing problem areas and for decision-making. The "evidence" label is applied to societal sectors (e.g. evidence-based healthcare and evidence-based social work), subject areas (e.g. evidence-based public health), specific practices (e.g. evidence-based mental health therapies) and actions of various kinds (such as evidence-based policy- or decision-making).

The argument that practice should be based on the most up-to-date, valid and reliable research findings "has an intuitive appeal and is so obviously sensible and rational that it is difficult to resist" (Trinder, 2000a, p. 3). The spread of the evidence model can only be described as a success story, with the concept of evidence having gained considerable "rhetorical power" across the world (Bohlin, 2011, p. 64). Today, the ideals and principles of the evidence model permeate healthcare and beyond. Activities involved in understanding, generating and applying evidence is part of many professionals' basic and continuing professional education.

The popularization of the evidence model has been facilitated by developments in information technology, especially electronic databases and the Internet, which have enabled practitioners, policy makers, researchers and others to readily identify, collate,

DOI: 10.4324/9781003318125-3

disseminate and access research on a global scale. The evidence movement also resonates with many contemporary societal issues and concerns, including the progress of New Public Management, which has highlighted issues of effectiveness, quality, accountability and transparency (Nilsen and Birken, 2020).

Practical application of the evidence model

Application of the evidence model can be described as a process in which different sources of knowledge are integrated for the best possible decisions for individuals, for example, patients in healthcare, clients in social work or students in school. According to a much-quoted definition by Sackett et al. (1996), practising in accordance with the evidence model means "a careful, openly reported and judicious use of the currently best evidence for decision-making on measures (interventions, programmes, etc.) to individuals, supplemented by professional expertise and the situation and wishes of the person concerned". Thus, they describe EBP in terms of the inter-weaving of three sources of knowledge: research-based knowledge, the practitioner's own experience and the preferences and values expressed by the client. This three-part model is usually illustrated with three overlapping circles, where the intersection is represented by EBP.

The actual application of the evidence model was originally described as a five-step critical appraisal procedure (Sackett et al., 1997): (1) formulate the need for information to answer questions; (2) look for the best available knowledge to answer the questions; (3) evaluate the knowledge available in terms of its scientific reliability and usefulness; (4) integrate this critical assessment with one's professional competence, the unique circumstances and wishes of the person concerned; (5) evaluate the action and effectiveness of performing the previous four steps and strive to improve the work.

The critical appraisal EBP procedure has also been described in terms of "5A" tasks to be carried out: assess; ask; acquire; appraise; apply. The practitioner must assess the client and the problem to determine the pertinent issues. A clear, answerable question must be asked before acquiring evidence from an appropriate knowledge source, for example, a systematic review, guideline or computerized decision support system. The evidence must be appraised to determine its validity and reliability. The process concludes by returning to the client; the practitioner has to decide whether it is appropriate to apply the evidence in the particular case or not (Gray, 2009; Hoffmann et al., 2010; Bergmark et al., 2011).

Applying the 5A procedure may be demanding in busy practice settings. Keeping abreast of research and reviewing it critically requires time and expertise. Research has shown considerable difficulties in realizing the evidence model according to this procedure. For this reason, simplified procedures have been described in the literature, starting from the fact that all five steps (or As) are not always needed. It is proposed that the procedure can be adapted to the specific circumstances (e.g. the problem the client has), the time available and the competence regarding the various steps (Gray, 2009; Bergmark et al., 2011).

Three variants for practising EBP have been described (Straus and McAlister, 2000): (1) "doing mode" is applicable when there are few time limits or other restrictions, making it possible to carry out at least steps 1–4 of the critical appraisal procedure; (2) "using mode" is applicable in more time-pressured contexts, proposing that step 3 can then be excluded and existing guidelines and other forms of knowledge compilations can be used; (3) "replicating mode" means relying on recommendations from "respected evidence-based opinion leaders", which is why steps 2 and 3 can be excluded.

In parallel with research that has pointed to barriers to the practical application of the evidence model, there has been an increase in the production of guidelines and other types of research summaries that condense research results and present various recommendations for practice, for example, clinical guidelines produced by the National Institute for Health and Care Excellence (NICE) in the United Kingdom or the national guidelines published by the National Board of Health and Welfare in Sweden. Guidelines are seen as a feasible way to achieve more EBP in many areas and activities.

Debate on the evidence model

Advocates of the evidence model argue that its successful spread is because the model is based on a fundamentally good idea, i.e. that practice and decisions in many settings and sectors of society should as far as possible rest on a scientific basis. This positive view of the evidence model is not shared by everyone, however. Many aspects of the evidence model have been, and continue to be, the subject of debate (Boaz et al., 2019; Palinkas, 2019). Several more or less overlapping themes can be identified in this debate.

Empiricism or rationalism?

The emphasis on evidence in the evidence model has led to EBM/EBP being considered an expression of an extreme form of empiricism (Greek *empeiria*, experience), i.e. the model is based on the assumption that knowledge of the world can best be obtained by observing reality (preferably in the form of randomized control trials [RCTs] or other types of experimental studies). Knowledge from empirical research is assigned greater importance than theories or reasoning, for example, assessment of what might be best for a client in a particular situation. The empiricism of the evidence model can be seen as a reaction against rationalism (Latin *ratio*, reason), which was expressed in terms of "intuition, unsystematic clinical experience, and pathophysiological explanations" in the original EBM proclamation (Evidence-Based Medicine Working Group, 1992, p. 2420). According to rationalism, existing knowledge of, for example, the physiology of the body, is sufficient for reasoning whether a particular intervention would be effective in treating a particular disease. The evidence model does not explicitly consider the interaction between observation and theory.

The evidence model has been critiqued for being unscientific due to its emphasis on empiricism at the expense of rationalism (Charlton and Miles, 1998; Miles et al., 2001). Theory facilitates interpretation and assessment of the credibility of evidence. For example, highly positive test results of a vaccine in an RCT gain more weight if there is also a plausible medical explanation for the result. Conversely, there may be greater reason to be sceptical of positive test results if theories raise doubts that a particular vaccine could have such effects (Sehon and Stanley, 2003).

Drawn to its extreme, empiricism means that one cannot conclude whether jumping with a parachute from an airplane is more effective for survival than jumping without a parachute unless this has been tested experimentally. However, Archie Cochrane, in his landmark book *Effectiveness and Efficiency: Random Reflections on Health Services* (1972), stated that treatments that have "immediate and up-to-date" effects, whether this has been tested in an RCT or not, have the greatest evidentiary value. He exemplified this with insulin for childhood diabetes.

What constitutes evidence?

To apply the evidence model, available evidence is needed that is ideally valid, reliable and unaffected by various kinds of bias. Questions about what constitutes "evidence" and what kind of research can produce trustworthy evidence are controversial in many areas (Greenhalgh, 2018). According to the most radical interpretation of the evidence model, only RCTs and summaries of such studies in systematic reviews can generate trustworthy evidence. In the book by Cochrane (1972), the RCT is highlighted as a gold standard for producing reliable knowledge. More pragmatic approaches consider different study designs and data to obtain evidence (Boaz et al., 2019). Alternative terms such as "evidence-informed practice" or "research-informed practice" have been proposed to emphasize this broader perspective.

If the starting point for the evidence model is that evidence requires RCTs, there are significant difficulties in many areas to realize EBP, for example, education, social work and public health, where it may be difficult to evaluate effects under experimental forms. However, many effective treatments in healthcare have never been tried in RCTs, for example, the Heimlich manoeuvre to remove objects that clog the airway or the defibrillator to send an electrical shock through the thorax to the heart's conduction system (Howick, 2011). In many areas, a broader perspective on what constitutes evidence is advocated today.

Do RCTs provide relevant answers?

Many researchers have criticized several aspects of RCTs for producing evidence. The methodological strength attributed to RCTs is questioned in areas where these types of experiments are considered too reductionist to adequately capture the complexity of reality. An RCT can provide answers to questions about whether a drug or treatment, for example, has an effect or not and how large these effects are. However, RCTs usually provide limited knowledge of the causal mechanisms that enable these effects. Thus, RCTs cannot answer questions such as "what makes it work?" or "what works, for whom, under what circumstances?" Furthermore, RCTs are difficult to carry out when the individual is not the most suitable unit of analysis. It may be difficult to involve sufficient numbers of study participants in randomization to intervention and control groups at aggregate levels of, for example, primary healthcare units, schools or local communities (Nilsen, 2006).

Criticism has been directed against the generalizability of the evidence produced in RCTs. This type of study has its main strength in terms of internal validity, that is, ensuring that the effects observed are indeed due to the intervention studied. Conclusions can be drawn about an intervention's efficacy (i.e. effects under ideal, controlled and research-driven conditions), but these studies provide less guidance on effectiveness (i.e. effects under realistic, everyday practice conditions). High internal validity is often achieved at the cost of poor external validity, that is, limited generalizability of the results to other contexts (Nilsen, 2006; Gray, 2009; Hoffmann et al., 2010). External validity is threatened by an atypical intervention (e.g. more extensive than what might be implementable in routine practice), an atypical delivery of the intervention (e.g. pre-training of healthcare professionals to deliver the intervention) and atypical patients (e.g. recruited from a homogeneous population) (Black, 1996).

Professional development or cookbook medicine?

Another debate concerns how the evidence model affects professional autonomy and development. Supporters of the evidence model believe that it contributes to the legitimization of the work of professionals. According to this perspective, increased transparency facilitates professionals' opportunities for critical reflection and learning, which benefits the development of professions (Trinder, 2000a).

However, critics instead see a risk that the evidence model contributes to increased control and standardization of work, which may lead to reduced professional autonomy. In many ways, the evidence model challenges activities and professions that have traditionally been regarded as an art, where factors such as the practitioner's "clinical eye" and his or her use of "illness scripts", rules of thumb and heuristics are considered important (Gabbay and Le May, 2011). The perceived devaluation of the professional's skills is one reason why the critics of the evidence model describe it as "cookbook medicine" and a "straitjacket" for professionals. It is argued that the application of the evidence model yields uniformity that does not promote professional development (Trinder, 2000b). According to some critics, there is even a risk of de-professionalization, because practitioners stagnate and lose their ability to use their critical judgement when it is more convenient to follow prepackaged guidelines and protocols (Bergmark et al., 2011).

Democratization or control?

It is difficult to object to the ideal or core message of the evidence model of creating a scientific basis for professional work so that it can live up to ethical expectations for different professions and activities. The evidence model implies a democratization of the knowledge base in contrast to authority- or eminence-based practice that is guided by individual authorities, traditions or ideologies (Bergmark et al., 2011).

This positive view of the evidence model as a democratic means is not shared by everyone. Regardless of the original intentions, critics argue that the evidence model has increasingly become a control instrument for authorities and decision-makers. EBM started on a small scale and inter-professional, in a kind of bottom-up process, but has developed into a worldwide evidence movement. Sackett and colleagues warned back in 1996 that the evidence model could be "hi-jacked" by decision-makers and become a tool for cutting healthcare costs. As pointed out by Cohen et al. (2004), the authors of EBM "have no control over how EBM is used and EBM supporters do not have the power to decide how society should apply EBM in the delivery of healthcare". Charlton and Miles (1998) describe the evidence movement as an "alliance of leaders and statistical technocrats" who are in turn ruled by "politicians, bureaucrats and statistical technicians". Hickey and Roberts (2011) consider "central control" to be the foundational philosophy of the evidence movement, and they see the pursuit of "administrative control" as the main driving force for the movement's spread.

What is the client's role?

Applying the evidence model is intended to ensure that clients receive the most effective practices possible and prevent them from being treated with ineffective or harmful practices. The evidence model makes clear, at least theoretically, the importance of the client's perception alongside the research evidence and the professional's assessment. Thus, there are strong arguments for the evidence model from a client perspective. At the same time, critics object that the model can be said to be based on a so-called ecological fallacy, that is, the conclusions of the research are drawn at the aggregate level, which are not necessarily true at the individual level. Thus, there is a built-in tension between the epidemiological approach of EBP, the implicit aim of which is the greatest possible benefit for the greatest possible number of individuals in a given population, and the individual professional's quest to achieve the greatest possible benefit for the individual in the client encounter.

Studies to produce evidence are often conducted on homogeneous populations of similar individuals, but individual clients are unique and are likely to deviate from the averages described in research. Although there is evidence that a particular drug or treatment cures or prevents disease in a particular population, it can be difficult to assess the extent to which this applies to specific individuals. There are examples where conclusions from experiments at the group level have been applied at the individual level with disastrous consequences; for example, the analgesic and anti-inflammatory drug rofecoxib (Vioxx, cardiovascular side effects) and the sleeping medication thalidomide (side effects in the form of birth defects).

A related question is what client involvement in EBP means in cases where the client's wishes conflict with the evidence and/or professional experience; for example, a client might prefer a particular therapeutic intervention that has been popularized in the media, without there being a reliable scientific basis. Bergmark et al. (2011) point to a dilemma in such situations: letting the client decide is contrary to the evidence model's assumption of applying the best available scientific evidence as a basis for decisions, but ignoring the client's wishes does not correspond with descriptions of how the evidence model should be applied in practice.

Is there evidence for the evidence model?

The evidence model, according to its advocates, is associated with a multitude of benefits. A paradox is that the empirical research support for the beneficial effects of applying EBM or EBP is limited. Thus, the evidence model may not be evidence-based, critics argue, because the model as a whole has not been tested in an RCT (or using other study designs) (Trinder, 2000b). The evidence model has been justified based on rationalism, that is, arguments and assumptions about its excellence.

Nevertheless, some studies have shown the benefits of evidence-based work in various settings and sectors of society by linking positive client outcomes to the application of the evidence model (i.e. working in accordance with the model). Compliance with recommendations in guidelines and standardized care plans, for example, has been shown to be associated with positive patient outcomes (Fritz et al., 2007; Ronellenfitsch et al., 2008; Rutten et al., 2010). However, critics argue that more extensive research is needed before it is possible to assert the existence of evidence for the evidence model (Trinder, 2000b; Hoffmann et al., 2010).

Can the evidence model be applied?

Ultimately, the question is whether the evidence model can be applied in routine practice in various settings and sectors of society. Both supporters and critics of the model recognize that the application of EBP in everyday practice is associated with difficulties. The ideal of practitioners who independently seek and scrutinize research in their field has proven difficult to achieve. Eight years after the first article on EBM, Guyatt et al. (2000) noted with some disappointment that clinicians would rather use guidelines and protocols of various kinds than carry out all the steps of the critical appraisal procedure. Upshur and Tracy (2004) noted a few years later that many clinicians had become "evidence consumers" rather than critically conscious evidence-based practitioners.

Implementation science has highlighted difficulties in achieving the evidence model's ideal of independent, critical practitioners who evaluate and use research in their daily activities. According to the research, there are significant problems with searching for and identifying relevant research studies (step 2 of the critical appraisal procedure) and evaluating the scientific reliability and usefulness of this research (step 3 of the procedure). Descriptions of EBP also do not provide any real guidance on how step 4 of the procedure should be performed; that is, integration of a critical evaluation of research with own professional competence and the client's conditions and wishes (Gabbay and Le May, 2011). These challenges have helped create demand for research on implementation issues and paved the way for implementation science.

Birth of implementation science

The evidence-based movement popularized the notion that research findings and empirically supported (i.e. evidence-based) interventions, programmes, services, etc. should be more widely spread and applied in various settings and sectors of society to improve the health and welfare of populations. It was recognized that implementation often produced suboptimal results, leading to many evidence-based interventions never making their way to the individuals who needed them. Implementation science can potentially produce knowledge that makes it possible to reduce or remove the gap between what has been proven to be an effective intervention and what is actually used and provided in various settings and sectors.

The field of implementation science has seen a surge of interest in the 2000s. The market for books, courses and conferences on the topic of implementation has increased multifold and there is a near-exponential growth in the number of articles on the topic of implementation science. Since the 2006 launch of *Implementation Science*, which was the first scientific journal to focus explicitly on implementation, several implementation-specific journals have emerged, including *Implementation Science Communications*, *Implementation Research and Practice*, *Global Implementation Research and Applications* and *Frontiers in Health Services* with a targeted section on implementation science research.

Although implementation science is an emerging field still under development, research on the challenges associated with how various forms of knowledge are translated into desired actions to address societal problems has a long history. Implementation science has been greatly influenced by innovation research concerning the spread of ideas, products and practices (Greenhalgh, 2018; Palinkas, 2019). This research originated in sociology in the early 1900s (Rogers, 2003). Everett Rogers collated different traditions and presented a conceptual apparatus for the spread and adoption of innovations in his ground-breaking book *Diffusion of Innovations*, which was first published in 1962. The theory originated from his own experience as a farmer and then as an investigator on the spread of agricultural innovations.

The notion of innovation attributes in the Theory of Diffusion (i.e. relative advantage, compatibility, complexity, trialability and observability; Rogers, 2003), has been widely applied in implementation science, both in individual studies (e.g. Aubert and Hamel, 2001; Foy et al., 2002; Völlink et al., 2002) and in determinant frameworks (e.g. Greenhalgh et al., 2005; Damschroder et al., 2009; Gurses et al., 2010) to assess the extent to which the characteristics of the implementation object (e.g. an evidence-based intervention) affect implementation outcomes. Furthermore, the Theory of Diffusion highlights the importance of intermediary actors (opinion leaders, change agents and gatekeepers) for successful adoption and implementation (Rogers, 2003), which is reflected in the roles described in numerous implementation determinant frameworks (e.g. Rycroft-Malone, 2010; Blase et al., 2012) and implementation strategy taxonomies (e.g. Oxman et al., 1995; Grimshaw et al., 2003; Walter et al., 2003).

Implementation science is also related to research on policy implementation, that is, the study of "how governments put policies into effect" (Howlett and Ramesh, 2003). This research rose to prominence in the 1970s during a period of increasing concern about the effectiveness of public policy. A policy is a plan or course of action intended to influence and determine decisions and actions. This research emerged from the insight that political intentions seldom resulted in the planned changes, which encouraged researchers to investigate what occurred in the policy process and how it affected the results (Cairney, 2012). The stage was set in 1973 by Jeffrey Pressman and Aaron Wildavsky with the publication of their book entitled *Implementation*, which investigated the implementation of a federal programme to increase employment among ethnic minority groups in Oakland, California (Pressman and Wildavsky, 1973). The study of policy implementation became a topic in public administration, a branch of political science that deals with the theory and practice of politics and political systems (Nilsen et al., 2013).

Implementation science also has many contact points with the study of research use (or research utilization). This research grew out of the social science research field of knowledge utilization in the 1970s; Robert Rich and Carol Weiss were prominent scholars (the term "knowledge utilization" has also been used as a collective name for all research relating to the use of knowledge). In the 1970s, well before the emergence of EBM or EBP, nursing researchers were building on concepts and theories from knowledge utilization in research to understand how nurses used research in their clinical practice. Many of the researchers who were active in the field of research use have gone on to research within implementation science (Nilsen and Birken, 2020).

References

Aubert, B.A., Hamel, G. (2001) Adoption of smart cards in the medical sector: the Canadian experience. *Social Science & Medicine* 53, 879–894. https://doi.org/10.1016/S0277-9536(00)00388-9

Bergmark, A., Bergmark, Å., Lundström, T. (2011). *Evidensbaserat socialt arbete*. Stockholm: Natur och Kultur.

Black, N. (1996) Why we need observational studies to evaluate the effectiveness of health care. *BMJ* 312, 1215–1218. https://doi.org/10.1136/bmj.312.7040.1215

Blase, K.A., Van Dyke, M., Fixsen, D.L., Bailey, F.W. (2012) Implementation science: key concepts, themes and evidence for practitioners in educational psychology. In: Kelly, B., Perkins, D.F. (Eds.), *Handbook of Implementation Science for Psychology in Education*. Cambridge: Cambridge University Press, pp. 13–34. https://doi.org/10.1017/CBO9781139013949.004

Boaz, A., Davies, H., Fraser, A., Nutley, S. (2019) What works now? An introduction. In: Boaz, A., Davies, H., Fraser, A., Nutley, S. (Eds.), *What Works Now? Evidence-Informed Policy and Practice*. Bristol: Policy Press, pp. 1–16. https://doi.org/10.56687/9781447345527-006

Bohlin, I. (2011) Evidensbaserat beslutsfattande i ett vetenskapsbaserat samhälle. Om evidensrörelsens ursprung, utbredning och gränser. In: Bohlin, I., Sager, M. (Eds.), *Evidensens många ansikten*. Lund: Arkiv, pp. 31–68.

Cairney, P. (2012) *Understanding Public Policy: Theories and Issues*. Basingstoke: Palgrave Macmillan. https://doi.org/10.1007/978-0-230-35699-3

Charlton B.G., Miles A. (1998) The rise and fall of EBM. *QJM* 91, 371–374. https://doi.org/10.1093/qjmed/91.5.371

Cochrane, A.L. (1972) *Effectiveness and Efficiency: Random Reflections on Health Services*. London: Nuffield Provincial Hospitals Trust.

Cohen, A.M., Stavri, P.Z., Hersh, W.R. (2004) A categorization and analysis of the criticisms of Evidence-Based Medicine. *International Journal of Medical Informatics* 73, 35–43. https://doi.org/10.1016/j.ijmedinf.2003.11.002

Damschroder, L.J., Aron, D.C., Keith, R.E., Kirsh, S.R., Alexander, J.A., Lowery, J.C. (2009) Fostering implementation of health services research findings into practice: a consolidated framework for advancing implementation science. *Implementation Science* 4, 50. https://doi.org/10.1186/1748-5908-4-50

Evidence Based Medicine Working Group (1992). Evidence-based medicine. A new approach to teaching the practice of medicine. *Journal of the American Medical Association* 268, 2420–2425. https://doi.org/10.1001/jama.268.17.2420

Foy, R., Maclennan, G., Grimshaw, J., Penney, G., Campbell, M., Grol, R. (2002) Attributes of clinical recommendations that influence change in practice following audit and feedback. *Journal of Clinical Epidemiology* 55, 717–722. https://doi.org/10.1016/S0895-4356(02)00403-1

Fritz, J., Cleland, J.A., Brennan, G.P. (2007) Does adherence to the guideline recommendation for active treatments improve the quality of care for patients with acute low back pain delivered by physical therapists? *Medical Care* 45, 973–980. https://doi.org/10.1097/MLR.0b013e318070c6cd

Gabbay, J., Le May, A. (2011) *Practice-Based Evidence for Healthcare: Clinical Mindlines*. Abingdon: Routledge. https://doi.org/10.4324/9780203839973

Gray, M. (2009) *Evidence-Based Healthcare and Public Health*. 3rd edition. Edinburgh: Churchill Livingstone Elsevier.

Greenhalgh, T. (2018) *How to Implement Evidence-Based Healthcare*. Hoboken, NJ: John Wiley.

Greenhalgh, T., Robert, G., Bate, P., Macfarlane, F., Kyriakidou, O. (2005) *Diffusion of Innovations in Service Organisations: A Systematic Literature Review*. Malden, MA: Blackwell Publishing. https://doi.org/10.1002/9780470987407

Grimshaw, J., McAuley, L.M., Bero, L.A., Grilli, R., Oxman, A.D., Ramsay, C., et al. (2003) Systematic reviews of effectiveness of quality improvement strategies and programmes. *Quality and Safety in Health Care* 12, 298–303. https://doi.org/10.1136/qhc.12.4.298

Gurses, A.P., Marsteller, J.A., Ozok, A.A., Xiao, Y., Owens, S., Pronovost, P.J. (2010) Using an interdisciplinary approach to identify factors that affect clinicians' compliance with evidence-based guidelines. *Critical Care Medicine* 38(8 Suppl), S282–S291. https://doi.org/10.1097/CCM.0b013e3181e69e02

Guyatt, G.H., Meade, M.O., Jaeschke, R.Z., Cook, D.J., Haynes, R.B. (2000) Practitioners of evidence based care: not all clinicians need to appraise evidence from scratch but all need some skills. *British Medical Journal* 320, 954–955. https://doi.org/10.1136/bmj.320.7240.954

Hickey, S., Roberts, H. (2011) *Tarnished Gold: The Sickness of Evidence-Based Medicine*. Self-published.

Hoffmann, T., Bennett, S., Del Mar, C. (2010) Introduction to evidence-based practice. In: Hoffmann, T., Bennett, S., Del Mar, C. (Eds.), *Evidence-Based Practice Across the Health Professions*. Chatswood, Australia: Elsevier, pp. 1–15.

Howick, J. (2011) *The Philosophy of Evidence-Based Medicine*. Oxford: BMJ. https://doi.org/10.1002/9781444342673

Howlett, M., Ramesh, M. (2003) *Studying Public Policy: Policy Cycles and Policy Subsystems*. Oxford: Oxford University Press.

Miles, A., Bentley, P., Polychronis, A., Grey, J., Meichiorri, C. (2001) Recent developments in the evidence-based healthcare debate. *Journal of Evaluation in Clinical Practice* 7, 85–89. https://doi.org/10.1046/j.1365-2753.2001.00301.x

Nilsen, P. (2006) *Opening the Black Box of Community-Based Injury Prevention Programmes*. PhD dissertation thesis, Linköping University, Linköping.

Nilsen, P., Birken, S.A. (2020) Prologue. In: Nilsen, P., Birken, S.A. (Eds.), *Handbook on Implementation Science*. Cheltenham: Edward Elgar. https://doi.org/10.4337/9781788975995.00006

Nilsen, P., Ståhl, C., Roback, K., Cairney, P. (2013) Never the twain shall meet? A comparison of implementation science and policy implementation research. *Implementation Science* 8, 63. https://doi.org/10.1186/1748-5908-8-63

Oxman, A.D., Thomson, M.A., Davis, D.A., Haynes, R.B. (1995) No magic bullets: a systematic review of 102 trials of interventions to improve professional practice. *CMAJ* 153, 1423–1431.

Palinkas, L.A. (2019) *Achieving Implementation and Exchange*. Bristol: Policy Press. https://doi.org/10.56687/9781447338147

Pressman, J.L., Wildavsky, A. (1973) *Implementation*. Berkeley, CA: University of California Press.

Rogers, E.M. (2003) *Diffusion of Innovations*. 5th edition. New York: Free Press.

Ronellenfitsch, U., Rossner, E., Jakob, J., Post, S., Hohenberger, P., Schwarzbach, M. (2008) Clinical pathways in surgery: Should we introduce them into clinical routine? A review article. *Langenbeck's Archives of Surgery* 393, 449–457. https://doi.org/10.1007/s00423-008-0303-9

Rutten, G.M., Degen, S., Hendriks, E.J., Braspenning, J.C., Harting, J., Oostendorp, R.A. (2010) Adherence to clinical practice guidelines for low back pain in physical therapy: do patients benefit? *Physical Therapy* 90, 1111–1122. https://doi.org/10.2522/ptj.20090173

Rycroft-Malone, J. (2010) Promoting Action on Research Implementation in Health Services (PARIHS). In: Rycroft-Malone, J., Bucknall, T. (Eds.), *Models and Frameworks for Implementing Evidence-Based Practice: Linking Evidence to Action*. Chichester: Wiley-Blackwell, pp. 109–136.

Sackett, D.L., Rosenberg, W.M., Gray, J.A., Haynes, R.B., Richardson, W.S. (1996) Evidence-based medicine: what it is and what it isn't. *British Medical Journal* 312, 71. https://doi.org/10.1136/bmj.312.7023.71

Sackett, D.L., Richardson, W.S., Rosenberg, W.M.C., Haynes, R.B. (1997) *Evidence-Based Medicine: How to Practice and Teach EBM*. London: Churchill Livingstone.

Sehon, S.R., Stanley D.E. (2003) A philosophical analysis of the evidence-based medicine debate. *BMC Health Services Research* 3, 14. https://doi.org/10.1186/1472-6963-3-14

Straus, S.E., McAlister, F.A. (2000) Evidence-based medicine: a commentary on common criticisms. *CMAJ* 163, 837–841.

Trinder, L. (2000a) Introduction: the context of evidence-based practice. In: Trinder, L., Reynolds, S. (Eds.), *Evidence-Based Practice*. Oxford: Blackwell, pp. 1–16. https://doi.org/10.1002/9780470699003.ch1

Trinder, L. (2000b) A critical appraisal of evidence-based practice. In: Trinder, L., Reynolds, S. (Eds.), Evidence-Based Practice. Oxford: Blackwell, pp. 212–241. https://doi.org/10.1002/9780470699003.ch10

Upshur, R.E.G., Tracy, C.S. (2004) Legitimacy, authority, and hierarchy: critical challenges for evidence-based medicine. *Brief Treatment and Crisis Intervention* 4, 197–204. https://doi.org/10.1093/brief-treatment/mhh018

Völlink, T., Meertens, R., Midden, C.J. (2002) Innovating 'diffusion of innovation' theory: innovation characteristics and the intention of utility companies to adopt energy conservation interventions. *Journal of Environmental Psychology* 22, 333–344. https://doi.org/10.1006/jevp.2001.0237

Walter, I., Nutley, S.M., Davies, H.T.O. (2003) Developing a taxonomy of interventions used to increase the impact of research. Discussion Paper 3. St. Andrews: Research Unit for Research Utilisation. University of St Andrews.

Wilson, P., Sheldon, T.A. (2019) Using evidence in health and healthcare. In: Boaz, A., Davies, H., Fraser, A., Nutley, S. (Eds.), *What Works Now? Evidence-Informed Policy and Practice*. Bristol: Policy Press, pp. 67–88. https://doi.org/10.51952/9781447345527.ch004

3 Fundamentals of implementation science

JoAnn E. Kirchner and Mark S. Bauer

The need for a science of implementation

Implementation science shares many characteristics, and the rigorous approach, of clinical research. However, it is distinct in that it attends to factors in addition to the effectiveness of the clinical innovation itself, to include identifying and addressing barriers and facilitators to the uptake of evidence-based clinical innovations. Throughout this chapter, the term innovation is used inclusively. In a clinical setting, this may be a new clinical intervention. It may be a prevention programme in a public health setting or a new model of service in a community setting.

The need for a science of implementation may be understood through a series of examples associated with the implementation of the Collaborative Chronic Care Model (CCM) within the US Department of Veteran Affairs. Thus, we start with a story (Box 3.1).

Box 3.1

It was, by all estimations, a successful research effort. We had mounted a randomized, controlled clinical trial across 11 sites in the US Department of Veterans Affairs (USVA), testing an organization of care called the Collaborative Chronic Care Model (CCM) for bipolar disorder versus treatment as usual (Bauer et al., 2006a) Over 3 years of follow-up, the CCM showed significant positive impact on weeks in mood episode, mental health quality of life, social role function, and satisfaction with care – all at no increased cost to the healthcare system (Bauer et al., 2006b). In parallel, a 2-year, four-site randomized controlled clinical trial of the bipolar CCM in the Group Health Cooperative of Puget Sound (now Kaiser Permanente), showed very similar outcomes at minimal cost, compared with treatment as usual (Simon et al., 2006). Both studies were published in the same year in mainstream psychiatric journals that are read and respected by mental health researchers, clinicians, and administrators. The CCM for bipolar disorders began to be endorsed by national clinical practice guidelines in the USVA and in Canada (Yatham et al., 2006), and the bipolar CCM was listed on the US Substance Abuse and Mental Health Services Administration's prestigious National Registry of Evidence-Based Programs and Practices. A worthwhile innovation in care? It was a no-brainer: improved outcome at little to no cost.

And yet, within a year of the end of the studies, none of the 15 sites had incorporated the CCM into their usual workflow. The clinicians who had participated in

---

DOI: 10.4324/9781003318125-4

the CCM went back to their usual duties, and the individuals with bipolar disorder went back to receiving their usual form of care. For all practical purposes, bipolar CCMs ceased to exist at these sites. Perhaps ironically, the only vestige of the CCM that remained 1 year after the study was that a group of patients at one of the sites continued to meet on their own to hold self-management skills groups (www. lifegoalscc.com), which were part of the CCM intervention.

Everything went right. What went wrong?

Unfortunately, this story is repeated frequently throughout healthcare. Clinical effectiveness, even when supported by numerous publications in peer-reviewed journals, does not ensure clinical uptake. Frequently noted studies indicate that it takes 17–20 years to get clinical innovations into practice; moreover, fewer than 50% of clinical innovations ever make it into general usage (Mosteller, 1981; Balas and Boren, 2000; Grant et al., 2003; Morris et al., 2011). The problem of non-uptake of effective clinical innovations is longstanding and persistent – and likely the rule rather than the exception. Reasons behind this problem lie beyond the clinical innovation and include contextual and other factors related to the use or non-use of the clinical innovation.

For instance, the first observation that citrus cures scurvy in the British Navy occurred in 1601; the first randomized controlled trial of citrus to treat scurvy was conducted in 1747. Yet the British Navy did not adopt routine use of citrus to prevent scurvy until 1795, and the British merchant marine not until 1865 (Mosteller, 1981). Similar instances of the lag between evidence and widespread usage are provided by Colditz and Emmons (2017). They contrast the slow uptake of the smallpox vaccine, penicillin, and insulin to the much more rapid uptake of anti-retroviral treatments for HIV/AIDS, making the point that contextual factors, not treatment effectiveness, play a dominant role in whether and how quickly a clinical innovation will become widely used. Similarly, Ferlie et al. (2005) studied non-adoption of eight hospital-based or primary care-based innovations in the United Kingdom. Their analysis demonstrated that, although the strength of the evidence contributed to the adoption of some clinical innovations, a more comprehensive explanation for non-adoption needed to also include contextual issues, such as the professional disciplines of the intended recipients.

Moving from establishing the efficacy of a clinical innovation to establishing its effectiveness in routine clinical settings

Given the need to support clinical uptake of efficacious innovations, researchers became aware of the necessity for studies, particularly clinical trials, that moved away from the highly structured environment of efficacy trials and into the routine clinical settings within which healthcare is delivered. With this transition, the focus of research broadened beyond internal validity (which prioritizes isolating treatment effects from all extraneous influences to determine whether an innovation has an impact) to also include considerations of external validity (which prioritizes the relevance and transferability of innovation effects from highly controlled experimental conditions into conditions under which the eventual end user of the innovation typically works). Trial designs were developed under the concept of "practice-based research" to expand the focus to include how a clinical innovation performed within the clinical settings in which it would potentially be used (Westfall et al., 2007). Thus, rather than focusing exclusively on the efficacy of a clinical innovation (internal validity, i.e. isolating and maximizing the impact of potential treatment), these designs also focused on effectiveness (external validity, i.e. generalizability to the practice settings in which the clinical innovation will be used).

However, as our story in Box 3.1 illustrates, even concerted effort at the effectiveness end of the trial design spectrum is not enough to guarantee routine usage of a clinical innovation. Moreover, although education and monitoring may be necessary to support the uptake of a new clinical innovation, they are rarely sufficient to change provider behaviour, as indicated by a meta-analysis by the Cochrane Collaboration which showed that audit and feedback only increased target provider behaviours by 4.3% (0.5%–16%) (Ivers et al., 2012). Thus, simply using traditional clinical trial approaches and pushing them further into real-world conditions is not sufficient to guarantee public health impact. Factors contributing to the non-adoption of evidence-based clinical innovations must be identified and addressed directly through promising methods and strategies that can be subjected to rigorous investigation in the emerging field of implementation science.

Answering the need: the emergence of implementation science

Implementation science is an inter-disciplinary field dedicated to studying how various evidence-based interventions or practices (e.g. innovations, programmes, services, policies, etc.) are best adopted and integrated into routine practice. Eccles and Mittman (2006) define it as "the scientific study of methods to promote the systematic uptake of research findings and other evidence-based practice into routine practice and, hence, to improve the quality and effectiveness of health services". In this definition, "methods" have since come to be referred to as "implementation strategies" (or merely "strategies"). The term, "implementation interventions", is also used to denote these methods although this term can cause confusion with clinical and other interventions directed at patients and other clients. The 2006 definition of implementation science emphasizes that research in this field investigates strategies to support implementation.

The concept of "implementation" is important in implementation science. The word is derived from the Latin *implere*, meaning to fulfil or carry into effect, which provides a basis for a similar definition of implementation. Weiner et al. (2023, p. 3) define implementation as "purposeful actions taken to put an evidence-based intervention into practice or into use".

Implementation science is sometimes confused with the evaluation of clinical interventions or practices. However, two features distinguish implementation science from this type of clinical evaluation: implementation science refers to the testing of implementation strategies for their effectiveness in supporting implementation and the use of theories, models and frameworks developed in implementation science or borrowed from other fields to understand and explain implementation processes and outcomes (Weiner et al., 2023).

The "implementation object", that is, the specific practice being implemented, is usually referred to as an evidence-based intervention (EBI) or an evidence-based practice (EBP). In health-related studies, both EBI and EBP may be considered shorthand terms for "programmes, practices, principles, procedures, products, pills and policies which have been found to be effective in improving health behaviours, health outcomes, or health-related environments in one or more well-designed research studies" (Leeman et al., 2017, p. 3). Similarly, Rabin and Brownson (2012, p. 24) define EBIs as "programmes, practices, processes, policies and guidelines". EBP can refer either to an individual intervention (i.e. an EBI) or to the overarching goal of striving for or attaining an EBP, which can be somewhat confusing. Further, the term "implementation object" usually refers to the use of an intervention or a practice.

Thus, the focus of implementation science is not to establish the health impact of a clinical innovation, but rather to identify and address the factors that affect its uptake into routine use. At the core of this rapidly growing science is the recognition that evidence-based clinical innovations must be complemented by evidence-based implementation strategies. Simply, the goal of implementation science is two-fold:

- Identify uptake barriers and facilitators across multiple levels of context (individuals in treatment, providers, professions, organizations, and other stakeholder groups).
- Develop, apply, and evaluate implementation strategies that overcome these barriers and enhance the facilitators to increase the uptake of evidence-based clinical innovations (Bauer and Kirchner, 2020).

Hence, in implementation science studies, the "intervention" under study is not the clinical innovation but rather the implementation strategies that support the uptake of that clinical innovation into routine clinical practice. Implementation strategies can be defined as methods to enhance the adoption, implementation, sustainment, and scale-up of an innovation (Proctor et al., 2013).

Implementation science lies at the applied end of the translational continuum, covering both research on dissemination (i.e. targeted transfer of knowledge to healthcare practitioners and other recipients) and implementation (i.e. active strategies to support implementation to achieve an EBP). In the USA, the term "dissemination and implementation" (D&I) research is common (Rabin and Brownson, 2012). This research calls out the need to explicitly study dissemination but it does not differ from research conducted under the implementation science banner.

In overly simplistic terms, the clinical researcher establishes the efficacy and then effectiveness of an innovation and then collaborates with the implementation science researcher to test ways of getting people to use it. This process as stated is overly simplistic because it suggests a unidimensional flow of tasks (Figure 3.1). In reality, the process is

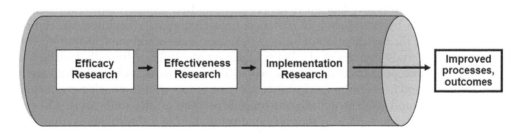

Figure 3.1 The traditional research pipeline.

Source: Curran et al. (2012)

much more iterative because implementation experience may suggest changes in the clinical innovation to increase its external validity (while also taking steps to ensure fidelity to its core components, supporting internal validity).

The scope of implementation science

Not surprisingly, implementation science involves investigation at more levels than just the individual patient/subject. Targets of investigation may also include the provider, clinic, facility, organization, community, and even the policy environment (Damschroder et al., 2009; Harvey and Kitson, 2015). Thus, also not surprisingly given the central role of context in implementation science, implementation science researchers include not just clinicians and clinical scientists but also social scientists, economists, systems engineers and health services researchers. In addition, special mention should be made of the relationship between implementation science researchers and their "operational partners" with whom a clinical innovation is to be deployed: healthcare system leaders, administrators, and staff who run and staff the clinics, facilities, and organizations (and sometimes also including policy makers).

Unlike clinical research, in which such individuals and structures play a primarily permissive or passively supportive role, in implementation research, operational colleagues need to be full partners in the research from study design to analysis, because implementation research aims to assess and actively intervene in their structures where they are the experts. Although there are cultural gaps between researchers and healthcare system leaders and staff that must be overcome (Kilbourne et al., 2012; Bauer et al., 2016), their participation is essential because an innovation will be implemented because of them, not in spite of them.

Optimizing the process: effectiveness-implementation hybrid designs

The shift in emphasis from clinical health outcomes to also include implementation strategies necessitates further development of trial designs. The development of hybrid effectiveness-implementation designs allows the study of both clinical and implementation outcomes. A comprehensive description of various common and emerging implementation science trial designs is beyond the scope of this chapter and can be found in other literature (Miller et al., 2023).

Approaching the development, evaluation, and implementation of a clinical innovation in discrete steps can be costly in terms of time, research costs and lost opportunities to improve healthcare. Curran et al. (2012) proposed an alternative approach to sequential studies by introducing effectiveness-implementation hybrid designs. Hybrid designs promote the examination of both clinical effectiveness and implementation outcomes within a study (Landes et al., 2019; Curran et al., 2022). Although described as a design, this concept has become more accepted as a framework within which a variety of randomized and non-randomized trial designs can be incorporated to document clinical effectiveness and implementation outcomes depending on the study aims. The primary aim of this framework is to support **rapid translation of a clinical innovation with** interventions in both the clinical and implementation domains tested simultaneously (Curran et al., 2012, 2022). Though the underlying premise of hybrid designs continues to evolve, current literature reflects three types of hybrid designs. These are described below with their associated aims in a table developed by Landes and colleagues (Table 3.1, Figure 3.2).

Table 3.1 Hybrid type and associated aims.

Study design	Hybrid type 1	Hybrid type 2	Hybrid type 3
Research aims	*Primary aim:* Determine the effectiveness of an intervention	*Primary aim:* Determine the effectiveness of an intervention	*Primary Aim:* Determine the impact of an implementation strategy
	Secondary aim: Better understand the context for implementation	*Co-primary aim (or secondary aim):* Determine feasibility and/or (potential) impact of an implementation strategy	*Secondary Aim:* Assess the clinical outcomes associated with implementation

Source: Landes et al. (2019)

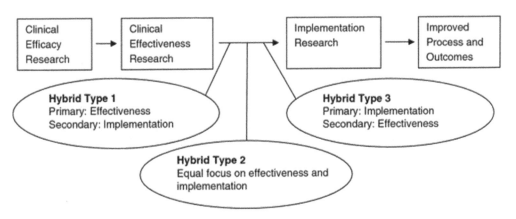

Figure 3.2 Hybrid type 1, 2 and 3 studies.
Source: Cully et al. (2012)

Let us continue the clinical story we began in Box 3.1 to illustrate the application of effectiveness-implementation hybrid designs (Box 3.2).

Box 3.2

Following the lack of sustained adoption of the bipolar CCM at the 15 sites described above, we partnered with the VA Office of Mental Health and Suicide Prevention (OMHSP) to support the implementation of cross-diagnosis CCM in VA general mental health clinics and conduct a randomized stepped-wedged trial testing the impact of CCM implementation support on the establishment of the CCM in participating clinics and on patient level outcomes (a hybrid type 2 design). This study applied an evidence-based implementation strategy, external facilitation (Kirchner et al., 2014), to support the uptake of CCM core elements in nine clinics

located in different VA medical centres (Bauer et al., 2016). One year of external facilitation support was associated with varying levels of implementation success but
overall improved clinician ratings of team-oriented variables (the implementation
outcome). This was also associated with a robust decrease in mental health hos-
pitalizations compared with non-participating clinics at the same medical centres;
mental health quality of life did not improve in the overall population of the clinics
but did for complex patients (those with three or more active psychiatric diagnoses)
(the effectiveness outcome).

Moving through the process: fidelity and adaptation in implementation science

A central concept within implementation science is the need to balance adaptation of a
clinical innovation to fit the context within which it is being implemented with fidelity
to the original clinical innovation. An example of this was the decision reflected in the
next phase of the CCM programme described in Box 3.2 to enlarge the target population
from individuals with bipolar disorder to the entire general mental health clinic population because it was recognized that there may not be a critical mass of individuals with
bipolar disorder to support a diagnosis-specific intervention in typical outpatient clinics.

Before adapting the clinical innovation to fit setting contextual factors, the core components of the clinical innovation must be defined. Fixsen et al. (2009) have defined
core components as the most essential and indispensable components of an intervention
practice or programme. These are the components without which the clinical innovation would not be able to achieve outcomes consistent with those achieved in clinical
trials. When considering what can be adapted and what should not, it can be helpful to
apply the Cancer Prevention and Control Research Network framework (Fernández et
al., 2014), which designates adaptations to the clinical innovation into three categories:

- Red light adaptations: things that probably cannot be modified.
- Yellow light adaptations: things that can probably be changed with caution.
- Green light adaptations: things that can probably be modified.

Green light (and at times yellow light) adaptations may enhance not only the uptake and
implementation of the clinical innovation but also the effectiveness within which it can
be delivered. In the case of the CCM programme, the CCM itself represented a red light,
because it was the core evidence-based innovation being studied. In contrast, broaden-
ing the target population was considered a yellow light, made credible by the extensive
evidence that indicated that the CCM could improve outcomes in the major diagnostic groups encountered in general mental health clinics (Woltmann et al., 2012; Miller
et al., 2013).

The goal of the process: sustainability

It is critical to recognize that the goal for implementation is not to simply implement
a clinical innovation but rather to have that innovation sustained long after the active implementation effort is completed; that is, to become "usual care". As noted by

implementation science researchers, "Sustainability has evolved from being considered as the endgame of a translational research process to a suggested 'adaptation phase' that integrates and institutionalizes interventions within local organizational and cultural contexts" (Chambers et al., 2013).

Clinical innovation sustainment is not something that should be considered at the end of implementation but rather should be addressed before and throughout the implementation process (Scheirer and Dearing, 2011). Successful sustainment of a clinical innovation should be viewed as a dynamic process that incorporates changes in organizational priorities, programme additions, and emerging evidence that naturally occurs over time (Shelton et al., 2020). Perhaps most critical is the need to realize that factors influencing the ability of a setting to sustain a clinical innovation may differ from those influencing successful implementation. Thus, there is a need to assess the capacity of the context in terms of the ability to institutionalize the clinical innovation. Identifying and addressing these factors can occur throughout the implementation process, but can also be accomplished through the development of a formal sustainability action plan (Scheirer and Dearing, 2011) that is created as part of the implementation process. This can be used to identify individuals responsible for actions that promote sustainability, including ongoing programme productivity assessment, adaptation and fidelity monitoring.

Let us return to the next phase of our CCM implementation story in terms of sustainability (Box 3.3).

Box 3.3

We investigated the sustainability of the CCM in general outpatient clinics in two ways. First, after the 1-year of implementation support ended, we assessed hospitalization rates in the subsequent year in the implementation clinics and controls (Bauer et al., 2021). The relative advantage of the CCM clinics disappeared during the second year when no implementation support was provided. Thus, we suspected that the CCM had not become "usual care" in these clinics.

In addition to this quantitative clinical outcome, a qualitative study (Miller et al., 2023) was undertaken 3 years after the end of implementation support to investigate the degree to which the various components of the CCM continued to be implemented by the nine clinics. As suspected, adoption was variable across CCM elements, with staff reporting that those CCM components that were most consistent with prevailing VA procedures or were championed by staff beyond the implementation clinics, were most likely to be sustained, whereas those viewed as more innovative were less so. Moreover, staff turnover represented a very significant barrier to sustainability, with some positions not filled when vacant, and often only a limited amount of education about the CCM when new staff were brought on board. Overall, results indicated that CCM implementation was most sustainable when it was pursued as a multi-level effort within the organization, with staff roles dedicated to CCM-consistent care practices within leadership and the front lines of direct clinical care.

Currently, a "second generation" randomized CCM implementation trial in VA general mental health clinics is under way that builds on the lessons of the work to date, aiming for sustained system change and sustained clinical outcomes.

Concluding remarks

In summary, implementation science seeks to "continue the job" of biomedical research, taking evidence-based clinical innovations and testing strategies to move them into wider practice. Given this goal, the principles and research methods of implementation science differ somewhat from clinical research. Most centrally, implementation science protocols do not ignore or control for context, but rather actively seek to intervene to change the context in which clinical innovations are used to enhance their uptake. Implementation science researchers interface closely with healthcare leaders and staff as partners, breaking down the research–practice divide to achieve the ultimate goal of increasing the public health impact of evidence-based innovations (Bauer and Kirchner, 2020).

Acknowledgement

This chapter builds upon an introductory manuscript for a special issue dedicated to introducing the principles and methods of implementation science to the non-specialist (Bauer and Kirchner, 2020).

References

Balas, E.A., Boren, S.A. (2000) Managing clinical knowledge for health care improvement. *Yearbook of Medical Informatics* (1), 65–70. https://doi.org/10.1055/s-0038-1637943

Bauer, M.S., Kirchner, J.E. (2020) Implementation science: what is it and why should I care? *Psychiatry Research* 283, 112376. https://doi.org/10.1016/j.psychres.2019.04.025

Bauer, M.S., McBride, L., Williford, W.O., Glick, H., Kinosian, B., Alshuler, L., et al. (2006a) Collaborative care for bipolar disorder: part I. Intervention and implementation in a randomized effectiveness trial. *Psychiatric Services* 57, 927–936. https://doi.org/10.1176/ps.2006.57.7.927

Bauer, M.S., McBride, L., Williford, W.O., Glick, H., Kinosian, B., Altshuler, L., et al. (2006b) Collaborative care for bipolar disorder, part II: impact on clinical outcome, function, and costs. *Psychiatric Services* 57, 937–945. https://doi.org/10.1176/ps.2006.57.7.937

Bauer, M.S., Miller, C.J., Kim, B., Lew, R., Weaver, K., Coldwell, C., et al. (2016) Partnering with health system operations leadership to develop a controlled implementation trial. *Implementation Science* 11, 22. https://doi.org/10.1186/s13012-016-0385-7

Bauer, M.S., Stolzmann, K., Miller, C.J., Kim, B., Connolly, S.L., Lew, R. (2021) Implementing the collaborative chronic care model in mental health clinics: achieving and sustaining clinical effects. *Psychiatric Services* 72, 586–589. https://doi.org/10.1176/appi.ps.202000117

Chambers, D.A., Glasgow, R.E., Stange, K.C. (2013) The dynamic sustainability framework: addressing the paradox of sustainment amid ongoing change. *Implementation Science* 8, 117. https://doi.org/10.1186/1748-5908-8-117

Colditz, G., Emmons, K. (2017) The promise and challenge of dissemination and implementation research. In: Brownson, R.C., Colditz, G.A., Proctor, E.K. (Eds.), *Dissemination and Implementation Research in Health*. 2nd edition. Oxford: Oxford University Press, pp. 1–18.

Cully, J.A., Armento, M.E.A., Mott, J., Nadorff, M.R., Naik, A.D., Stanley, M.A., Sorocco, K.H., Kunik, M.E., Petersen, N.J., Kauth, M.R. (2012). Brief cognitive behavioral therapy in primary care: a hybrid type 2 patient-randomized effectiveness-implementation design. *Implementation Science* 7, 64. https://doi.org/10.1186/1748-5908-7-64

Curran, G.M., Bauer, M.S., Mittman, B., Pyne, J.M., Stetler, C. (2012) Effectiveness-implementation hybrid designs: combining elements of clinical effectiveness and implementation research to enhance public health impact. *Medical Care* 50, 217–226. https://doi.org/10.1097/MLR.0b013e3182408812

Curran, G.M., Landes, S.J., McBain, S.A., Pyne, J.M., Smith, J.D., Fernandez, M.E., et al. (2022) Reflections on 10 years of effectiveness-implementation hybrid studies. *Frontiers in Health Services* 2, 1053496. https://doi.org/10.3389/frhs.2022.1053496

Damschroder, L.J., Aron, D.C., Keith, K.E., Kirsh, S.R., Alexander, J.A., Lowery, J.C. (2009) Fostering implementation of health services research findings into practice: a consolidated framework for advancing implementation science. *Implementation Science* 4, 50. https://doi.org/10.1186/1748-5908-4-50

Eccles, M.P., Mittman, B.S. (2006) Welcome to implementation science. *Implementation Science* 1, 1. https://doi.org/10.1186/1748-5908-1-1

Ferlie, E., Fitzgerald, L., Wood, M., Hawkins, C. (2005) The nonspread of innovations: the mediating role of professionals. *Academy of Management Journal* 48, 117–134. https://doi.org/10.5465/amj.2005.15993150

Fernández, M.E., Melvin, C.L., Leeman, J., Ribisl, K.M., Allen, J.D., Kegler, M.C., et al. (2014) The cancer prevention and control research network: an interactive systems approach to advancing cancer control in implementation research and practice. *Cancer Epidemiology, Biomarkers & Prevention* 23, 2512–2521. https://doi.org/10.1158/1055-9965.EPI-14-0097

Fixsen, D.L., Blasé, K.A., Naoom, S.F., Wallace, F. (2009) Core implementation components. *Research on Social Work Practice* 19, 531–540. https://doi.org/10.1177/1049731509335549

Grant, J., Green, L., Mason, B. (2003) Basic research and health: a reassessment of the scientific basis for the support of biomedical science. *Research Evaluation* 12, 217–224. https://doi.org/10.3152/147154403781776618

Harvey, G., Kitson, A. (2015) Translating evidence into healthcare policy and practice: single versus multi-faceted implementation strategies – is there a simple answer to a complex question? *International Journal of Health Policy and Management* 4, 123–126. https://doi.org/10.15171/ijhpm.2015.54

Ivers, N., Jamtvedt, G., Flottorp, S., Young, J.M., Odgaard-Jensen, J., French, S.D., et al. (2012) Audit and feedback: effects on professional practice and healthcare outcomes. *Cochrane Database of Systematic Reviews* (6), CD000259. https://doi.org/10.1002/14651858.CD000259.pub3

Kilbourne, A.M., Williams, M., Bauer, M.S., Arean, P. (2012) Implementation research: reducing the research-to-practice gap in depression treatment. *Depression Research and Treatment* 2012, 1–2. https://doi.org/10.1155/2012/476027

Kirchner, J.E., Kearney, L.K., Ritchie, M.J., Dollar, K.M., Swensen, A.B., Schohn, M. (2014) 'Research & services partnerships: lessons learned through a national partnership between clinical leaders and researchers. *Psychiatric Services* 65, 577–579. https://doi.org/10.1176/appi.ps.201400054

Landes, S.J., McBain, S.A., Curran, G.M. (2019) An introduction to effectiveness-implementation hybrid designs. *Psychiatry Research* 280, 112513. https://doi.org/10.1016/j.psychres.2019.112513

Leeman, J., Birken, S.A., Powell, B.J., Rohweder, C., Shea, C.M. (2017). Beyond "implementation strategies". Classifying the full range of strategies used in implementation science and practice. *Implementation Science* 12, 125. https://doi.org/10.1186/s13012-017-0657-x

Miller, C.J., Grogan-Kaylor, A., Perron, B.E., Kilbourne, A.M., Woltmann, E., Bauer, M.S. (2013) Collaborative chronic care models for mental health conditions: cumulative meta-analysis and metaregression to guide future research and implementation. *Medical Care* 51, 922–930. https://doi.org/10.1097/MLR.0b013e3182a3e4c4

Miller, C.J., Kim, B., Connolly, S.L., Spitzer, E.G. Brown, M., Bailey, H.M., et al. (2023) Sustainability of the collaborative chronic care model in outpatient mental health teams three years post-implementation: a qualitative analysis. *Administration and Policy in Mental Health and Mental Health Services Research* 50, 151–159. https://doi.org/10.1007/s10488-022-01231-0

Morris, Z.S., Wooding, S., Grant, J. (2011) The answer is 17 years, what is the question: understanding time lags in translational research. *Journal of the Royal Society of Medicine* 104, 510–520. https://doi.org/10.1258/jrsm.2011.110180

Mosteller, F. (1981) Innovation and evaluation. *Science* 211, 881–886. https://doi.org/10.1126/science.6781066

Proctor, E.K., Powell, B.J., McMillen, J.C. (2013) Implementation strategies: recommendations for specifying and reporting. *Implementation Science* 8, 139. https://doi.org/10.1186/1748-5908-8-139

Rabin, B.A., Brownson, R.C. (2012) Developing the terminology for dissemination and implementation research. In: Brownson, R.C., Colditz, G.A., Proctor, E.K. (Eds.), *Dissemination and Implementation Research in Health*. Oxford: Oxford University Press, pp. 23–51.

Scheirer, M.A., Dearing, J.W. (2011) An agenda for research on the sustainability of public health programs. *American Journal of Public Health* 101, 2059–2067. https://doi.org/10.2105/AJPH.2011.300193

Shelton, R.C., Chambers, D.A., Glasgow, R.E. (2020) An extension of RE-AIM to enhance sustainability: addressing dynamic context and promoting health equity over time. *Frontiers in Public Health* 8, 134. https://doi.org/10.3389/fpubh.2020.00134

Simon, G.E., Ludman, E.J., Bauer, M.S., Unützer, J., Operskalski, B. (2006) Long-term effectiveness and cost of a systematic care program for bipolar disorder. *Archives of General Psychiatry* 63, 500. https://doi.org/10.1001/archpsyc.63.5.500

Weiner, B.J., Lewis, C.C., Sherr, K. (2023). Introducing Implementation Science. In: *Practical Implementation Science*, eds Weiner BJ, Lewis CC, Sherr K. New York: Springer Publishing. Pp: 1–22.

Westfall, J.M., Mold, J., Fagnan, L. (2007) Practice-based research – "blue highways" on the NIH roadmap. *JAMA*, 297(4), p. 403. https://doi.org/10.1001/jama.297.4.403.

Woltmann, E., Grogan-Kaylor, A., Perron, B., Georges, H., Kilbourne, A.M., Bauer, M.S. (2012) Comparative effectiveness of collaborative chronic care models for mental health conditions across primary, specialty, and behavioral health care settings: systematic review and meta-analysis. *American Journal of Psychiatry* 169, 790–804. https://doi.org/10.1176/appi.ajp.2012.11111616

Yatham, L.N., Kennedy, S.H., Parikh, S.V., Schaffer, A., Bond, D.J., Frey, B.N., et al. (2006) Canadian Network for Mood and Anxiety Treatments (CANMAT) guidelines for the management of patients with bipolar disorder: update 2007: CANMAT guidelines for bipolar disorder. *Bipolar Disorders* 8, 721–739. https://doi.org/10.1111/j.1399-5618.2006.00432.x

4 A taxonomy of theories, models and frameworks in implementation science

Per Nilsen

Introduction

Implementation science began largely as a field of "trial and error". Studies often lacked theoretical rationale for the selection and use of specific implementation strategies (Eccles et al., 2005). Mixed results on achieving an evidence-based practice (EBP) in various settings were commonly attributed to a limited theoretical basis (Kitson et al., 1998; Davies et al., 2003; Eccles et al., 2005; Michie et al., 2005; Sales et al., 2006). Poor theoretical underpinning makes it difficult to understand and explain how and why implementation succeeds or fails, thus restricting opportunities to identify factors that predict the likelihood of implementation success and developing improved strategies to support implementation.

Despite the field's empirically driven start, implementation science has become increasingly based on theory over time. There is now wide recognition of the importance of establishing the theoretical bases of implementation strategies to understand the how and why of changing practice. There are now so many theoretical approaches that some researchers have complained about the difficulties of choosing the most appropriate (ICEBeRG, 2006; Godin et al., 2008; Mitchell et al., 2010; Rycroft-Malone and Bucknall, 2010; Cane et al., 2012; Martinez et al., 2014).

Theories, models and frameworks in implementation science

Theories in implementation science aim to explain the causal mechanisms of implementation. Models in implementation science are commonly used to describe and/or guide the process of translating research into practice rather than to predict or analyse what factors influence implementation outcomes. Determinant frameworks in implementation science often have a descriptive purpose by pointing to factors believed or found to influence implementation outcomes.

In general, models can be described as theories with a more narrowly defined scope of explanation; a model is descriptive, whereas a theory is explanatory as well as descriptive (Frankfort-Nachmias and Nachmias, 1996). A model typically involves a deliberate simplification of a phenomenon or a specific aspect of a phenomenon. Models need not be completely accurate representations of reality to have value (Carpiano, 2006; Cairney, 2012). A framework usually denotes a structure, overview, outline, system or plan consisting of various descriptive categories, for example, concepts, constructs or variables, and the relations between them that are presumed to account for a phenomenon (Sabatier, 1999).

DOI: 10.4324/9781003318125-5

A key difference between models and frameworks in implementation science is that the former recognize a temporal sequence of implementation endeavours, whereas frameworks do not explicitly take a process perspective of implementation. However, the terms "theories", "models" and "frameworks" are not used consistently in the field; they are often used interchangeably (Estabrooks et al., 2006; Kitson et al., 2008; Rycroft-Malone and Bucknall, 2010).

Three overarching aims of the use of theories, models and frameworks in implementation science can be identified:

- Describing and/or guiding the process of translating research into practice.
- Understanding and/or explaining what influences implementation outcomes.
- Evaluating implementation.

Based on descriptions of their origins, how they were developed, what knowledge sources they drew on, stated aims and applications in implementation science, theoretical approaches that aim at understanding and/or explaining influences on implementation outcomes (i.e. the second aim) can be further broken down into:

- Determinant frameworks.
- Classic theories.
- Implementation theories.

Thus, five categories of theoretical approaches used in implementation science can be delineated, as shown in Figure 4.1. This five-category taxonomy has been referred to as "Nilsen's Taxonomy" (KTDRR, 2022) and "Nilsen's Schema" (Washington University, 2022).

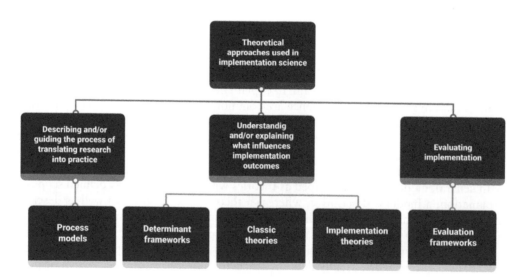

Figure 4.1 Three aims of the use of theoretical approaches in implementation science and the five categories of theories, models and frameworks.

Descriptions of the five categories

Process models

Process models specify steps (stages, phases) in the process of translating research into practice, including the implementation and use of research. The aim of process models is to describe and/or guide the process of translating research into practice. An action model is a type of process model that provides practical guidance in the planning and execution of implementation endeavours and/or implementation strategies to facilitate implementation. The terms "model" and "framework" are both used, but the former appears to be the more common.

Examples of process models include models by Landry et al. (2001), Davis et al. (2007) and Majdzadeh et al. (2008). Other examples are the CIHR (Canadian Institutes of Health Research) Model of Knowledge Translation (Canadian Institutes of Health Research, 2014), the K2A (Knowledge-to-Action) Framework (Wilson et al., 2011), the Stetler Model (Stetler, 2010), the ACE (Academic Center for Evidence-Based Practice) Star Model of Knowledge Transformation (Stevens, 2013), the Knowledge-to-Action Model (Graham et al., 2006), the Iowa Model (Titler et al., 1994), the Ottawa Model (Logan and Graham, 1998) and the Quality Implementation Framework (Meyers et al., 2012). Four process models are described in Chapter 5.

Determinant frameworks

Determinant frameworks specify types (also known as classes or domains) of determinants and individual determinants, which act as barriers and enablers (independent variables) that influence implementation outcomes (dependent variables). Some frameworks also specify relationships between some types of determinants. The overarching aim is to understand and/or explain influences on implementation outcomes, for example, predicting outcomes or interpreting outcomes retrospectively.

Examples of determinant frameworks include EPIS (Exploration-Preparation-Implementation-Sustainment) (Aarons et al., 2011), i-PARIHS (integrated-Promoting Action on Research Implementation in Health Services) (Harvey and Kitson, 2016), PARIHS (Promoting Action on Research Implementation in Health Services) (Kitson et al., 1998), Active Implementation Frameworks (Blase et al., 2012), Understanding-User-Context Framework (Jacobson et al., 2003), Conceptual Model (Greenhalgh et al., 2005), framework by Grol et al. (2005), framework by Cochrane et al. (2007), Ecological Framework by Durlak and DuPre (2008), CFIR (Consolidated Framework for Implementation Research) (Damschroder et al., 2009), framework by Gurses et al. (2010), Theoretical Domains Framework (Michie et al., 2014), TICD (Tailored Implementation for Chronic Disease) (Flottorp et al., 2013).

Classic theories

Classic theories is a label used for theories that originate from fields external to implementation science (e.g. psychology, sociology and organizational theory) that can be applied to provide understanding and/or explanation of aspects of implementation. These theories have been referred to as "classic" (or "classic change") theories to distinguish them from research-to-practice models (Graham et al., 2009). An important example is the Theory of Diffusion (Rogers, 2003) but there are also countless individual-level, group-level and organizational-level theories and concepts, some of which are described in Chapter 8.

Implementation theories

Implementation theories are theories that have been developed by implementation researchers (from scratch or by adapting existing theories and concepts) to provide understanding and/or explanation of aspects of implementation. Examples include Absorptive Capacity (Zahra and George, 2002), Organizational Readiness (Weiner, 2009), COM-B (Capacity Opportunities Motivation – Behaviour) (Michie et al., 2011) and Normalization Process Theory (May and Finch, 2009). Three implementation theories are described in Chapter 7.

Evaluation frameworks

Evaluation frameworks specify aspects of implementation that could be evaluated to determine implementation success. Two prime examples are Reach, Effectiveness, Adoption, Implementation and Maintenance (RE-AIM) (Glasgow et al., 1999) and the outcome framework developed by Proctor et al. (2010), both of which are described in Chapter 9. RE-AIM has evolved over time and is not only used for evaluation purposes. Theories, models and frameworks from the other four categories can also function as "evaluation frameworks" because they specify concepts and constructs that may be operationalized and measured. For instance, the Theoretical Domains Framework (e.g. Fleming et al., 2014; Phillips et al., 2015) and Normalization Process Theory (McEvoy et al., 2014) and COM-B (e.g. Connell et al., 2015; Praveen et al., 2014) have all been widely used as evaluation frameworks.

Many theories, models and frameworks have spawned instruments that serve evaluation purposes, for example, tools linked to PARIHS (Estabrooks et al., 2009; McCormack et al., 2009), CFIR (Damschroder and Lowery, 2013) and the Theoretical Domains Framework (Dyson et al., 2013). Other examples include the EBP Implementation Scale to measure the extent to which EBP is implemented (Melnyk et al., 2008) and instruments to operationalize theories such as Implementation Climate (Jacobs et al., 2014) and Organizational Readiness (Gagnon et al., 2011).

Concluding remarks

The proposed taxonomy distinguishes between five categories of theoretical approaches in implementation science, yet there is considerable overlap between some of the categories of the taxonomy. Thus, determinant frameworks, classic theories and implementation theories can also help guide an implementation effort (i.e. functioning as process models) because they identify potential barriers and enablers that might be important to address when undertaking an implementation endeavour. They can also be used for evaluation because they describe aspects that might be important to evaluate (i.e. functioning as evaluation frameworks).

Some frameworks combine determinant framework and process model characteristics, thus aiming to both provide guidance for the implementation process and identify potentially important determinants. A good example of such a framework/model is

EPIS; it highlights four temporal phases in the process of implementation, providing information to guide this process (i.e. a process model trait), and it identifies a number of determinants that may be relevant to consider in these four phases (i.e. a determinant framework trait) (Aarons et al., 2011; Moullin et al., 2019). Somewhat similarly, a determinant framework such as the Active Implementation Framework (Holmes et al., 2012) also appears to have a dual aim of providing hands-on support to implement something and identifying determinants of this implementation that need to be addressed.

Despite the overlap between different theories, models and frameworks used in implementation science, knowledge about the five categories of theoretical approaches is important to identify and select relevant approaches in various situations. Most determinant frameworks provide limited "how-to" support for carrying out implementation endeavours because the determinants may be too generic to provide sufficient detail for guiding users through an implementation process. Conversely, the relevance of addressing barriers and enablers to translating research into practice is mentioned in many process models, yet these models do not identify or systematically structure specific determinants associated with implementation success.

The five categories of the taxonomy are not always recognized as separate types of approaches in the literature. For instance, systematic reviews and overviews by Graham and Tetroe (2007), Mitchell et al. (2010), Flottorp et al. (2013), Meyers et al. (2012) and Tabak et al. (2012) have not distinguished between process models, determinant frameworks or classic theories because they all deal with factors believed or found to have an impact on implementation processes and outcomes. However, what matters most is not necessarily how an individual approach is labelled, but it is important to recognize that these theories, models and frameworks differ in terms of their assumptions, aims and other characteristics that have implications for their use.

Acknowledgement

This chapter builds upon Per Nilsen's paper "Making sense of implementation theories, models and frameworks", published 2015 in *Implementation Science*, Vol. 10, 53.

References

Aarons, G.A., Hurlburt, M., Horwitz, S.M. (2011) Advancing a conceptual model of evidence-based practice implementation in public service sectors. *Administration and Policy in Mental Health and Mental Health Services Research* 38, 4–23. https://doi.org/10.1007/s10488-010-0327-7

Blase, K.A., Van Dyke, M., Fixsen, D.L., Bailey, F.W. (2012) Implementation science: key concepts, themes and evidence for practitioners in educational psychology. In: Kelly, B., Perkins, D.F. (Eds.), *Handbook of Implementation Science for Psychology in Education*. Cambridge: Cambridge University Press, pp. 13–34. https://doi.org/10.1017/CBO9781139013949.004

Cairney, P. (2012) *Understanding Public Policy: Theories and Issues*. Basingstoke: Palgrave Macmillan. https://doi.org/10.1007/978-0-230-35699-3_1

Canadian Institutes of Health Research (CIHR). About knowledge translation. Retrieved from www.cihr-irsc.gc.ca/e/29418.html (accessed 18 December 2014).

Cane, J., O'Connor, D., Michie, S. (2012) Validation of the theoretical domains framework for use in behaviour change and implementation research. *Implementation Science* 7, 37. https://doi.org/10.1186/1748-5908-7-37

Carpiano, R.M. (2006) A guide and glossary on postpositivist theory building for population health. *Journal of Epidemiology and Community Health* 60, 564–570. https://doi.org/10.1136/jech.2004.031534

Cochrane, L.J., Olson, C.A., Murray, S., Dupuis, M., Tooman, T., Hayes, S. (2007) Gaps between knowing and doing: understanding and assessing the barriers to optimal health care. *Journal of Continuing Education in the Health Professions* 27, 94–102. https://doi.org/10.1002/chp.106

Connell, L.A., McMahon, N.E., Redfern, J., Watkins, C.L., Eng, J.J. (2015) Development of a behaviour change intervention to increase upper limb exercise in stroke rehabilitation. *Implementation Science* 10, 34. https://doi.org/10.1186/s13012-015-0223-3

Damschroder, L.J., Lowery, J.C. (2013) Evaluation of a large-scale weight management program using the consolidated framework for implementation research (CFIR). *Implementation Science* 8, 51. https://doi.org/10.1186/1748-5908-8-51

Damschroder, L.J., Aron, D.C., Keith, R.E., Kirsh, S.R., Alexander, J.A., Lowery, J.C. (2009) Fostering implementation of health services research findings into practice: a consolidated framework for advancing implementation science. *Implementation Science* 4, 50. https://doi.org/10.1186/1748-5908-4-50

Davies, P., Walker, A., Grimshaw, J. (2003) Theories of behavior change in studies of guideline implementation. *Proceedings of the British Psychological Society* 11, 120.

Davis, S.M., Peterson, J.C., Helfrich, C.D., Cunningham-Sabo, L. (2007) Introduction and conceptual model for utilization of prevention research. *American Journal of Preventive Medicine* 33(1 Suppl), S1–S5. https://doi.org/10.1016/j.amepre.2007.04.004

Durlak, J.A., DuPre, E.P. (2008) Implementation matters: a review of research on the influence of implementation on program outcomes and the factors affecting implementation. *American Journal of Community Psychology* 41, 327–350. https://doi.org/10.1007/s10464-008-9165-0

Dyson, J., Lawton, R., Jackson, C., Cheater, F. (2013) Development of a theory-based instrument to identify barriers and levers to best hand hygiene practice among healthcare practitioners. *Implementation Science* 8, 111. https://doi.org/10.1186/1748-5908-8-111

Eccles, M.P., Grimshaw, J., Walker, A., Johnston, M., Pitts, N. (2005) Changing the behavior of healthcare professionals: the use of theory in promoting the uptake of research findings. *Journal of Clinical Epidemiology* 58, 107–112. https://doi.org/10.1016/j.jclinepi.2004.09.002

Estabrooks, C.A., Thompson, D.S., Lovely, J.J., Hofmeyer, A. (2006) A guide to knowledge translation theory. *Journal of Continuing Education in the Health Professions* 26, 25–36. https://doi.org/10.1002/chp.48

Estabrooks, C.A., Squires, J.E., Cummings, G.G., Birdsell, J.M., Norton, P.G. (2009) Development and assessment of the Alberta Context Tool. *BMC Health Services Research* 9, 234. https://doi.org/10.1186/1472-6963-9-234

Fleming, A., Bradley, C., Cullinan, S., Byrne, S. (2014) Antibiotic prescribing in long-term care facilities: a qualitative, multidisciplinary investigation. *BMJ Open* 4, e006442. https://doi.org/10.1136/bmjopen-2014-006442

Flottorp, S.A., Oxman, A.D., Krause, J., Musila, N.R., Wensing, M., Godycki-Cwirko, M., et al. (2013) A checklist for identifying determinants of practice: a systematic review and synthesis of frameworks and taxonomies of factors that prevent or enable improvements in healthcare professional practice. *Implementation Science* 8, 35. https://doi.org/10.1186/1748-5908-8-35

Frankfort-Nachmias, C., Nachmias, D. (1996) *Research Methods in the Social Sciences*. London: Arnold.

Gagnon, M., Labarthe, J., Légaré, F., Ouimet, M., Estabrooks, C.A., Roch, G., et al. (2011) Measuring organizational readiness for knowledge translation in chronic care. *Implementation Science* 6, 72. https://doi.org/10.1186/1748-5908-6-72

Glasgow, R.E., Vogt, T.M., Boles, S.M. (1999) Evaluating the public health impact of health promotion interventions: the RE-AIM framework. *American Journal of Public Health* 89, 1322–1327. https://doi.org/10.2105/AJPH.89.9.1322

Godin, G., Bélanger-Gravel, A., Eccles, M., Grimshaw, J. (2008) Healthcare professionals' intentions and behaviours: a systematic review of studies based on social cognitive theories. *Implementation Science* 3, 36. https://doi.org/10.1186/1748-5908-3-36

Graham, I.D., Tetroe, J. (2007) Some theoretical underpinnings of knowledge translation. *Academic Emergency Medicine* 14, 936–941.

Graham, I.D., Logan, J., Harrison, M.B., Straus, S.E., Tetroe, J., Caswell, W., et al. (2006) Lost in knowledge translation: time for a map? *Journal of Continuing Education in the Health Professions* 26, 13–24. https://doi.org/10.1002/chp.47

Graham, I.D., Tetroe, J., KT Theories Group. (2009) Planned action theories. In: Straus, S.E., Tetroe, J., Graham, I.D. (Eds.), *Knowledge Translation in Health Care: Moving from Evidence to Practice*. Chichester: Wiley-Blackwell/BMJ, pp. 185–195.

Greenhalgh, T., Robert, G., Bate, P., Macfarlane, F., Kyriakidou, O. (2005) *Diffusion of Innovations in Service Organisations: A Systematic Literature Review*. Malden, MA: Blackwell. https://doi.org/10.1002/9780470987407

Grol, R., Wensing, M., Eccles, M. (2005) *Improving Patient Care: The Implementation of Change in Clinical Practice*. Edinburgh: Elsevier Butterworth Heinemann.

Gurses, A.P., Marsteller, J.A., Ozok, A.A., Xiao, Y., Owens, S., Pronovost, P.J. (2010) Using an interdisciplinary approach to identify factors that affect clinicians' compliance with evidence-based guidelines. *Critical Care Medicine* 38(8 Suppl), S282–S291. https://doi.org/10.1097/CCM.0b013e3181e69e02

Harvey, G., Kitson. A. (2016) PARIHS revisited: from heuristic to integrated framework for the successful implementation of knowledge into practice. *Implementation Science* 11, 33. https://doi.org/10.1186/s13012-016-0398-2

Holmes, B.J., Finegood, D.T., Riley, B.L., Best, A. (2012) Systems thinking in dissemination and implementation research. In: Brownson, R.C., Colditz, G.A., Proctor, E.K. (Eds.), *Dissemination and Implementation Research in Health*. Oxford: Oxford University Press, pp. 192–212. https://doi.org/10.1093/acprof:oso/9780199751877.003.0009

ICEBeRG. (2006) Designing theoretically-informed implementation interventions. *Implementation Science* 1, 4. https://doi.org/10.1186/1748-5908-1-4

Jacobs, S.R., Weiner, B.J., Bunger, A.C. (2014) Context matters: measuring implementation climate among individuals and groups. *Implementation Science* 9, 46. https://doi.org/10.1186/1748-5908-9-46

Jacobson, N., Butterill, D., Goering, P. (2003) Development of a framework for knowledge translation: understanding user context. *Journal of Health Services Research Policy* 8, 94–99. https://doi.org/10.1258/135581903321466067

Kitson, A.L., Harvey, G., McCormack, B. (1998) Enabling the implementation of evidence based practice: a conceptual framework. *Quality and Safety in Health Care* 7, 149–158. https://doi.org/10.1136/qshc.7.3.149

Kitson, A.L., Rycroft-Malone, J., Harvey, G., McCormack, B., Seers, K., Titchen, A. (2008) Evaluating the successful implementation of evidence into practice using the PARiHS framework: theoretical and practical challenges. *Implementation Science* 3, 1. https://doi.org/10.1186/1748-5908-3-1

KTDRR (Center on Knowledge Translation for Disability and Rehabilitation Research) (2022). The rise of implementation science. Available from: https://ktdrr.org/products/kt-implementation/rise-of-implementation-science.html Accessed 20 July 2022.

Landry, R., Amara, N., Lamari, M. (2001) Climbing the ladder of research utilization: evidence from social science research. *Science Communication* 22, 396–422. https://doi.org/10.1177/1075547001022004003

Logan, J., Graham, I.D. (1998) Toward a comprehensive interdisciplinary model of health care research use. *Science Communication* 20, 227–246. https://doi.org/10.1177/1075547098020002004

Majdzadeh, R., Sadighi, J., Nejat, S., Mahani, A.S., Gholami, J. (2008) Knowledge translation for research utilization: design of a knowledge translation model at Tehran University of Medical Sciences. *Journal of Continuing Education in the Health Professions* 28, 270–277.

Martinez, R.G., Lewis, C.C., Weiner, B.J. (2014) Instrumentation issues in implementation science. *Implementation Science* 9, 118. https://doi.org/10.1186/s13012-014-0118-8

May, C., Finch, T. (2009) Implementing, embedding, and integrating practices: an outline of normalization process theory. *Sociology* 43, 535–554. https://doi.org/10.1177/0038038509103208

McCormack, B., McCarthy, G., Wright, J., Coffey, A. (2009) Development and testing of the Context Assessment Index (CAI). *Worldviews on Evidence-Based Nursing* 6, 27–35. https://doi.org/10.1111/j.1741-6787.2008.00130.x

McEvoy, R., Ballini, L., Maltoni, S., O'Donnell, C.A., Mair, F.S., Macfarlane, A. (2014) A qualitative systematic review of studies using the normalization process theory to research implementation processes. *Implementation Science* 9, 2. https://doi.org/10.1186/1748-5908-9-2

Melnyk, B.M., Fineout-Overholt, E., Mays, M.Z. (2008) The Evidence-Based Practice Beliefs and Implementation Scales: psychometric properties of two new instruments. *Worldviews on Evidence-Based Nursing* 5, 208–216. https://doi.org/10.1111/j.1741-6787.2008.00126.x

Meyers, D.C., Durlak, J.A., Wandersman, A. (2012) The Quality Implementation Framework: a synthesis of critical steps in the implementation process. *American Journal of Community Psychology* 50, 462–480. https://doi.org/10.1007/s10464-012-9522-x

Michie, S., Johnston, M., Abraham, C., Lawton, R., Parker, D., Walker, A. (2005) Making psychological theory useful for implementing evidence based practice: a consensus approach. *Quality and Safety in Health Care* 14, 26–33. https://doi.org/10.1136/qshc.2004.011155

Michie, S., Stralen, M.M., West, R. (2011) The behaviour change wheel: a new method for characterising and designing behaviour change interventions. *Implementation Science* 6, 42. https://doi.org/10.1186/1748-5908-6-42

Michie, S., Atkins, L., West, R. (2014) *The Behaviour Change Wheel: A Guide to Designing Interventions*. London: Silverback.

Mitchell, S.A., Fisher, C.A., Hastings, C.E., Silverman, L.B., Wallen, G.R. (2010) A thematic analysis of theoretical models for translational science in nursing: mapping the field. *Nursing Outlook* 58, 287–300. https://doi.org/10.1016/j.outlook.2010.07.001

Moullin, J.C., Dickson, K.S., Stadnick, N.A., Rabin, B., Aarons, G.A. (2019) Systematic review of the Exploration, Preparation, Implementation, Sustainment (EPIS) framework. *Implementation Science* 14, 1. https://doi.org/10.1186/s13012-018-0842-6

Phillips, C.J., Marshall, A.P., Chaves, N.J., Lin, I.B., Loy, C.T., Rees, G., et al. (2015) Experiences of using Theoretical Domains Framework across diverse clinical environments: a qualitative study. *Journal of Multidisciplinary Healthcare* 8, 139–146. https://doi.org/10.2147/JMDH.S78458

Praveen, D., Patel, A., Raghu, A., Clifford, G.D., Maulik, P.K., Abdul, A.M., et al. (2014) SMART-Health India: development and field evaluation of a mobile clinical decision support system for cardiovascular diseases in rural India. *JMIR MHealth and UHealth* 2, e54. https://doi.org/10.2196/mhealth.3568

Proctor, E., Silmere, H., Raghavan, R., Hovmand, P., Aarons, G., Bunger, A., et al. (2010) Outcomes for implementation research: conceptual distinctions, measurement challenges, and research agenda. *Administration and Policy in Mental Health and Mental Health Services Research* 38, 65–76. https://doi.org/10.1007/s10488-010-0319-7

Rogers, E.M. (2003) *Diffusion of Innovations*. 5th edition. New York: Free Press.

Rycroft-Malone, J., Bucknall, T. (2010) Theory, frameworks, and models: laying down the groundwork. In: Rycroft-Malone, J., Bucknall, T. (Eds.), *Models and Frameworks for Implementing Evidence-Based Practice: Linking Evidence to Action*. Chichester: Wiley-Blackwell, pp. 23–50.

Sabatier, P.A. (1999) *Theories of the Policy Process*. Boulder, CO: Westview Press.

Sales, A., Smith, J., Curran, G., Kochevar, L. (2006) Models, strategies, and tools: theory in implementing evidence-based findings into health care practice. *Journal of General Internal Medicine* 21(Suppl 2), S43–S49. https://doi.org/10.1111/j.1525-1497.2006.00362.x

Stetler, C.B. (2010) Stetler model. In: Rycroft-Malone, J., Bucknall, T. (Eds.), *Models and Frameworks for Implementing Evidence-Based Practice: Linking Evidence to Action*. Chichester: Wiley-Blackwell, pp. 51–82.

Stevens, K.R. (2013) The impact of evidence-based practice in nursing and the next big ideas. *The Online Journal of Issues in Nursing* 18(2), 4. https://doi.org/10.3912/OJIN.Vol18No02Man04

Tabak, R.G., Khoong, E.C., Chambers, D.A., Brownson, R.C. (2012) Bridging research and practice: models for dissemination and implementation research. *American Journal of Preventive Medicine* 43, 337–350. https://doi.org/10.1016/j.amepre.2012.05.024

Titler, M.G., Kleiber, C., Steelman, V., Goode, C., Rakel, B., Barry-Walker, J., et al. (1994) Infusing research into practice to promote quality care. *Nursing Research* 43, 307–313. https://doi.org/10.1097/00006199-199409000-00009

Washington University (2022). Pick a theory, model or framework. Retrieved from https://impsciuw.org/implementation-science/research/frameworks/ (accessed 20 July 2022).

Weiner, B.J. (2009) A theory of organizational readiness for change. *Implementation Science* 4, 67. https://doi.org/10.1186/1748-5908-4-67

Wilson, K.M., Brady, T.J., Lesesne, C., on behalf of the NCCDPHP Work Group on Translation. (2011) An organizing framework for translation in public health: the knowledge to action framework. *Preventing Chronic Disease* 8, A46.

Zahra, S.A., George, G. (2002) Absorptive capacity: a review, reconceptualization, and extension. *Academy of Management Review* 27, 185–203. https://doi.org/10.2307/4134351

5   Process models

Per Nilsen and Julia E. Moore

What are process models?

The aim of process models is to delineate and/or guide the process of translating research into practice, thus providing support for "how-to" implement. They usually describe specific activities to be carried out in a number of temporal stages (phases, stages, steps, etc.) of the research-to-practice process. Process models can be used both prospectively to plan and execute implementation and retrospectively to identify activities that contributed to implementation success (or lack thereof). The stages are often presented in a sequential graphic format, either cyclical or linear, from development and/or review of research to implementation and use of research in the form of various evidence-based practices.

The terminology of process models is somewhat inconsistent because some of the models that aim to facilitate implementation are referred to as frameworks, for example, the Knowledge-to-Action Framework (KTA) (Graham et al., 2006) and Quality Implementation Framework (QIF) (Meyers et al., 2012a). Some process models have been labelled "action models" and "planned action models" (Graham and Tetroe, 2010). Action models have been described as "active" because they are used to "guide or cause change" (Graham et al., 2009, p. 185).

Many of the process models originate from nursing-led research on research utilization (or knowledge utilization), a line of research that focuses on the application of research-based knowledge in nurses' clinical practice (Stetler, 2001). Examples include the Stetler Model (Stetler, 1994), the Academic Center for Evidence-Based Practice (ACE) Star Model of Knowledge Transformation (Stevens, 2013), KTA (Graham et al., 2006), the Iowa Model (Titler et al., 1994) and the Ottawa Model (Logan and Graham, 1998). Studies on research utilization began in the 1970s, predating the emergence of the evidence-based movement and implementation science. There are also numerous examples of similar models that have been developed in implementation science, including models by Grol and Wensing (2004), Pronovost et al. (2008), QIF (Meyers et al., 2012a) and the Implementation Process Model (IMP) (Parker et al., 2021). Four process models are described in this chapter.

One aspect of process models that is often overlooked is that there are two distinct types of process model that serve different purposes: "precursor" models used to design an evidence-based practice (e.g. an intervention or a programme) to be implemented and "planning" models used to plan for implementation of an existing practice. Precursor-type process models focus primarily on understanding knowledge-doing gaps, needs and various problems concerning the current way of working (e.g. not using sufficiently

DOI: 10.4324/9781003318125-6

evidence-based practices), identifying evidence-based practices to address these problems, understanding barriers and facilitators to implement these practices and selecting implementation strategies to address these barriers and facilitators. Planning-type process models to plan implementation assume that all this work has already been completed and shift the emphasis to considering how to implement the practice in different settings. Neglecting the existence of these distinct purposes and their corresponding process models can result in the utilization of inappropriate process models, which can be counterproductive and may instil doubt regarding the usefulness of process models, possibly prompting individuals to abandon their use.

Precursor-type process models for designing evidence-based practices (e.g. an intervention) for implementation describe the procedural steps involved in selecting implementation strategies to implement the practice in question. These models are valuable for researchers engaged in designing an evidence-based practice to evaluate its efficacy and effectiveness, as well as for implementers planning for the implementation of a practice. These process models typically involve defining the long-term goals, defining those being asked to change and clarifying expected behavioural changes, understanding barriers and facilitators to making these changes (also referred to as determinants), and then selecting implementation strategies. The Stetler Model (Stetler, 2001) and KTA (Graham et al., 2006) are examples of this type of model.

Process models that help with planning for the implementation of a specific evidence-based practice delineate the steps involved in getting this practice into routine use. The practice could have been designed using a precursor-type process model. Activities in implementation planning process models often include assessing readiness and context, planning for adaptations, implementation and sustainability, building implementation teams, assessing fidelity, and evaluation. QIF (Meyers et al., 2012b) is an example of this type of process model. However, many process models address both types of activities but place greater emphasis on one type over the other. As a result, there is often overlap between the two types of process models, contributing to some confusion regarding the use of process models. For example, the KTA (Graham et al., 2006) acknowledges the need to plan for implementation and sustainability but does not address these in detail.

The Stetler Model

The Stetler Model by Cheryl Stetler is one of the earliest process models. It was originally referred to as the Stetler/Marram Model when it was introduced in 1976 (Stetler and Marram, 1976). The aim was to provide guidance for nurses' assessment of the applicability of research findings and their use of these findings in clinical practice. The model was based on the authors' own experiences and did not have "any specific basis in research", according to Stetler (1994, p. 15). The model is an example of a precursor-type model that focuses primarily on designing the practice intended for implementation, for example, selecting evidence for the practice being implemented and then selecting implementation strategies to address barriers and facilitators to change.

The emergence in the early 1990s of the evidence-based movement prompted a refinement of the original Stetler/Marram model in 1994. Stetler (1994) linked the concept of research utilization with the new concept of evidence-based practice by recognizing that the systematic use of research was a prerequisite for achieving an evidence-based practice. The original model's three phases (Validation; Evaluation; Decision making) were extended to six phases (Preparation; Validation; Comparative evaluation; Decision making; Translation/application; Evaluation). At the same time, conceptual underpinnings and a set of assumptions were added to provide a more solid scientific foundation (Stetler, 1994).

The model was refined again in 2001 based on the continuing experience of using the model with nurses (Stetler, 2001). The previous versions had a focus on individual practitioners, but the new version was intended to provide "explicit direction both for individuals and for individuals operating within groups responsible for research utilization/evidence-based practice" (Stetler, 2001, p. 278). Six phases became five as the new model merged two of the phases of the 1994 model (Stetler, 2001):

1 Preparation: this phase involves specifying the purpose of the research review, for example, wanting to solve a particular clinical problem. The user of the model should consider environmental factors that can influence potential application of the research and personal factors that can diminish objectivity when interpreting research.

2 Validation: the aim of this phase is to assess the strengths and weaknesses of the research; the end points are either accepting or rejecting the research for potential use.

3 Comparative evaluation/decision making: assuming the outcome of phase 2 is acceptance, in the third phase, the findings are synthesized and assessed with regard to feasibility, fit with current practice and setting as well as other criteria. This phase concludes with a decision to either use, consider using or not using the research in practice.

4 Translation/application: this phase is the "how-to" of implementation of the synthesized findings, which might require developing a guideline, policy or action plan to facilitate implementation unless the research is easy to implement.

5 Evaluation: The practitioner of the research use evaluates this against the goals for this use.

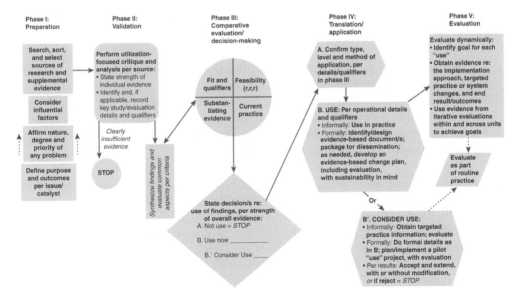

Figure 5.1 The 2001 Stetler Model.

Source: Stetler (2001); reproduced with permission from Cheryl B. Stetler

Knowledge-to-Action Framework

The KTA framework was developed by Ian Graham and colleagues to achieve "conceptual clarity" and "offer a framework to help elucidate what we believe to be the key elements of the KTA process" (Graham et al., 2006, p. 14). The ambition was to construct an "elegant, usable model that would resonate with potential users by balancing practicality and level of detail" (Graham and Tetroe, 2010, p. 213). The focus of KTA is primarily on designing the practice intended for implementation, for example, selecting evidence for the practice being implemented and then selecting implementation strategies to address barriers and facilitators to change.

KTA was developed as part of a project intended to define concepts associated with the knowledge-to-action process (e.g. knowledge translation, knowledge transfer, knowledge exchange, dissemination and implementation) and a review of so-called planned action theories, models and frameworks (or change theories/models) of relevance for the process. A planned action theory, model or framework was defined by Graham and Tetroe (2010) as a set of logically inter-related concepts that explain how change occurs, predict how various forces in an environment will react in specified change situations and help planners or change agents control variables that increase or decrease the likelihood of the occurrence of change. The model also drew on the authors' experience of implementing research (Graham and Tetroe, 2010).

The term "action" was chosen purposively instead of "practice" (i.e. "knowledge-to-practice") because the authors considered the former term to be more generic, encompassing the use of knowledge by practitioners, patients, the public and policymakers. After the 2006 publication, KTA was elaborated on in 2009 in the book *Knowledge Translation in Health Care*, edited by Sharon Straus, Jacqueline Tetroe and Ian Graham and in 2010 in the book *Models and Frameworks for Implementing Evidence-Based Practice: Linking Evidence to Action*, edited by Jo Rycroft-Malone and Tracey Bucknell.

KTA divides the knowledge-to-action process into two parts, Knowledge Creation and Action Cycle, with each part consisting of a number of activities. Knowledge Creation comprises the following three phases (Graham et al., 2006):

1 Knowledge inquiry: first-generation knowledge that is largely unrefined, for example, primary studies and information of variable quality.
2 Knowledge synthesis: second-generation knowledge represents the aggregation of existing knowledge, for example, systematic reviews and meta-analyses.
3 Knowledge tools/products: third-generation knowledge consists of knowledge tools and products such as guidelines, decision aids and rules.

Knowledge becomes more refined and useful to stakeholders as it progresses from inquiry to synthesis and tools/products. At each phase of knowledge creation, knowledge producers can tailor their activities to the needs of the potential users, for example, tailoring their research questions to address the problems identified by users and customize the message for the users (Graham et al., 2006).

The Action Cycle was derived from a review of planned action theories by Graham and colleagues in 2006. They identified 31 theories, models and frameworks published between 1983 and 2006 which were analysed in relation to the activities of the Action Cycle. This cycle consists of seven phases (Graham et al., 2006):

1 Identify a problem that needs addressing and identify, review and select the knowledge relevant to the problem: the initial phase involves a group or individuals identifying

that there is a problem that deserves attention and searching for knowledge that might address the problem. Relevant research needs to be critically appraised to determine its validity and usefulness for the problem identified.

2 Adapt the knowledge that has been identified to the local context: the second phase concerns the process that individuals or groups go through as they make decisions about the value, usefulness and appropriateness of particular knowledge to their setting and circumstances.

3 Assess barriers to using the knowledge: the next phase involves the assessment of potential barriers to make it possible to target, overcome or diminish these barriers using appropriate strategies in the subsequent phase.

4 Select, tailor and implement strategies to promote the use of knowledge: this phase focuses on the planning and execution of strategies to facilitate implementation of the knowledge.

5 Monitor knowledge use: this phase is necessary to determine how and the extent to which knowledge has been put to use and if the strategies have been sufficient to bring about the desired change.

6 Evaluate the outcomes of using the knowledge: the aim of this phase is to determine the impact of using the knowledge, for example, whether the knowledge makes a difference in terms of health and practitioner outcomes.

7 Sustain ongoing knowledge use: the last phase concerns the sustainment of knowledge. The barriers to ongoing use of the knowledge may be different from the barriers that existed when the knowledge was first introduced.

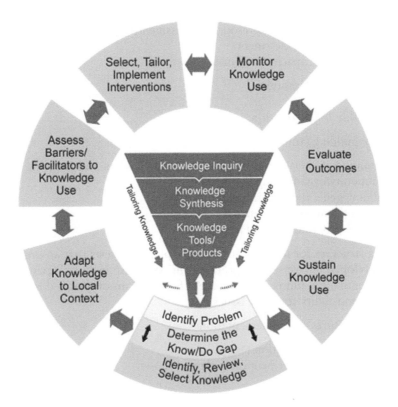

Figure 5.2 Knowledge-to-Action (KTA).

Source: Graham et al. (2006); reproduced with permission from Ian D. Graham

Quality Implementation Framework

QIF was developed by Duncan Meyers and colleagues to achieve improved understanding of "the nature of the implementation process" (Meyers et al., 2012b, p. 482). The authors posited that "quality implementation" is "putting an innovation into practice in such a way that it meets the necessary standards to achieve the innovation's desired outcomes" (Meyers et al., 2012b, p. 482). Unlike the Stetler Model and KTA, QIF is a process model focused on planning for implementation, and it is based on the assumption that implementation strategies have already been selected.

The authors examined 25 theories, models and frameworks across multiple research and practice areas, including three determinant frameworks described in Chapter 6, Promoting Action on Research Implementation in Health Services (PARIHS) (Kitson et al., 1998), Consolidated Framework for Implementation Research (CFIR) (Damschroder et al., 2009) and Practical, Robust Implementation and Sustainability Model (PRISM) (Feldstein and Glasgow, 2008). A synthesis of the frameworks yielded 14 activities (referred to as steps) to be carried out in the implementation process. These steps were clustered into a four-phase temporal sequence (Meyers et al., 2012a):

I Initial consideration regarding the host setting: work in the first phase of implementation focuses primarily on the ecological fit between the innovation and the host setting.

- Assessment strategies:

    1 Conducting a needs and resources assessment.
    2 Conducting a fit assessment.
    3 Conducting a capacity/readiness assessment.

- Decisions about adaptation:

    4 Possibility for adaptation.

- Capacity-building strategies:

    5 Obtaining explicit buy-in from critical stakeholders and fostering a supportive community/organizational climate.
    6 Building general/organizational capacity.
    7 Staff recruitment/maintenance.
    8 Effective pre-innovation staff training.

II Creating a structure for implementation: this phase suggests that an organized structure be developed to oversee the process. This structure includes having a clear plan for implementing the innovation and identifying a team of qualified individuals who will take responsibility for these issues.

- Structural features for implementation:

    9 Creating implementation teams.
    10 Developing an implementation plan.

III Ongoing structure once implementation begins: The actual implementation begins in this phase. There are three important tasks in this phase (see below).

- Ongoing implementation support strategies:

  11 Technical assistance/coaching/supervision.
  12 Process evaluation.
  13 Supportive feedback mechanism.

IV Improving future applications: the final phase indicates that retrospective analysis and self-reflection coupled with feedback from the host setting can identify particular strengths and weaknesses that occurred during implementation.

  14 Learning from experience.

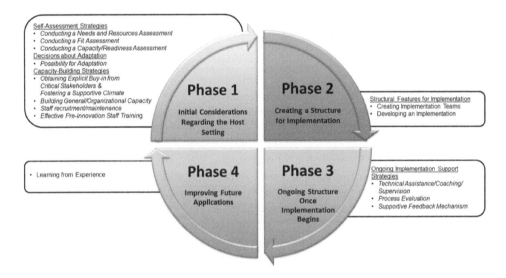

Figure 5.3 Quality Implementation Framework (QIF).

Source: Meyers et al. (2012a); reproduced with permission from Duncan C. Meyers, Abraham Wandersman and Joseph A. Durlak

Based on QIF, Meyers et al. (2012b) constructed the Quality Implementation Tool (QIT). They wanted to turn QIF into a user-friendly tool, with the ambition "to assist stakeholders in community/organizations in their efforts to implement with quality" (Meyers et al., 2012b, p. 481). The tool is more specific and detailed than QIF. It identifies six goals (referred to as components), each consisting of a number of activities to be carried out, in total 29 activities (referred to as action steps) (Meyers et al., 2012b):

1 Develop an implementation team.

  1.1 Decide on the structure of the team overseeing implementation (e.g. steering committee, advisory board, community coalition, etc.).
  1.2 Identify an implementation team leader.

1.3   Identify and recruit content area specialists as team members.

1.4   Identify and recruit other agencies and/or community members such as family members and business leaders as team members.

1.5   Assign team members roles, processes and responsibilities.

2   Foster supportive organization-/community-wide climate and conditions.

2.1   Identify and foster a relationship with a champion for the innovation.

2.2   Communicate the perceived need for the innovation within the organization/community.

2.3   Communicate the perceived benefit of the innovation within the organization/community.

2.4   Establish practices that counterbalance stakeholder resistance to change.

2.5   Create policies that enhance accountability.

2.6   Create policies that foster shared decision making and effective communication.

2.7   Ensure that the innovation has adequate administrative support.

3   Develop an implementation plan.

3.1   List tasks required for implementation.

3.2   Establish a timeline for implementation tasks.

3.3   Assign implementation tasks to specific stakeholders.

4   Receive training and technical assistance (TA).

4.1   Determine specific needs for training and/or TA.

4.2   Identify and foster relationship with a trainer(s) and/or TA provider(s).

4.3   Ensure that trainer(s) and/or TA provider(s) have sufficient knowledge about the organization/community's needs and resources.

4.4   Ensure that trainer(s) and/or TA provider(s) have sufficient knowledge about the organization/community's goals and objectives.

4.5   Work with TA providers to implement the innovation.

5   Practitioner-developer collaboration in implementation.

5.1   Collaborate with expert developers (e.g. researchers) about factors that have an impact on the quality of implementation in the organization/community.

5.2   Engage in problem solving.

6   Evaluate the effectiveness of the implementation.

6.1   Measure the fidelity of implementation.

6.2   Measure the dosage of the innovation (i.e. how much of the innovation was actually delivered).

6.3   Measure the quality of the innovation's delivery (e.g. implementer enthusiasm, leader preparedness and other qualitative aspects).

6.4   Measure participant responsiveness to the implementation process (i.e. degree to which participants are engaged in the activities of the innovation).

6.5   Measure the degree of programme differentiation (i.e. the extent to which the targeted innovation differs from other innovations in the organization/community).

6.6   Measure the reach of the programme (i.e. the extent to which the innovation is delivered to the people it was designed to reach).

6.7   Document all adaptations that are made to the innovation (i.e. extent to which adjustments were made to the original innovation to fit the host setting's needs, resources, preferences or other important characteristics).

Implementation Process Model

The IMP was first described in 2021 by Gillian Parker and colleagues (Parker et al., 2021). It was developed based on a two-stage online Delphi process to "reach agreement on the key elements in healthcare implementation processes" (Parker et al., 2021, p. 2). According to the authors, the motivation for developing IMP was the lack of consensus on "the key elements of the implementation process that are essential to successful implementation" (Parker et al., 2021, p. 2). The model built on previous work by Kastner et al. (2020), which also involved Ian Graham and Sharon Straus, who are behind other process models. This process model focuses on planning for implementation, assuming that the implementation strategies have been selected.

Fifty-four individuals (10% of 534 approached) responded to the Delphi survey in the first round. Of these, 41% lived in Canada and 39% in the United States; 83% were researchers and 59% were female. The response rate for the second Delphi round was 59%, which meant that 32 people responded to both surveys.

IMP highlights two main components (referred to as domains) of relevance for the entire implementation and sustainability process (Parker et al., 2021):

- Stakeholder engagement: this is an iterative process of actively soliciting the knowledge, experience, judgement and values of individuals selected to represent a broad range of interests in a particular issue. The purpose is to create a shared understanding and to make relevant, transparent and effective decisions.
- Context: this can be the environment, setting or organizational structure and can act as either a barrier or facilitator to implementation.

The domains feature three sub-domains (which are overarching activities) of which the first includes seven more specific activities (referred to as elements) (Parker et al., 2021):

1 Develop an implementation and sustainability plan: create a plan for implementation according to identified implementation objectives and readiness, and sustainability assessment:

   1.1   Identify the purpose of the implementation of the intervention/innovation.
   1.2   Identify additional stakeholders that should be part of the implementation.
   1.3   Assess the fit and effectiveness of the potential intervention/innovation and then select the most appropriate intervention/innovation.
   1.4   Define the scope of implementation and sustainability.
   1.5   Identify the determinants of implementation and sustainability.
   1.6   Assess the context and characteristics of the adopter environment including its capacity to sustain the intervention/innovation.
   1.7   Develop a monitoring and evaluation plan.

2 Implement the intervention/innovation.
3 Monitor and evaluate the implementation and sustainability of the intervention/innovation.

Concluding remarks

This chapter has described four process models. There are many other process models, but most share many characteristics with the models presented here. In many ways, these models present an ideal view of implementation as a structured, linear process that proceeds stepwise, in an orderly fashion. However, authors behind many models empha-size that the actual process is not necessarily sequential. For example, Parker et al. (2021, p. 8) recognize that "implementation is a dynamic process which does not unfold in a linear fashion". Similarly, Meyers et al. (2012a, p. 474) observe that "quality implemen-tation does not always occur in the exact sequence of [the steps]". Graham et al. (2006, p. 18) state that the seven action phases of KTA can occur sequentially or simultaneously because the boundaries between the stages are "fluid and permeable".

An important feature of many process models is the assessment of barriers and facilita-tors to implementation, that is, determinants of implementation, as one of the stages of the implementation process. This means that they combine the process perspective with features of determinant frameworks, which are used in implementation science to analyse determinants of implementation outcomes. However, the emphasis in process models is very much on the research-to-practice process, and the assessment of the determinants is merely one of many stages. This appraisal is not as comprehensive as in determinant frameworks, which explains why determinant frameworks are often used in conjunction with process models.

The process models vary with regard to how they were developed. Models such as the Stetler Model and the Iowa Model (Titler et al., 1994) are largely based on the authors' own experiences of implementing research in various settings. Models such as KTA and QIF also drew on the authors' experience but combined this with knowledge gained from literature reviews of theories, models, frameworks and individual studies to identify key features of successful implementation processes. The Delphi-based IMP represents a third option although it is likely that the experts' opinions were formed from both research-based and experience-based knowledge.

Some of the process models have been used extensively in implementation science re-search. KTA appears to be the most widely applied process model (Birken et al., 2017). A systematic review of the KTA literature by Field et al. (2014) identified 146 studies de-scribing varying degrees of KTA use. The model has been particularly popular in Canada where it was developed. Similarly, there are many studies describing the use of QIF; for example, studies on the implementation of a primary healthcare system improvement ini-tiative in South Africa (Eboreime et al., 2018), electronic medical records for clinical and research purposes in Malaysia (Nor et al., 2018), an oral screening tool for paediatric cardiologists in the United States (McCargar et al., 2020) and a mindfulness-informed social and emotional learning programme in elementary schools in England (Delaney et al., 2022). QIF has been translated into Swedish by the Public Health Agency of Swe-den, which has the national responsibility for public health issues in Sweden, and into Danish by the Center for Innovation and Methodology, a public organization operated by six municipalities in Denmark.

The Stetler Model has also been used widely in empirical research. In contrast, there are few studies describing the use of IMP, but this model was published in 2021, which restricts opportunities for broader use. The extent to which the process models are actually used by practitioners, for example, in clinical settings, is unknown, but it is likely to be limited in comparison with the use of quality improvement tools such as Plan-Do-Study-Act, Root Cause Analysis, Process Mapping or Pareto Chart (Nilsen et al., 2022).

In many ways, process models could be viewed as a form of implementation strat-egy because their use is intended to support implementation by identifying important activities that need to be accomplished when planning and executing implementation.

Therefore, studies comparing implementation guided by process models with "standard implementation" (i.e. without the use of process models) would be relevant to investigate whether or to what extent the use of process models contributes to better results.

References

Birken, S.A., Powell, B.J., Shea, C.M., Haines, E.R., Kirk, M.A., Leeman, J., Rohweder, C., Damschroder, L., Presseau, J. (2017) Criteria for selecting implementation science theories and frameworks: results from an international survey. *Implementation Science* 12, 124. https://doi.org/10.1186/s13012-017-0656-y

Damschroder, L.J., Aron, D.C., Keith, R.E., Kirsh, S.R., Alexander, J.A., Lowery, J.C. (2009) Fostering implementation of health services research findings into practice: a consolidated framework for advancing implementation science. *Implementation Science* 4, 50. https://doi.org/10.1186/1748-5908-4-50

Delaney, A., Crooks, C.V., Bax, K., Savage, S., Spencer, T. (2022) Partnering to support a mindfulness-informed social and emotional learning program in elementary schools: Strategies aligned with the Quality Implementation Framework. *Canadian Journal of Community Mental Health* 41, 103–121. https://doi.org/10.7870/cjcmh-2022-022

Eboreime, E.A., Eyles, J., Nxumalo, N., Eboreime, O.L., Ramaswamy, R. (2018) Implementation process and quality of a primary health care system improvement initiative in a decentralized context: a retrospective appraisal using the quality implementation framework. *International Journal of Health Planning and Management* 34, e369–e386. https://doi.org/10.1002/hpm.2655

Feldstein, A.C., Glasgow, R.E. (2008) A practical, robust implementation and sustainability model (PRISM) for integrating research findings into practice. *Joint Commission Journal on Quality and Patient Safety* 34, 228–243. https://doi.org/10.1016/S1553-7250(08)34030-6

Field, B., Booth, A., Ilott, I., Gerrish, K. (2014) Using the Knowledge to Action Framework in practice: a citation analysis and systematic review. *Implementation Science* 9, 172. https://doi.org/10.1186/s13012-014-0172-2

Graham, I.D., Tetroe, J.M. (2010) The Knowledge To Action framework. In: Rycroft-Malone, J., Bucknall, T. (Eds.), *Models and Frameworks for Implementing Evidence-Based Practice: Linking Evidence to Action*. Chichester: Wiley-Blackwell, pp. 207–222.

Graham, I.D., Logan, J., Harrison, M.B., Straus, S.E., Tetroe, J., Caswell, W., et al. (2006) Lost in knowledge translation: time for a map? *Journal of Continuing Education in the Health Professions* 26, 13–24. https://doi.org/10.1002/chp.47

Graham, I.D., Tetroe, J., KT Theories Group. (2009) Planned action theories. In: Straus, S.E., Tetroe, J., Graham, I.D. (Eds.), *Knowledge Translation in Health Care: Moving from Evidence to Practice*. Chichester: Wiley-Blackwell/BMJ, pp. 185–195.

Grol, R., Wensing, M. (2004) What drives change? Barriers to and incentives for achieving evidence-based practice. *Medical Journal of Australia* 180, S57–S60. https://doi.org/10.5694/j.1326-5377.2004.tb05948.x

Kastner, M., Makarski, J., Hayden, L., Lai, Y., Chan, J., Treister, V., et al. (2020). Improving KT tools and products: development and evaluation of a framework for creating optimized, Knowledge-activated Tools (KaT). *Implementation Science Communications* 1, 47. https://doi.org/10.1186/s43058-020-00031-7

Kitson, A.L., Harvey, G., McCormack, B. (1998) Enabling the implementation of evidence based practice: a conceptual framework. *Quality and Safety in Health Care* 7, 149–158. https://doi.org/10.1136/qshc.7.3.149

Logan, J., Graham, I.D. (1998) Toward a comprehensive interdisciplinary model of health care research use. *Science Communication* 20, 227–246. https://doi.org/10.1177/1075547098020002004

McCargar, S.I., Olsen, J., Steelman, R.J., Huang, J.H., Palmer, E.A., Burch, G.H., et al. (2020). Implementation of a standardized oral screening tool by paediatric cardiologists. *Cardiology in the Young* 30, 1815–1820. https://doi.org/10.1017/S1047951120002826

Meyers, D.C., Durlak, J.A., Wandersman, A. (2012a) The Quality Implementation Framework: a synthesis of critical steps in the implementation process. *American Journal of Community Psychology* 50, 462–480. https://doi.org/10.1007/s10464-012-9522-x

Meyers, D.C., Katz, J., Chien, V., Wandersman, A., Scaccia, J.P., Wright, A. (2012b). Practical implementation science: developing and piloting the Quality Implementation Tool. *American Journal of Community Psychology* 50, 481–496. https://doi.org/10.1007/s10464-012-9521-y

Nilsen, P., Thor, J., Bender, M., Leeman, J., Andersson-Gäre, B., Sevdalis, N. (2022). Bridging the silos: a comparative analysis of implementation science and improvement science. *Frontiers in Health Services* 1, 1–13. https://doi.org/10.3389/frhs.2021.817750

Nor, N.A.M., Taib, N.A., Saad, M., Zaini, H.S., Ahmad, Z, Ahmad, Y., et al. (2018) Development of electronic medical records for clinical and research purposes: the breast cancer module using an implementation framework in a middle income country – Malaysia. *BMC Bioinformatics* 19(Suppl 13), 402. https://doi.org/10.1186/s12859-018-2406-9

Parker G., Kastner, M., Born, K., Berta, W. (2021) Development of an implementation process model: a Delphi study. *BMC Health Services Research* 21, 558. https://doi.org/10.1186/s12913-021-06501-5

Pronovost, P.J., Berenholtz, S.M., Needham, D.M. (2008) Translating evidence into practice: a model for large scale knowledge translation. *BMJ* 337, a1714. https://doi.org/10.1136/bmj.a1714

Stetler, C.B. (1994) Refinement of the Stetler/Marram model for application of research findings to practice. *Nursing Outlook* 42, 15–25. https://doi.org/10.1016/0029-6554(94)90067-1

Stetler, C.B. (2001). Updating the Stetler model of research utilization to facilitate evidence-based practice. *Nursing Outlook* 49, 272–279. https://doi.org/10.1067/mno.2001.120517

Stetler, C.B., Marram, G. (1976). Evaluating research findings for applicability in practice. *Nursing Outlook* 24, 559–563.

Stevens, K.R. (2013) The impact of evidence-based practice in nursing and the next big ideas. *Online Journal of Issues in Nursing* 18(2), 4. https://doi.org/10.3912/OJIN.Vol18No02Man04

Titler, M.G., Kleiber, C., Steelman, V., Goode, C., Rakel, B., Barry-Walker, J., et al. (1994) Infusing research into practice to promote quality care. *Nursing Research* 43, 307–313. https://doi.org/10.1097/00006199-199409000-00009

6 Determinant frameworks

Per Nilsen

What are determinant frameworks?

"In all implementation efforts, there is a need for someone somewhere to do something differently", noted Wilson and Kislov (2022, p. 7). "In order to achieve this, a clear understanding is required of what needs to change and the factors that are likely to help or hinder any change to occur." These influencing factors are usually termed determinants in implementation science. Determinant frameworks describe different types of determinants, typically divided into barriers and facilitators that are hypothesized or have been found to influence implementation outcomes; for example, healthcare professionals' use of an evidence-based practice or adherence to recommendations in a clinical guideline. Each type of determinant usually comprises a number of individual barriers (hindrances, impediments) and/or facilitators (enablers), which are seen as independent variables that have an impact on implementation outcomes (i.e. the dependent variable). Some frameworks hypothesize relationships between these determinants (e.g. Greenhalgh et al., 2004; Durlak and DuPre, 2008; Gurses et al., 2010; Aarons et al., 2011), whereas others recognize such relationships without clarifying them (e.g. Cochrane et al., 2007).

Determinant frameworks can be used to inform the choice of implementation strategies that may best address the barriers and facilitators. They can also be used to retrospectively explain implementation outcomes by assessing differences in determinants across implementation settings (Damschroder et al., 2022). These frameworks do not explain how change takes place and do not describe causal mechanisms, underscoring that they are not theories. Six common determinant frameworks are presented in this chapter.

Promoting Action on Research Implementation in Health Services and integrated-Promoting Action on Research Implementation in Health Services

The Promoting Action on Research Implementation in Health Services (PARIHS) framework emerged from the observation that successful implementation in healthcare is often a complex and challenging process. An important influence was the authors' interest in experiential learning, enabling change and empowering clinical staff to take ownership and control (Harvey and Kitson, 2020). Linked to this was a particular interest in facilitation as a mechanism for enabling implementation and improvement (Kitson et al., 1996). The team behind PARIHS drew on their experience across a range of projects, including clinical audit, quality improvement, practice development and clinical guideline development, to map out what appeared to be the key determinants of successful implementation (Harvey and Kitson, 2020).

DOI: 10.4324/9781003318125-7

PARIHS was first published in 1998 (Kitson et al., 1998), although at that time it was not labelled as the PARIHS framework. That came later at the first public road test of the framework at a conference (which happened to be in Paris) (Harvey and Kitson, 2020). The original PARIHS framework proposition was that successful implementation (of research evidence) was a function of the dynamic inter-play between three types of determinants, referred to as constructs (each of which consists of a number of sub-constructs) (Rycroft-Malone, 2010):

- Evidence: the nature and strength of the evidence, comprising research, clinical, patient and local experience.
- Context: characteristics of the environment or setting in which the proposed change is to be implemented; context is subdivided into the prevailing culture, leadership roles and the organization's approach to evaluation.
- Facilitation: the type of support needed to help people change their attitudes, habits, skills and ways of thinking and working.

After the initial publication of the (then unnamed) PARIHS framework, the researchers moved from an inductive phase to a more deductive testing and refinement phase, which produced the first revision of the framework (Rycroft-Malone et al., 2002). This resulted in a number of journal publications and generated considerable interest in PARIHS. Published papers from other users of the framework suggested a high level of face and content validity (Helfrich et al., 2010). At the same time, the PARIHS team continued to work on the framework. This led to the most recent revision, the integrated or i-PARIHS framework (Harvey and Kitson, 2016).

i-PARIHS shares the same underlying philosophy as the original PARIHS framework, but the meaning of the Evidence and Context constructs was broadened and a fourth type of determinant was added, Recipients. The expanded view of evidence was due to the recognition that evidence is often adapted in a process of aligning external explicit evidence with local priorities and practice, which enhances the compatibility of a proposed change, as recognized in the innovation literature. The term innovation replaced evidence to reflect that innovation is a broader concept. Context was broadened to also encompass meso- and macro-level influences on implementation, with reference to their inclusion in other determinant frameworks such as the Consolidated Framework for Implementation Research (CFIR). The Recipients construct was added in response to feedback that insufficient attention had been paid in the original framework to the actors involved in implementation. The new Recipients construct encompasses the people who are affected by and influence implementation at both the individual and collective team levels (Figure 6.1).

The revised i-PARIHS framework posits that successful implementation results from the facilitation of an innovation (with different levels of evidence) with the intended recipients in their context. Thus, the four constructs of i-PARIHS are (Harvey and Kitson, 2020):

- Recipients: characteristics of individuals, teams and other stakeholders engaged and owning the innovation.
- Innovation: characteristics of what is being implemented.
- Context: characteristics of the inner context (the immediate, local setting for implementation) and the outer context (the wider health system, including policies, regulatory frameworks and political environment).
- Facilitation: an enabling process comprising facilitation roles and strategies to assess, align and manage features of the recipients, innovation and context.

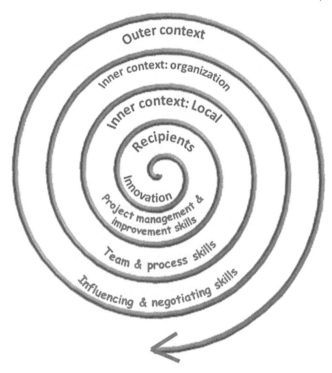

Figure 6.1 Integrated-Promoting Action on Research Implementation in Health Services (i-PARIHS).

Source: Harvey and Kitson (2016)

PARIHS and the extended i-PARIHS have been widely used in research studies. A citation analysis of PARIHS in 2019 identified over 1050 published articles that cited the framework. Of these, 259 papers reported using PARIHS to inform an implementation study in some way; for example, framing the overall design, planning a strategy and/or structuring the analysis and evaluation (Bergstrom et al., 2020).

Theoretical Domains Framework

The framework that became known as the Theoretical Domains Framework (TDF) was first described in 2005 by Michie and colleagues. They developed the framework in a collaborative effort with a cross-disciplinary group of 64 health psychology theorists, health services researchers and health psychologists. The aim was to simplify psychological theory relevant to behaviour change to make it accessible to researchers involved in implementation science (Michie et al., 2005).

TDF was constructed based on a synthesis of 128 theoretical constructs found in 33 behaviour change theories, including many cognitive/motivation theories; for example, Theory of Planned Behaviour, Theory of Reasoned Action, Health Belief Model, Social Cognitive Theory and Self-Determination Theory (Michie et al., 2005; Cane et al., 2012). Of the 128 constructs, 17 were prioritized as relevant for inter-disciplinary research to understand and change behaviours. The resulting consensus identified 12 theoretical domains that should be considered when seeking to explain why implementation of evidence-based practices succeeds or fails and for designing strategies to achieve improved implementation. Although TDF is based on many theories that specify causal mechanisms of behaviour change, the framework does not account for such mechanisms, instead treating the determinant domains as independent variables and behaviour change as a dependent variable (Michie et al., 2005).

TDF subsequently underwent a validation exercise with an independent group of behavioural experts to investigate the optimal structure and content of the framework (Cane et al., 2012). This resulted in a new version of TDF, which had similar structure and content as the original but it featured 14 domains covering 84 theoretical constructs. This version of TDF includes the following types of determinants, that is, domains (Michie et al., 2014):

- Knowledge: an awareness of the existence of something.
- Skills: an ability or proficiency acquired through practice.
- Memory, attention and decision processes: the ability to retain information, focus selectively on aspects of the environment and choose between two or more alternatives.
- Behavioural regulation: anything aimed at managing or changing objectively observed or measured actions.
- Social/professional role and identity: a coherent set of behaviours and displayed personal qualities of an individual in a social or work setting.
- Beliefs about capabilities: acceptance of truth, reality or validity about an ability, talent or facility that a person can put to constructive use.
- Optimism: the confidence that things will happen for the best or that desired goals will be attained.
- Beliefs about consequences: acceptance of the truth, reality or validity about outcomes of a behaviour in a given situation.
- Intentions: a conscious decision to perform a behaviour or a resolve to act in a certain way.
- Goals: mental representations of outcomes or end states that the individual wants to achieve.
- Reinforcement: increasing the probability of a response by arranging a dependent relationship, or contingency, between the response and a given stimulus.
- Emotion: a complex reaction pattern, involving experiential, behavioural and physiological elements, by which the individual attempts to deal with a personally significant matter or event.
- Environmental context and resources: any circumstance of a person's situation or environment that discourages or encourages the development of skills and abilities, independence, social competence and adaptive behaviour.
- Social influences: those inter-personal processes that can cause individuals to change their thoughts, feelings or behaviours.

TDF can be used in combination with Capability Opportunity Motivation – Behaviour (COM-B) (described in Chapter 8 on implementation science theories because it specifies causal mechanisms). Each domain of the TDF relates to one of the three components (C, O, M) of COM-B. An analysis based on COM-B can be used as a screening tool to indicate which domains to explore in more detail if it is not feasible to assess all 14 domains of TDF. The TDF tends to be the tool of choice when the focus is on understanding an implementation problem in depth, as opposed to conducting a behavioural diagnosis as the starting point (D'Lima et al., 2020).

TDF and COM-B are part of the Behaviour Change Wheel, which is an integrated approach to identify and match determinants with appropriate implementation strategies in the form of intervention functions and policies. Intervention functions are activities (e.g. education, persuasion, coercion and training) aimed at changing behaviour by influencing capability, opportunity and/or motivation. Policies are decisions made by authorities (e.g. issuing guidelines, regulations and legislation) that can support the delivery of intervention functions to increase the likelihood of implementation success. Nine intervention functions and seven policy categories are featured in the Behaviour Change Wheel (Michie et al., 2014). The fundamentals of the Behaviour Change Wheel approach are addressed in Chapter 9.

TDF has been widely applied in implementation science research to identify barriers and facilitators to implementation, both in interview studies and questionnaire surveys. Validated questionnaire measures of the TDF have been published. TDF is also applicable to other research designs; for example, structured observations, documentary analysis and case study designs. Furthermore, TDF can be used to inform systematic reviews by providing a structure for classifying barriers and facilitators (D'Lima et al., 2020). A website for the Behaviour Change Wheel approach, including TDF (www.behaviour changewheel.com), provides information about TDF for researchers, practitioners and policy makers and others with an interest in implementation issues.

Practical, Robust Implementation and Sustainability Model

The Practical, Robust Implementation and Sustainability Model (PRISM) is a determinant framework developed by Feldstein and Glasgow (2008). The framework is intended to guide the planning, implementation and evaluation of evidence-based programmes and interventions (McCreight et al., 2019). PRISM draws on a literature review that aimed to identify studies concerning determinants of implementation success. This was combined with the authors' own experience regarding concepts that they considered relevant for the development of the framework. Many aspects were derived from research concerning the diffusion of innovations, social ecology, quality improvement and the PRECEDE/ PROCEED model (Predisposing, Reinforcing and Enabling Constructs in Educational Diagnosis and Evaluation/Policy, Regulatory and Organizational Constructs in Educational and Environmental Development). The framework also borrows from the Chronic Care Model of effective chronic disease management (Feldstein and Glasgow, 2008).

PRISM was developed with special attention paid to multi-level contextual influences of relevance for the five types of outcomes specified in the Reach, Effectiveness, Adoption, Implementation and Maintenance (RE-AIM) framework (Rabin et al., 2022), which is described in Chapter 9. PRISM used an inclusive definition of context, defining it as any determinants (e.g. policies, organization climate and workflow) that are not part of the programme or intervention being implemented (McCreight et al., 2019). The following types of determinants, referred to as elements, are described in PRISM (Figure 6.2) (Feldstein and Glasgow, 2008):

- Programme (intervention), organizational perspective: characteristics such as organizational readiness for the programme, the programme's evidence strength and proposed implementation strategy.

- Programme (intervention), patient perspective: characteristics such as the programme's patient-centredness, patient barriers and service and access, and feedback of results.
- External environment: characteristics such as market forces, regulatory environment and community resources.
- Implementation and sustainability infrastructure: characteristics such as adopter training and support, dedicated team for implementation and plan for sustainability.
- Recipients, organizational characteristics: characteristics that affect organizations' ability to successfully change behaviours in a given clinical area; for example, clinical leadership, management support and communication, and expectation of sustainability; these factors can be considered at the levels of top management, middle managers and frontline teams.
- Recipients, patient characteristics: characteristics of the targeted patients; for example, age, gender, socioeconomic status, health literacy and culture.

Since the original 2008 publication, PRISM has been used across diverse topics, populations and settings. A 2022 scoping review by Rabin et al. (2022) identified nearly 200 articles referencing PRISM to inform or direct the research or integrate it within the research design. The studies reflected a diverse body of literature that applied PRISM

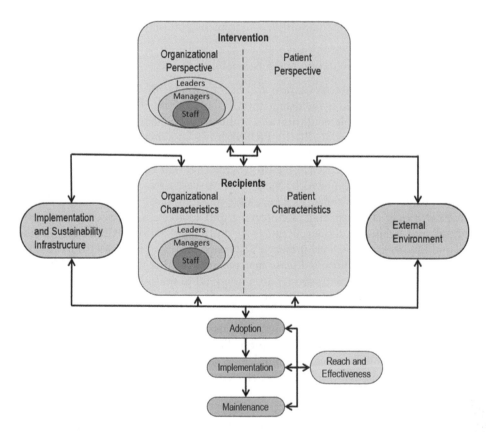

Figure 6.2 Practical, Robust Implementation and Sustainability Model (PRISM).

Source: Feldstein and Glasgow (2008)

across the stages of intervention planning, implementation and evaluation. Twenty-three studies integrated PRISM within their research methodology, but very few used PRISM in combination with RE-AIM outcomes. A website devoted to PRISM and RE-AIM (https://re-aim.org) features descriptions of the two frameworks and provides information and tools for users.

Consolidated Framework for Implementation Research

The CFIR was designed to be a "one stop shop" for clearly labelled and defined theoretical constructs to describe determinants that are associated with implementation success (Damschroder et al., 2009). The framework was designed to implement evidence-based practices into physical clinical settings although it has also found use in many other contexts. The authors sought to develop a collection of constructs that were easy to understand and apply by implementation practitioners (to guide implementation) and implementation science researchers (to study implementation) (Damschroder et al., 2020).

CFIR was based on 19 theories, models and frameworks, including the two previously described determinant frameworks PARIHS and PRISM as well as process models such as the Stetler Model (Stetler, 2001) and the Ottawa Model (Graham and Logan, 2004). The framework also drew on Greenhalgh and colleagues' compilation based on their review of 500 published sources across 13 scientific disciplines (Greenhalgh et al., 2004).

The framework comprises five types of determinants, referred to as domains, each of which consists of a number of sub-domains (Figure 6.3) (Damschroder et al., 2022):

- Innovation domain: characteristics of the innovation; for example, relative advantage, adaptability, trialability and complexity (this domain was previously named intervention characteristics).
- Outer setting domain: characteristics of the setting in which the inner setting exists; for example, patient needs, resources, external policies and incentives.
- Inner setting domain: characteristics of the setting in which the innovation is implemented; for example, structural characteristics and culture of the setting.
- Individuals domain: characteristics of the individuals delivering the innovation; for example, their knowledge and self-efficacy.
- Implementation process domain: the activities and strategies used to implement the innovation; for example, planning and executing.

Damschroder et al. (2009) have emphasized that the boundaries between the domains are fuzzy and dynamic. For example, innovations can fit poorly with local settings and be resisted by individuals who will be affected by the innovation, but an active process to adapt the innovation and engage individuals might contribute to successful implementation.

In 2022, Damschroder and colleagues updated CFIR based on a literature review of studies that featured feedback on CFIR and a survey of authors who had used CFIR in a published study. This led to some revisions of construct names and definitions. The name of the domain intervention characteristics was changed to the innovation domain. The individuals who should benefit from the innovation were referred to as recipients (instead of patients). Also, the term deliverers was introduced to refer to the individuals delivering the innovation.

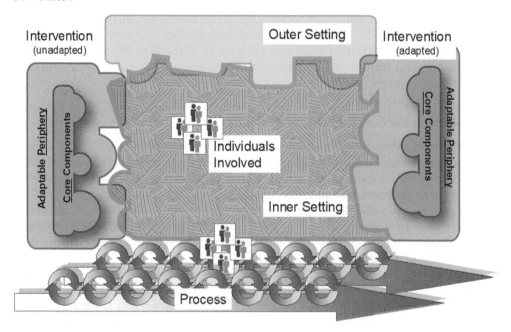

Figure 6.3 Consolidated Framework for Implementation Research (CFIR).
Source: Damschroder et al. (2009)

CFIR is one of the most widely used determinant frameworks in implementation science. Over 1000 articles citing the CFIR have been indexed in PubMed and the original 2009 CFIR paper has been consistently listed in the top five most frequently accessed articles in the *Implementation Science* journal in the decade since its publication. The framework has been used broadly, not only in healthcare settings but also in settings and environments such as schools (Leeman et al., 2018), farms (Tinc et al., 2018), communityhealth settings (Stanhope et al., 2018) and global health settings (Naidoo et al., 2018; Soi et al., 2018). CFIR has also been used in an effort (Waltz et al., 2019) to match CFIR-derived barriers with implementation strategies based on a taxonomy of 72 strategies described in the Expert Recommendations for Implementing Change (ERIC) (Powell et al., 2015). This matching is described in Chapter 9. A website (https://cfirguide.org) has been developed to provide information, tools, measures and other resources to help researchers who use CFIR.

Exploration Preparation Implementation Sustainment framework

The Exploration, Preparation, Implementation and Sustainment (EPIS) framework was initially developed to identify and illustrate implementation, determinants, mechanisms, and processes in public sector service systems in the United States (Aarons et al., 2011). EPIS is both a process model and a determinant framework. EPIS takes its name from the four, non-linear/recursive phases of the implementation: exploration, preparation, implementation, sustainment. As a process model, EPIS acknowledges that implementers must often revisit implementation activities over time to mitigate emergent, real-world challenges in the implementation and sustainment process. As a determinant framework, EPIS describes a set of variables whose relationships to each other and implementation success evolve across the four phases of implementation.

EPIS' namesake phases include (Aarons et al., 2011):

- Exploration: a period of appraisal when health needs of patients, clients or communities are considered to identify the best evidence-based practices, programmes or policies (i.e. the innovation) to address those needs.
- Preparation: focuses on identifying potential determinants and mechanisms (i.e. barriers/facilitators) of implementation and assessing whether adaptations are needed at the system, organization, and/or individual-level, and/or to the innovation itself.
- Implementation: the innovation use is initiated and integrated into the system, organization(s) or providers' practice. Ongoing monitoring of implementation strategies, target participants and outcomes is necessary to adjust efforts to overcome unplanned barriers or nonoptimal progress during the implementation phase.
- Sustainment: the outer and inner context structures, processes and supports are established so that the innovation continues to be delivered as part of routine practice to maintain the desired implementation, service and health outcomes.

EPIS describes four domains of determinants, referred to as factors in the framework (Figure 6.4). Each factor includes multiple constructs to help researchers and practitioners investigate relevant determinants that influence implementation progress and success over time. The strength of any determinant or mechanism can vary across implementation phases. EPIS also includes the importance of inter-connections and linkages of organizations and individuals in dynamic interactions that can facilitate or impede implementation and sustainment (Aarons et al., 2011).

- Outer context factors: the multi-level environmental determinants that are external to the specific implementing organization(s); the outer context includes multi-level leadership, service and policy environments, funding, inter-organizational networks, advocacy groups, and characteristics of patients/clients who are the intended recipients of the innovation.
- Inner context factors: the multi-level context where the focal innovation is being implemented; the inner context includes organizational leadership, organizational characteristics (e.g. climate, structure, receptivity), quality and fidelity monitoring/support, staffing processes, and individual characteristics of providers of the innovation (e.g. values, attitudes, motivations).
- Bridging factors: formal arrangements (e.g. contracts), relational ties (e.g. partnerships), and processes (e.g. data sharing processes) that span and align the outer and inner contexts; bridging factors have functions and forms; functions specify the purpose of each bridging factor relevant to the implementation effort, and forms explain the specific structures and activities that the bridging factor offers to align outer and inner contexts and facilitate implementation success.
- Innovation factors: characteristics of the innovation developers, characteristics of the innovation (e.g. components, complexity, cost) and its fit, or how well it meets the needs of the population or setting where it is implemented.

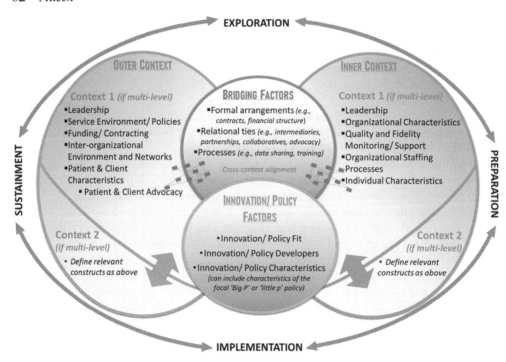

Figure 6.4 Exploration, Preparation, Implementation and Sustainment (EPIS) framework.
Source: Moullin et al. (2019); Crable et al. (2022b)

Since its development, EPIS has guided research and practice in a variety of settings and countries (Moullin et al., 2019) and has been referenced in more than 1600 peer-reviewed publications. EPIS-guided research studies span a variety of public sectors (e.g. public health, child welfare, mental or behavioural health, education, medical, criminal-legal) and levels, ranging from implementation efforts at the national policy level to service systems and the organizational level. Researchers have demonstrated the usefulness of EPIS for guiding research on elements of power and equity (Stanton et al., 2022), policy (Willging et al., 2015; Crable et al., 2022a) and team effectiveness (Aarons et al., 2014; Willging et al., 2017) across multi-level, cross-context dissemination and implementation efforts.

The EPIS framework is dynamic and continues to evolve. A global systematic review of EPIS-guided research helped generate refined definitions of EPIS phases, domains and constructs (Moullin et al., 2019) and specify distinct functions and forms of bridging factors that align outer and inner contexts (Lengnick-Hall et al., 2021). D&I researchers and practitioners continue to develop and advance the original framework by improving operationalization and measurement of EPIS determinants and mechanisms, enhancing the breadth and depth of EPIS applications and improving the intervention planning and implementation processes. In addition, EPIS constructs have been used to inform qualitative approaches for collecting and analysing data describing implementation experiences (Aarons et al., 2014; Beidas et al., 2016; Willging et al., 2017, 2018; Crable et al., 2022b). An EPIS framework website (www.EPISframework.com) has been developed as a resource for users by providing information about EPIS to facilitate informed decisions about how to apply it.

Tailored Implementation for Chronic Diseases

The Tailored Implementation for Chronic Diseases (TICD) checklist was developed as part of a European research project, funded under the European Community Seventh Framework during 2011–2015. A study protocol was published in 2011, advocating the use of tailoring of strategies (referred to as "implementation interventions") to match identified determinants of implementation (Wensing et al., 2011). The aim of the project was to assess tailored implementation programmes to improve healthcare for patients with chronic diseases, predominantly in primary healthcare settings (Wensing, 2017). Five programmes were studied in five European countries, focusing on multimorbidity, vascular conditions, chronic obstructive pulmonary disease and obesity. The project was informed by reviews of published studies on tailored implementation and a Cochrane review on tailored strategies was updated as part of the project (Baker et al., 2015).

The contents of TICD were first published in 2013 by Flottorp et al. (2013). A systematic review was conducted of determinant frameworks, referred to as "checklists", which resulted in retrieval of 87 potentially relevant papers. The final selection of frameworks was based on assessment of several criteria, including the frameworks' comprehensiveness, relevance, applicability, simplicity, clarity and usefulness. This process led to the inclusion of 12 frameworks, including three described in this chapter, namely PARIHS, TDF and CFIR. Based on a synthesis of the 12 frameworks, TICD included 57 potential determinants of practice, which were classified into seven domains (Flottorp et al., 2013). The domains are the following, with examples of the contents (i.e. underlying constructs) of each domain:

- Guideline factors: intervention/innovation characteristics, e.g. its trialability, compatibility, relative advantage and scientific basis.
- Individual health professional factors: knowledge, skills, attitudes, etc. of the individuals.
- Patient factors: patients' knowledge, skills, attitudes, adherence, etc.
- Professional interactions: culture, teamwork, communication and other inner setting influences.
- Incentives and resources: inner setting influences such as funding availability, monitoring and feedback mechanisms.
- Capacity for organizational change: inner setting influences such as learning climate, readiness for implementation and structural features of the organization.
- Social, political and legal factors: economic and political context in the external environment.

TICD is the most recently published determinant framework of the six ones presented in this chapter. It integrates aspects of other frameworks, which was considered a key strength when used in a study by Haverhals et al. (2022), who stated, "It combines aspects of both the CFIR and the TDF, in that it covers both organizational and individual determinants of implementation in a parsimonius manner" (Haverhals et al., 2022, p. 05). The use of TICD has not been documented in a review, but 20 published papers have been collected and are available through the *Implementation Science* journal website (www.biomedcentral.com/collections/TICD). The collection encompasses protocol papers, process evaluations and summative evaluations for the five implementation programmes as well as other methodological and process elements.

Concluding remarks

This chapter has presented six common determinant frameworks in implementation science. Although these frameworks may seem superficially quite disparate, with a broad range of terms, concepts and constructs, there is considerable convergence on many features. The frameworks are multi-level, identifying determinants at different levels, from the individual implementer (e.g. healthcare practitioners) to the organization and beyond. Hence, these frameworks recognize that implementation is a multidimensional phenomenon, with multiple interacting influences. The frameworks imply a systems approach to implementation. A system can be understood only as an integrated whole because it is composed not only of the sum of its components but also of the relationships among those components (Holmes et al., 2012). However, determinants are often assessed individually in implementation studies (e.g. Légaré et al., 2008; Johnson et al., 2010; Broyles et al., 2012; Verweij et al., 2012), implicitly assuming a linear relationship between the determinants and the outcomes, thus ignoring the fact that individual barriers and facilitators may interact in various ways that can be difficult to predict.

Strategies are not always explicitly accounted for in determinant frameworks. For example, they are not mentioned in TDF or EPIS, but they are addressed in some form in PARIHS and i-PARIHS (facilitation construct), CFIR (process domain) and PRISM (implementation and sustainability infrastructure element). The frameworks describe a range of implementation objects, with different terms being used; for example, innovation (i-PARIHS, CFIR and EPIS), evidence (PARIHS) and programme and intervention (PRISM). The outcome of interest is the use of these objects, regardless of whether they are physical objects such as medical technologies (e.g. a digital health tool) or immaterial practices (e.g. providing cognitive behaviour therapy sessions). The relevance of the end-users (e.g. patients, clients or community residents) of the implemented object is not always addressed explicitly in determinant frameworks although end-user perspectives seem to be increasingly recognized in implementation science.

The context is an integral part of all the determinant frameworks. Described as "an important but poorly understood mediator of change and innovation in health care organizations" (Dopson and Fitzgerald, 2006, p. 79), the context lacks a unifying definition in implementation science (and related fields such as organizational behaviour and quality improvement). However, context is generally understood as the conditions or surroundings in which implementation occurs, typically referring to circumstances beyond the direct influence of individuals. Hence, although implementation science researchers agree that the context is a critically important concept for understanding and explaining implementation, there is a lack of consensus regarding how this concept should be interpreted, in what ways the context is manifested and how contextual influences might be captured in research.

In summary, determinant frameworks are similar with regard to the general types of determinants they feature. Figure 6.5 highlights five types of determinants accounted for in many determinant frameworks:

- Characteristics of the implementation object (i.e. an evidence-based practice).
- Influences of the implementers (e.g. healthcare practitioners or community social workers).
- End-user influences (e.g. patients, clients or community residents).
- Contextual influences.
- Effectiveness of implementation strategies used to support implementation.

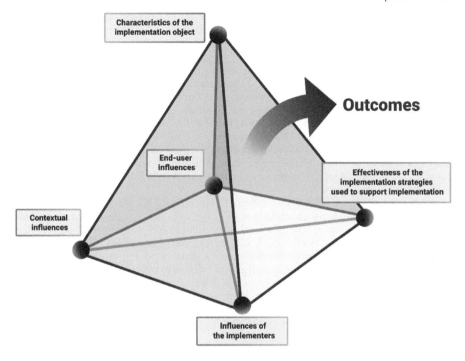

Figure 6.5 Synthesis of numerous determinant frameworks, illustrating interdependent influences on implementation success

The arrow in the figure represents the implementation outcomes that result from the five types of determinants. The links between the nodes depict the inter-dependency between the different types of determinants to underscore that they should ideally be assessed holistically rather than in isolation from each other. There could be synergistic effects such that two seemingly minor barriers constitute an important obstacle to successful outcomes if they interact or potentially strong facilitators may combine to generate weak effects.

Ultimately, determinant frameworks share many commonalities and researchers in implementation science largely agree on what the main influences on implementation outcomes are, albeit to a lesser extent on which terms are best used to describe these determinants. Several determinant frameworks have undergone revisions to account for lessons learned from the use of the frameworks and in response to changing circumstances. This trend suggests that knowledge about implementation determinants is still evolving.

Acknowledgement

Thanks to Kristin Thomas for her constructive ideas, and to Caroline Karlsson for designing Figures 6.5 and 4.1.

References

Aarons, G.A., Hurlburt, M., Horwitz, S.M. (2011) Advancing a conceptual model of evidence-based practice implementation in public service sectors. *Administration and Policy in Mental Health and Mental Health Services Research* 38, 4–23. https://doi.org/10.1007/s10488-010-0327-7

Aarons, G.A., Fettes, D.L., Hurlburt, M.S., Palinkas, L.A., Gunderson, L., Willging, C.E. (2014) Collaboration, negotiation, and coalescence for interagency-collaborative teams to scale-up evident-based practice. *Journal of Clinical Child & Adolescent Psychology* 43, 915–928. https://doi.org/10.1080/15374416.2013.876642

Baker, R., Camosso-Stefinovic, J., Gillies, C., Shaw, E.J., Cheater, F., Flottorp, S., Robertson, N., Wensing, M., Fiander, M., Eccles, M.P., Godycki-Cwirko, M., van Lieshout, J., Jäger, C., Cochrane Effective Practice and Organisation of Care Group (2015). Tailored interventions to address determinants of practice. Cochrane Database of Systematic Reviews 2015, Issue 4. Art. No.: CD005470. https://doi.org/10.1002/14651858.CD005470.pub3

Beidas, R.S., Stewart, R.E., Adams, D.R., Fernandez, T., Lustbader, S., Powell, B.J., et al. (2016) A multi-level examination of stakeholder perspectives of implementation of evidence-based practices in a large urban publicly-funded mental health system. *Administration and Policy in Mental Health and Mental Health Services Research* 43, 893–908. https://doi.org/10.1007/s10488-015-0705-2

Bergstrom, A., Ehrenberg, A., Eldh, A., Graham, I., Gustafsson, K., Harvey, G., et al. (2020) The use of the PARIHS framework in implementation research and practice - a citation analysis of the literature. *Implementation Science* 15, 68. https://doi.org/10.1186/s13012-020-01003-0

Broyles, L., Rodriguez, K.L., Kraemer, K.L., Sevick, M., Price, P.A., Gordon, A.J. (2012) A qualitative study of anticipated barriers and facilitators to the implementation of nurse-delivered alcohol screening, brief intervention, and referral to treatment for hospitalized patients in a Veterans Affairs medical center. *Addiction Science & Clinical Practice* 7, 7. https://doi.org/10.1186/1940-0640-7-7

Cane, J., O'Connor, D., Michie, S. (2012) Validation of the theoretical domains framework for use in behaviour change and implementation research. *Implementation Science* 7, 37. https://doi.org/10.1186/1748-5908-7-37

Cochrane, L.J., Olson, C.A., Murray, S., Dupuis, M., Tooman, T., Hayes, S. (2007) Gaps between knowing and doing: understanding and assessing the barriers to optimal health care. *Journal of Continuing Education in the Health Professions* 27, 94–102. https://doi.org/10.1002/chp.106

Crable, E.L., Lengnick-Hall, R., Stadnick, N., Moullin, J.C., Aarons, G. (2022a) Where is "policy" in dissemination and implementation science? Recommendations to advance theories, models, and frameworks: EPIS as a case example. *Implementation Science* 17, 80. https://doi.org/10.1186/s13012-022-01256-x

Crable, E.L., Benintendi, A., Jones, D.K., Walley, A.Y., Hicks, J.M., Drainoni, M.L. (2022b) Translating Medicaid policy into practice: policy implementation strategies from three US states' experiences enhancing substance use disorder treatment. *Implementation Science* 17, 3. https://doi.org/10.1186/s13012-021-01182-4

D'Lima, D., Lorencatto, F., Michie, S. (2020) The Behaviour Change Wheel approach. In: Nilsen, P., Birken, S.A. (Eds.), *Handbook on Implementation Science*. Cheltenham: Edward Elgar, pp. 168–214. https://doi.org/10.4337/9781788975995.00014

Damschroder, L., Aron, D., Keith, R., Kirsh, S., Alexander, J., Lowery, J. (2009) Fostering implementation of health services research findings into practice: a consolidated framework for advancing implementation science. *Implementation Science* 4, 50. https://doi.org/10.1186/1748-5908-4-50

Damschroder, L., Reardon, C.M., Lowery, J.C. (2020) The consolidated framework for implementation research (CFIR). In: Nilsen, P., Birken, S.A. (Eds.), *Handbook on Implementation Science*. Cheltenham: Edward Elgar, pp. 88–113. https://doi.org/10.4337/9781788975995.00011

Damschroder, L., Reardon, C.M., Opra Widerquist, M.A., Lowery, J. (2022) The updated Consolidated Framework for Implementation Research based on user feedback. *Implementation Science* 17, 75. https://doi.org/10.1186/s13012-022-01245-0

Dopson, S., Fitzgerald, L. (2006) The active role of context. In: Dopson, S., Fitzgerald, L. (Eds.), *Knowledge to Action? Evidence-Based Health Care in Context*. Oxford: Oxford University Press, p. 223. https://doi.org/10.1093/acprof:oso/9780199259014.003.0005

Durlak, J.A., DuPre, E.P. (2008) Implementation matters: a review of research on the influence of implementation on program outcomes and the factors affecting implementation. *American Journal of Community Psychology* 41, 327–350. https://doi.org/10.1007/s10464-008-9165-0

Feldstein, A.C., Glasgow, R.E. (2008) A practical, robust implementation and sustainability model (PRISM) for integrating research findings into practice. *Joint Commission Journal on Quality and Patient Safety* 34, 228–243. https://doi.org/10.1016/S1553-7250(08)34030-6

Flottorp, S., Oxman, A.D., Krause, J., Musila, N.R., Wensing, M., Godycki-Cwirko, M., Baker, R., Eccles, M.P. (2013). A checklist for identifying determinants of practice. A systematic review and synthesis of frameworks and taxonomies of factors that prevent or enable improvements in healthcare professional practice. *Implementation Science* 8, 35. https://doi.org/10.1186/1748-5908-8-35

Graham, I.D., Logan, J. (2004) Innovations in knowledge transfer and continuity of care. *Canadian Journal of Nursing Research* 36, 89–103.

Greenhalgh, T., Robert, G., Macfarlane, F., Bate, P., Kyriakidou, O. (2004) Diffusion of innovations in service organizations: systematic review and recommendations. *Milbank Quarterly* 82, 581–629. https://doi.org/10.1111/j.0887-378X.2004.00325.x

Gurses, A.P., Marsteller, J.A., Ozok, A.A., Xiao, Y., Owens, S., Pronovost, P.J. (2010) Using an interdisciplinary approach to identify factors that affect clinicians' compliance with evidence-based guidelines. *Critical Care Medicine* 38(8 Suppl), S282–S291. https://doi.org/10.1097/CCM.0b013e3181e69e02

Harvey, G., Kitson, A. (2016) PARIHS revisited: from heuristic to integrated framework for the successful implementation of knowledge into practice. *Implementation Science* 11, 33. https://doi.org/10.1186/s13012-016-0398-2

Harvey, G., Kitson, A. (2020) Promoting action on research implementation in health services: the integrated-PARIHS framework (i-PARIHS). In: Nilsen, P., Birken, S.A. (Eds.), *Handbook on Implementation Science*. Cheltenham: Edward Elgar, pp. 114–143. https://doi.org/10.4337/9781788975995.00012

Haverhals, L.M., Magid, K.H., Kononowech, J. (2022). Applying the Tailored Implementation in Chronic Diseases framework to inform implementation of the preferences elicited and respected for seriously ill veterans through enhanced decision-making program in the United States Veterans Health Administration. *Frontiers in Health Services* 2, 2 September 2022. https://doi.org/10.3389/frhs.2022.935341

Helfrich, C., Damschroder, L., Hagedorn, H., Daggett, G., Sahay, A., Ritchie, M., et al. (2010) A critical synthesis of literature on the Promoting Action on Research Implementation in Health Services (PARIHS) framework. *Implementation Science* 5, 82. https://doi.org/10.1186/1748-5908-5-82

Holmes, B.J., Finegood, D.T., Riley, B.L., Best, A. (2012) Systems thinking in dissemination and implementation research. In: Brownson, R.C., Colditz, G.A., Proctor, E.K. (Eds.), *Dissemination and Implementation Research in Health*. Oxford: Oxford University Press, pp. 192–212. https://doi.org/10.1093/acprof:oso/9780199751877.003.0009

Johnson, M., Jackson, R., Guillaume, L., Meier, P., Goyder, E. (2010) Barriers and facilitators to implementing screening and brief intervention for alcohol misuse: a systematic review of qualitative evidence. *Journal of Public Health* 33, 412–421. https://doi.org/10.1093/pubmed/fdq095

Kitson, A., Ahmed, L.B., Harvey, G., Seers, K., Thompson, D.R. (1996) From research to practice: one organizational model for promoting research-based practice. *Journal of Advanced Nursing* 23, 430–440. https://doi.org/10.1111/j.1365-2648.1996.tb00003.x

Kitson, A., Harvey, G., McCormack, B. (1998) Enabling the implementation of evidence based practice: a conceptual framework. *Quality in Health Care* 7, 149–159. https://doi.org/10.1136/qshc.7.3.149

Leeman, J., Wiecha, J.L., Vu, M., Blitstein, J.L., Allgood, S., Lee, S., et al. (2018) School health implementation tools: a mixed methods evaluation of factors influencing their use. *Implementation Science* 13, 48. https://doi.org/10.1186/s13012-018-0738-5

Légaré, F., Ratté, S., Gravel, K., Graham, I.D. (2008) Barriers and facilitators to implementing shared decision-making in clinical practice: update of a systematic review of health professionals' perceptions. *Patient Education and Counseling* 73, 526–535. https://doi.org/10.1016/j.pec.2008.07.018

Lengnick-Hall, R., Stadnick, N.A., Dickson, K.S., Moullin, J.C., Aarons, G.A. (2021) Forms and functions of bridging factors: specifying the dynamic links between outer and inner contexts during implementation and sustainment. *Implementation Science* 16, 34. https://doi.org/10.1186/s13012-021-01099-y

McCreight, M.S., Rabin, B.A., Glasgow, R.E., Ayele, R.A., Leonard, C.A., Gilmartin, H.M., et al. (2019) Using the Practical, Robust Implementation and Sustainability Model (PRISM) to qualitatively assess multilevel contextual factors to help plan, implement, evaluate, and disseminate health services programs. *Translational Behavioral Medicine* 9, 1002–1011. https://doi.org/10.1093/tbm/ibz085

Michie, S., Johnston, M., Abraham, C., Lawton, R., Parker, D., Walker, A. (2005) Making psychological theory useful for implementing evidence based practice: a consensus approach. *BMJ Quality & Safety* 14, 26–33. https://doi.org/10.1136/qshc.2004.011155

Michie, S., Atkins, L., West, R. (2014) *The Behaviour Change Wheel. A Guide to Designing Interventions.* 1st edition. London: Silverback, pp. 1003–1010.

Moullin, J.C., Dickson, K.S., Stadnick, N.A., Rabin, B., Aarons, G.A. (2019) Systematic review of the Exploration, Preparation, Implementation, Sustainment (EPIS) framework. *Implementation Science* 14, 1. https://doi.org/10.1186/s13012-018-0842-6

Naidoo, N., Zuma, N., Khosa, N.S., Marincowitz, G., Railton, J., Matlakala, N., et al. (2018) Qualitative assessment of facilitators and barriers to HIV programme implementation by community health workers in Mopani district, South Africa. *PLoS One* 13, e0203081. https://doi.org/10.1371/journal.pone.0203081

Powell, B., Waltz, T., Chinman, M., Damschroder, L.J., Smith, J.L., Matthieu, M.M., et al. (2015) A refined compilation of implementation strategies: results from the Expert Recommendations for Implementing Change (ERIC) project. *Implementation Science* 10, 21. https://doi.org/10.1186/s13012-015-0209-1

Rabin, B.A., Cakici, J., Golden, C.A., Estabrooks, P.A., Glasgow, R.E., Gaglio, B. (2022) A citation analysis and scoping systematic review of the operationalization of the Practical, Robust Implementation and Sustainability Model (PRISM). *Implementation Science* 17, 62. https://doi.org/10.1186/s13012-022-01234-3

Rycroft-Malone, J. (2010). Promoting Action on Research Implementation in Health Services (PARIHS). In: Rycroft-Malone, J., Bucknall, T. (Eds.), *Models and Frameworks for Implementing Evidence-Based Practice: Linking Evidence to Action.* Chichester: Sigma Theta Tau International, pp: 109–136.

Rycroft-Malone, J., Kitson, A., Harvey, G. (2002) Ingredients for change: revisiting a conceptual framework. *Quality & Safety in Health Care* 11, 174–180. https://doi.org/10.1136/qhc.11.2.174

Soi, C., Gimbel, S., Chilundo, B., Muchanga, V., Matsinhe, L., Sherr, K. (2018) Human papillomavirus vaccine delivery in Mozambique: identification of implementation performance drivers using the Consolidated Framework for Implementation Research (CFIR). *Implementation Science* 13, 151. https://doi.org/10.1186/s13012-018-0846-2

Stanhope, V., Manuel, J.I., Jessell, L., Halliday, T.M. (2018) Implementing SBIRT for adolescents within community mental health organizations: a mixed methods study. *Journal of Substance Abuse Treatment* 90, 38–46. https://doi.org/10.1016/j.jsat.2018.04.009

Stanton, M.C., Ali, S.B., The Sustain Center Team. (2022) A typology of power in implementation: building on the exploration, preparation, implementation, sustainment (epis) framework to advance mental health and HIV health equity. *Implementation Research and Practice* 3, 26334895211064250. https://doi.org/10.1177/26334895211064250

Stetler, C.B. (2001) Updating the Stetler Model of research utilization to facilitate evidence-based practice. *Nursing Outlook* 49, 272–279. https://doi.org/10.1067/mno.2001.120517

Tinc, P.J., Gadomski, A., Sorensen, J.A., Weinehall, L., Jenkins, P., Lindvall, K. (2018) Applying the Consolidated Framework for implementation research to agricultural safety and health: barriers, facilitators, and evaluation opportunities. *Safety Science* 107, 99–108. https://doi.org/10.1016/j.ssci.2018.04.008

Verweij, L.M., Proper, K.I., Leffelaar, E.R., Weel, A.N., Nauta, A.P., Hulshof, C.T., et al. (2012) Barriers and facilitators to implementation of an occupational health guideline aimed at preventing weight gain among employees in the Netherlands. *Journal of Occupational and Environmental Medicine* 54, 954–960. https://doi.org/10.1097/JOM.0b013e3182511c9f

Waltz, T.J., Powell, B.J., Fernández, M.E., Abadie, B., Damschroder, L.J. (2019) Choosing implementation strategies to address contextual barriers: diversity in recommendations and future directions. *Implementation Science* 14, 42. https://doi.org/10.1186/s13012-019-0892-4

Wensing, M. (2017). The Tailored Implementation in Chronic Diseases (TICD) project: Introduction and main findings. *Implementation Science* 12, 5. https://doi.org/10.1186/s13012-016-0536-x

Wensing, M., Oxman, A., Baker, R., Godycki-Cwirko, M., Flottorp, S., Szecsenyi, J., Grimshaw, J., Eccles, M. (2011). Tailored implementation for chronic diseases (TICD): A project protocol. *Implementation Science* 6, 103. https://doi.org/10.1186/1748-5908-6-103

Willging, C.E., Green, A.E., Gunderson, L., Chaffin, M., Aarons, G.A. (2015) From a "perfect storm" to "smooth sailing": policymaker perspectives on implementation and sustainment of an evidence-based practice in two states. *Child Maltreatment* 20, 24–36. https://doi.org/10.1177/1077559514547384

Willging, C.E., Trott. E.M., Fettes, D., Gunderson, L., Green, A.E., Hurlburt, M.S., et al. (2017) Research-supported intervention and discretion among frontline workers implementing home visitation services. *Research on Social Work Practice* 27, 664–675. https://doi.org/10.1177/1049731515601897

Willging, C.E., Gunderson, L., Green, A.E., Jaramillo, E.T., Garrison, L., Ehrhart, M.G., et al. (2018) Perspectives from community-based organizational managers on implementing and sustaining evidence-based interventions in child welfare. *Human Service Organizations: Management, Leadership & Governance* 42, 359–379. https://doi.org/10.1080/23303131.2018.1495673

Wilson, P., Kislov, R. (2022) *Implementation Science.* Cambridge: Cambridge University Press. https://doi.org/10.1017/9781009237055

7   Implementation theories

Kristin Thomas and Per Nilsen

Introduction

A theory is usually defined in terms of being a set of analytical principles or statements designed to structure our observation, understanding and explanation of the world (Wacker, 1998; Carpiano and Daley, 2006). Scholars typically point to a theory as being made up of definitions of variables, a domain where the theory applies, a set of relationships between the variables and specific predictions (Bunge, 1967; Reynolds, 1971; Dubin, 1978). A "good theory" provides a clear explanation of how and why specific relationships lead to specific events. Theories are often described in an abstraction-continuum. High abstraction level theories (general or grand theories) have an almost unlimited scope, middle abstraction level theories explain limited sets of phenomena and lower-level abstraction theories are empirical generalizations of more limited scope and application (Merton, 1968; Wacker, 1998). Theories within implementation science are usually middle-range theories and are thus restricted in their area of application.

The label "implementation theories" was given by Nilsen (2015) to theories developed specifically for use in research on implementation of evidence-based practices by researchers active in the field of implementation science (although these theories may be used beyond implementation science). Implementation theories differ from the process models and determinant frameworks also used in implementation science. Theories in implementation science imply some predictive capacity and attempt to explain the causal mechanisms of implementation. This is not the case with process models and determinant frameworks; they point to factors believed or found to influence implementation processes and outcomes, but unlike theories, they do not specify the mechanisms of change. Thus, neither process models nor determinant frameworks provide explanations; they only describe empirical phenomena by fitting them into a set of categories (Nilsen, 2015). In general, theories can offer a common language for researchers and practitioners. For implementation science, this could be especially important considering its interdisciplinary nature and the importance of bringing together multiple perspectives in the endeavour to understand and explain implementation.

Normalization Process Theory

The Normalization Process Theory (NPT) (May et al., 2009) began life in the early 2000s as a model constructed on the basis of empirical studies of the implementation of new technologies (May, 2006; May et al., 2007). The model was subsequently expanded and

DOI: 10.4324/9781003318125-8

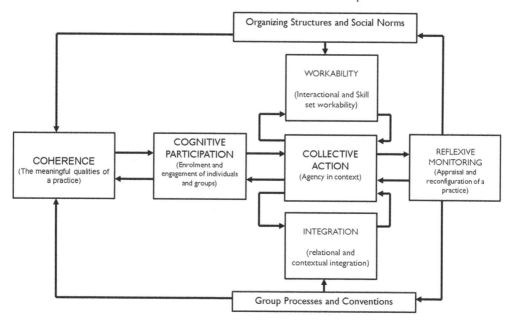

Figure 7.1 The implementation core of Normalization Process Theory (NPT).
Source: May and Finch (2009)

developed into a theory as change mechanisms and inter-relations between various constructs were delineated (May and Finch, 2009; May et al., 2009). NPT was first described as a theory in 2009 in articles in *Sociology* (May and Finch, 2009) and *Implementation Science* (May et al., 2009) (Figure 7.1).

NPT "identifies factors that promote and inhibit the routine incorporation of complex interventions into everyday practice" (Murray et al., 2010, p. 2). The theory focuses on the work that individuals and groups do to enable an intervention to become normalized, which is defined as "the embedding of a technique, technology or organizational change as a routine and taken-for-granted element of clinical practice" (May, 2006, p. 2). Thus, the NPT is concerned with what people do (e.g. implementers, healthcare providers, patients and other end-users) when implementing change, rather than individuals' attitudes, knowledge or beliefs about the change.

The theory identifies four social mechanisms of embedding (i.e. normalizing) complex interventions in practice and the relationships between these.

- Coherence: the process of making sense of and understanding a new practice, for example, a new evidence-based treatment method. Coherence-building is proposed to be done on both individual and collective levels through:

  - Differentiation: understanding how a new practice differ from current practice.
  - Communal specification: building a shared understanding of the objectives, benefits and value of the new practice.
  - Individual specification: understanding specific tasks and responsibilities connected to the new practice.
  - Internalization: understanding the value, benefits and importance of the new practice.

- Cognitive participation: the relational work that individuals and groups do to engage in, create and maintain a community of commitment around a new practice; this work includes:

  - Initiation: bringing implementation forward.
  - Enrolment: the organization and re-organization of relationships to promote commitment and engagement.
  - Legitimation: building trust and confidence among key stakeholders.
  - Activation: shared definitions of actions and procedures needed to sustain commitment and engagement.

- Collective action: the operational work that individuals and groups do to incorporate a new practice in everyday practice. This can be understood as how individuals and groups operationalize and realize a new practice in an everyday setting through mobilizing resources and skills. Collective action includes:

  - Interactional workability: operationalizing intervention components within everyday practice.
  - Relational integration: build and maintain accountability and confidence in the practice and other users.
  - Skill set workability: assigning roles and responsibilities when operationalizing the practice to everyday practice.
  - Contextual integration: resource allocation and execution of protocols, policies and procedures.

- Reflexive monitoring: the appraisal work that individuals and groups do to assess and understand how a new practice may influence current practice. This work can be formal, casual or informal with the ultimate goal of appraising the impact and effect of a new practice. This appraisal work includes:

  - Systematization: assessment of how effective and useful the new practice is for me and others around me.
  - Communal appraisal: assessment by individuals on their own and together through interaction and negotiation of the value, benefit and the workings of the new practice.
  - Individual appraisal: individual-level appraisal of the worth and impact of the new practice on current work.
  - Reconfiguration: appraisal work done by individuals or groups whereby the new practice is refined and modified to make it realistic and fit current practice.

NPT has been widely used to study the implementation of a broad range of interventions within various settings and sectors, including healthcare, social care and education (McEvoy et al., 2014; May et al., 2018). A systematic review of published NPT studies in 2018 (May et al., 2018) identified 108 discrete studies that had used NPT. The review concluded that 10% of the papers featured critique of some aspect of NPT, primarily the terminology, which many felt can be difficult to understand. A website (https://normali zation-process-theory.northumbria.ac.uk) provides information to guide the use of NPT in both qualitative and quantitative studies. A 23-item questionnaire instrument, the Normalisation MeAsure Development (NoMAD), can be used to measure the constructs of NPT (Finch et al., 2018; Rapley et al., 2018).

Organization readiness for change

The construct of organizational readiness for change (ORC) is acknowledged as an important determinant for implementation and a potential mediator of implementation strategy effectiveness (Figure 7.2) (Weiner, 2020). The construct is included in frameworks and models within implementation science such as the Consolidated Framework for Implementation Research (CFIR) (Damschroder et al., 2009) and the Quality Implementation Framework (QIF) (Meyers et al., 2012). Weiner expanded on the construct when he developed the theory of ORC. In the ORC theory, the construct is defined as the shared psychological and behavioural preparedness among organizational members (i.e. individuals and groups involved in an implementation) to implement a specific change. Simply put, organizational readiness for change is conceptualized as the collective state of being willing and able to implement a new practice, for example, an intervention or technology (Weiner, 2009).

The ORC theory posits that organizational readiness for change consists of two facets:

- Change commitment: this refers to the shared resolve among members of an organization to implement a specific change. It concerns the extent to which individuals and groups are willing to engage in actions and behaviours that are required to successfully implement the change.
- Change efficacy: this refers to the shared beliefs among individuals and groups in an organization regarding their joint ability to carry out the implementation. Change efficacy represents the extent to which organizational members perceive there is enough knowledge and sufficient resources and capability to implement a specific change.

Change commitment and change efficacy are conceptually inter-related. Lack of confidence in one's capabilities to execute a course of action can impair one's motivation to engage in that course of action. Similarly, fear and other negative emotions can lead one to question or downplay one's capabilities. These two facets of organizational readiness tend to covary but not perfectly (Weiner, 2020).

When organizational readiness is high, organizational members will go "above and beyond the call of duty" by taking action to support implementation that exceeds job requirements or role expectations. High organizational readiness to change increases the likelihood of change being initiated and persisting, with more cooperative

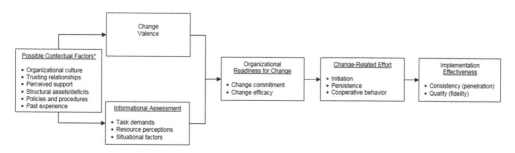

Figure 7.2 Organizational readiness for change (ORC).

Source: adapted from Weiner (2009)

behaviour (e.g. volunteering for problem-solving teams). Thus, initiation, persistence and cooperative behaviour mediate between organizational readiness for change and implementation effectiveness.

An organization's readiness for change is influenced by:

- Change valence: the shared belief that a change is needed, important, beneficial and worthwhile. Individuals and groups within an organization can perceive a change as important for different reasons; for example, the change is urgently needed, the change resonates with core values or respected peers value the change. However, the key aspect here is the shared view that a particular change is meaningful for the organization.
- Informational assessment: the assessment made by individuals and groups regarding their joint implementation capability. It involves their shared assessments on what the change will involve and require (task demand), what resources there are to implement the change (resource perceptions) and what the local conditions are for implementation (situational factors).

Change valence and informational assessment are proposed to be influenced by contextual factors such as organizational culture and climate, previous experiences of implementing change, policies and procedures, as well as organizational resources and structures. These contextual factors are thought to be less change-specific and thus more stable over time.

Readiness for change at an organizational level has not been the subject of as much empirical research as individual readiness for change (Weiner, 2020). Three reviews have shown that most measures of organizational readiness for change have limited reliability or validity (Holt et al., 2007; Weiner et al., 2008; Gagnon et al., 2014). However, Shea et al. (2014) has developed the Organizational Readiness for Implementing Change (ORIC), which has been shown to be valid and reliable. ORIC is a 12-item measure of change commitment and change efficacy based on the theory described here.

Capability Opportunity Motivation – Behavior

Capability Opportunity Motivation – Behaviour (COM-B) was introduced as part of a 2011 paper that introduced the Behaviour Change Wheel (Michie et al., 2011), described in Chapter 9, which addresses matching of determinants (i.e. barriers and facilitators) with implementation strategies. The theory draws on two somewhat unusual sources: a US consensus meeting of behavioural theorists in 1991 and a principle of US criminal law dating back many centuries that considers prerequisites for performance of specified volitional behaviours (Michie et al., 2011, 2014).

COM-B posits that for behaviour change to occur, individuals need to perceive that they are psychologically and physically able to perform the behaviour (i.e. capability), perceive that they have the social and physical opportunity to engage in the behaviour (i.e. opportunity) and perceive that they want or need to carry out the behaviour more than other competing behaviours (i.e. motivation). The three components are interlinked. The single-headed and double-headed arrows in Figure 7.3 represent potential influences between the components in the COM-B system (Michie et al., 2011, 2014).

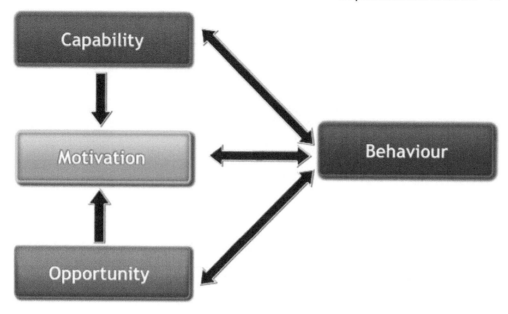

Figure 7.3 Capability Opportunity Motivation – Behaviour (COM-B).
Source: Michie et al. (2011)

Each of the three components of COM-B is divided into two types:

- Capability: an individual's perceived physical and psychological ability to accomplish, perform or take part in a behaviour.
  - Psychological capability: knowledge, skills and stamina to engage in a behaviour.
  - Physical capability: physical strength, skills and stamina.
- Opportunity: external factors that make a behaviour possible.
  - Physical opportunity: opportunities or restraints within the environment, such as time, location and resources.
  - Social opportunity: opportunities connected to social factors, such as cultural norms, social cues and access to networks.
- Motivation: conscious and unconscious cognitive processes that can direct and inspire a behaviour:
  - Reflective motivation: making plans and evaluating things that have already happened.
  - Automatic motivation: primarily automatic processes, such as desires, impulses and inhibitions.

COM-B is linked to the Theoretical Domains Framework (TDF), as shown in Table 7.1. A key difference between COM-B and TDF is that the former specifies causal mechanisms, which TDF does not. This is why COM-B should be considered a theory, whereas TDF is a determinant framework (even though it is based on theories).

Table 7.1 Alignment of Capability Opportunity Motivation – Behaviour (COM-B) and the Theoretical Domains Framework (TDF).

COM-B	TDF
Physical capability	Physical skills
Psychological capability	Knowledge
	Memory, attention and decision processes
	Behavioural regulation
Reflective motivation	Professional/social role and identity
	Beliefs about capabilities
	Optimism
	Beliefs about consequences
	Intentions
	Goals
Automatic motivation	Reinforcement
	Emotion
Physical opportunity	Environmental context and resources
Social opportunity	Social influences

Source: Michie et al. (2014)

Since its introduction in 2011, COM-B has become widely used in implementation science. It has been shown to be useful in investigating conditions (i.e. barriers and facilitators) for implementing change and for developing implementation strategies to address barriers and facilitators. COM-B has been applied to many different health-related areas, in both individual studies and systematic reviews (e.g. Alexander et al., 2014; McDonagh et al., 2018; Atkins et al., 2020; Rosário et al., 2021; Timlin et al., 2021). It is used both as a standalone theory and as part of the Behaviour Change Wheel tool (described in Chapter 9).

Concluding remarks

This chapter has described three theories developed within implementation science. They can be used in research (e.g. to generalize empirical knowledge across settings) and in implementation efforts (e.g. to generate theory-informed implementation strategies). NPT and ORC emphasize the collective nature of implementation and thus conceptualize implementation as a team effort (e.g. collective action in NPT and shared resolve in ORC). In contrast, COM-B conceptualizes implementation from the perspective of individuals' behaviours, although the three components of the theory can be construed at individual, group and societal levels (Michie et al., 2014).

It can be difficult to select an appropriate theoretical approach due to the sheer number of theories, models and frameworks in implementation science. Chapter 12 provides input on how to choose between different theoretical approaches. Selecting one theory means placing weight on some aspects (e.g. certain causal factors or the individual level rather than the collective level) at the expense of others, thus offering only partial understanding. It is important to be aware of the underlying assumptions of the theories at one's disposal. Combining the merits of multiple theories may offer more complete understanding and explanation, yet such combinations may mask contrasting assumptions regarding key issues. For instance, are people driven primarily by their individual beliefs and motivation or does a pervasive professional or organizational culture impose norms, values and expectations that regulate how people behave, thus making individual traits relatively unimportant? Is a particular clinical behaviour primarily influenced by reflective thought processes or is it an automatically enacted habit?

Development of theories (and models and frameworks) has been important in implementation science to understand and explain how and why implementation succeeds or fails. The use of theories was debated more often at the early stages of implementation science, when some critics (e.g. Oxman, 2005; Bhattacharyya et al., 2006) argued that theory was not necessarily better than common sense for guiding implementation. Common sense has been defined as a group's shared tacit knowledge concerning a phenomenon (Fletcher, 1984). It could be argued that common sense about how or why something works (or does not) also constitutes a theory, albeit an informal and non-codified one. In either case, empirical research is important to study how and the extent to which the use of implementation theories (and models and frameworks) contributes to more effective implementation. It is also important to explore how the current theories can be further developed to better address implementation challenges. Hence, implementation science benefits from both inductive construction of new or expanded theories and deductive application of theories.

Although the use of theory does not necessarily yield more effective implementation than using common sense, there are certain advantages to applying formal theory over common sense (i.e. informal theory). Theories are explicit and open to question and examination; common sense usually consists of implicit assumptions, beliefs and ways of thinking and is therefore more difficult to challenge. If deductions from a theory are incorrect, the theory can be adapted, extended or abandoned. Theories are more consistent with existing facts than common sense, which typically means that a hypothesis based on an established theory is a more educated guess than one based on common sense. Furthermore, theories give individual facts a meaningful context and contribute towards building an integrated body of knowledge, whereas common sense is more likely to produce isolated facts (Cacioppo, 2004).

References

Alexander, K.E., Brijnath, B., Mazza, D. (2014). Barriers and enablers to delivery of the Healthy Kids Check: an analysis informed by the Theoretical Domains Framework and COM-B model. *Implementation Science* 9, 60. https://doi.org/10.1186/1748-5908-9-60

Atkins, L., Sallis, A., Chadborn, T., Shaw, K., Schneider, A., Hopkins, S. et al. (2020). Reducing catheter-associated urinary tract infections: a systematic review of barriers and facilitators and strategic behavioural analysis of interventions. *Implementation Science* 15, 44. https://doi.org/10.1186/s13012-020-01001-2

Bhattacharyya, O. Reeves, S., Garfinkel, S., Zwarenstein, M. (2006). Designing theoretically-informed implementation interventions: fine in theory, but evidence of effectiveness in practice is needed. *Implementation Science* 1, 5. https://doi.org/10.1186/1748-5908-1-5

Bunge, M. (1967). *Quantum Theory and Reality: Studies in the Foundations Methodology, and Philosophy of Science*. Berlin: Springer-Verlag.

Cacioppo, J. (2004). Common sense, intuition and theory in personality and social psychology. *Personality and Social Psychology Review* 8, 114–122. https://doi.org/10.1207/s15327957pspr0802_4

Carpiano, R. M. and Daley, D. M. (2006). A guide and glossary on postpositivist theory building for population health. *Journal of Epidemiology and Community Health* 60, 564–570. https://doi.org/10.1136/jech.2004.031534

Damschroder, L.J., Aron, D.C., Keith, R.E., Kirsh, S.R., Alexander, J.A., Lowery, J.C. (2009). Fostering implementation of health services research findings into practice: a consolidated framework for advancing implementation science. *Implementation Science* 4, 50. https://doi.org/10.1186/1748-5908-4-50

Dubin, R. (1978). *Theory Building: A Practical Guide to the Construction and Testing of Theoretical Models*. New York: Free Press.

Finch, T.L., Girling, M., May, C.R., Mair, F.S., Murray, E., Treweek, S., et al. (2018). Improving the normalization of complex interventions : part 2 - validation of the NoMAD instrument for assessing implementation work based on normalization process theory (NPT). *BMC Medical Research Methodology* 18, 135. https://doi.org/10.1186/s12874-018-0591-x.

Fletcher, G.J. (1984). Psychology and common sense. *American Psychologist* 39, 203–213.

Gagnon, M.P., Attieh, R., Ghandour, elK., Légaré, F., Ouimet, M., Estabrooks, C.A., et al. (2014). A systematic review of instruments to assess organizational readiness for knowledge translation in health care. *PLoS ONE* 9, e114338. https://doi.org/10.1371/journal.pone.0114338

Holt, D.T., Armenakis, A.A., Feild, H.S., Harris, S.G. (2007). Readiness for organizational change: the systematic development of a scale. *Journal of Applied Behavioral Science* 43, 232–255. https://doi.org/10.1177/0021886306295295

May, C. (2006). A rational model for assessing and evaluating complex interventions in health care. *BMC Health Services Research* 6, 86. https://doi.org/10.1186/1472-6963-6-86

May, C., Finch, T. (2009). Implementing, embedding, and integrating practices: an outline of normalization process theory. *Sociology* 43, 535–554. https://doi.org/10.1177/0038038509103208

May, C., Finch, T., Mair, F., Ballini, L., Dowrick, C., Eccles, M., et al. (2007). Understanding the implementation of complex interventions in health care : the normalization process model. *BMC Health Services Research* 7, 148. https://doi.org/10.1186/1472-6963-7-148

May, C.R., Mair, F., Finch, T., MacFarlane, A., Dowrick, C., Treweek, S., et al. (2009). Development of a theory of implementation and integration: Normalization Process Theory. *Implementation Science* 4, 29. https://doi.org/10.1186/1748-5908-4-29

May, C.R., Cummings, A., Girling, M., Bracher, M., Mair, F.S., May, C.M., et al. (2018). Using Normalization Process Theory in feasibility studies and process evaluations of complex healthcare interventions: a systematic review. *Implementation Science* 13, 80. https://doi.org/10.1186/s13012-018-0758-1

McDonagh, L.K., Saunders, J.M., Cassell, J., Curtis, T., Bastaki, H., Hartney, T., et al. (2018). Application of the COM-B model to barriers and facilitators to chlamydia testing in general practice for young people and primary care practitioners: A systematic review. *Implementation Science* 13, 130. https://doi.org/10.1186/s13012-018-0821-y

McEvoy, R., Ballini, L., Maltoni, S., O'Donnell, C.A., Mair, F.S., Macfarlane, A. (2014). A qualitative systematic review of studies using the normalization process theory to research implementation processes. *Implementation Science* 9. 2. https://doi.org/10.1186/1748-5908-9-2

Merton, S. (1968). *Social Theory and Social Structure*. New York: Free Press.

Meyers, D.C., Durlak, J.A., Wandersman, A. (2012). The Quality Implementation Framework: a synthesis of critical steps in the implementation process. *American Journal of Community Psychology* 50, 462–480. https://doi.org/10.1007/s10464-012-9522-x

Michie, S., Atkins, L., West, R. (2014) *The Behaviour Change Wheel: A Guide to Designing Interventions*. Sutton: Silverback Publishing.

Michie, S., van Stralen, M.M., West, R. (2011). The behaviour change wheel: a new method for characterising and designing behaviour change interventions. *Implementation Science* 6, 42. https://doi.org/10.1186/1748-5908-6-42

Murray, E., Treweek, S., Pope, C., MacFarlane, A., Ballini, L., Dowrick, C., et al. (2010). Normalisation process theory: a framework for developing, evaluating and implementing complex interventions. *BMC Medicine* 8, 63. https://doi.org/10.1186/1741-7015-8-63

Nilsen, P. (2015). Making sense of implementation theories, models and frameworks. *Implementation Science* 10, 53. https://doi.org/10.1186/s13012-015-0242-0

Oxman, A.D. (2005). The OFF theory of research utilization. *Journal of Clinical Epidemiology* 58, 113–116. https://doi.org/10.1016/j.jclinepi.2004.10.002

Rapley, T. et al. (2018). Improving the normalization of complex interventions: Part 1 - Development of the NoMAD instrument for assessing implementation work based on normalization process theory (NPT). *BMC Medical Research Methodology* 18, 133. https://doi.org/10.1186/s12874-018-0590-y

Reynolds, P. (1971) *A Primer in Theory Construction*. New York: Bobbs-Merrill.

Rosário, F., Santos, M.I., Angus, K., Pas, L., Ribeiro, C., Fitzgerald, N., et al. (2021). Factors influencing the implementation of screening and brief interventions for alcohol use in primary care practices: a systematic review using the COM-B system and Theoretical Domains Framework. *Implementation Science* 16, 6. https://doi.org/10.1186/s13012-020-01073-0

Shea, C.M., Jacobs, S.R., Esserman, D.A., Bruce, K., Weiner, B.J., et al. (2014). Organizational readiness for implementing change: a psychometric assessment of a new measure. *Implementation Science* 9, 7. https://doi.org/10.1186/1748-5908-9-7

Timlin, D., McCormack, J.M., Simpson, E.E.A. (2021). Using the COM-B model to identify barriers and facilitators towards adoption of a diet associated with cognitive function (MIND diet). *Public Health Nutrition* 24, 1657–1670. https://doi.org/10.1017/S1368980020001445

Wacker, J.G. (1998). A definition of theory: research guidelines for different theory-building research methods in operations management. *Journal of Operations Management* 16, 361–385. https://doi.org/10.1016/s0272-6963(98)00019-9

Weiner, B.J. (2009). A theory of organizational readiness for change. *Implementation Science* 4, 67. https://doi.org/10.1186/1748-5908-4-67

Weiner, B.J. (2020). A theory of organizational readiness for change. In: Nilsen, P., Birken, S.A. (Eds.), *Handbook on Implementation Science*. Cheltenham: Edward Elgar, pp. 215–231. https://doi.org/10.4337/9781788975995.00015

Weiner, B.J., Amick, H., Lee, S.D. (2008). Measurement of organizational services research and other fields *Medical Care Research and Review* 65, 379–436 https://doi.org/10.1177/1077558708317802

8 Theories and concepts from other fields of potential utility for implementation science

Per Nilsen

Individual-level theories

Implementation science uses many of the theories from psychology on individuals' health-related and consumer behaviours; psychology is traditionally the study of the individual. The assumption is that it is ultimately the individual, for example, the physician, nurse, social worker or teacher, who makes a decision to use an evidence-based intervention or not, thus making the individual a relevant unit of analysis to understand and explain how and why implementation succeeds or fails. Four types of individual-level theories are described here: behaviourism; social-cognitive theories; dual-process theories; and learning theories.

Behaviourism

Behaviourism is based on the premise that behaviours can be studied in a systematic manner. The sources of behaviour are assumed to be external and behaviours are learned through interaction with the environment. Thus, interest is directed towards externally observable and measurable behaviours. The term "behaviourism" was coined in 1913 by John Watson in his paper "Psychology as the behaviorist views it" and in 1924, he published his book entitled *Behaviorism*. In the 1930s, Skinner developed operant conditioning as a method of learning that occurs by means of reinforcement and punishment. Through operant learning, an association is made between a behaviour and consequences for that behaviour; when a desirable result follows an action, the behaviour becomes more likely to be repeated. Conversely, responses followed by adverse outcomes are less likely to be repeated (Hunt, 2007).

Behaviourist principles are evident in implementation strategies that involve the use of financial incentives to encourage practitioners to change an existing practice, for example, reducing antibiotic prescription by offering funds for hospital investment if specific prescribing targets have been met. Another example is the audit and feedback strategy, whereby the audit is a review of performance based on explicit criteria or standards that is subsequently fed back to the practitioners in a structured manner. Building on operant learning theory, organizational behaviour management (OBM) is an established approach to achieve behaviour change in organizations. OBM involves examination of target behaviours in terms of their antecedent stimuli that may correlate with the behaviour and consequences that may affect the behaviours in question (Diener et al., 2009; Wilder et al., 2009; Cunningham and Geller, 2012). OBM-informed antecedent and consequence-based strategies were used in a study that sought to reduce low-value care to achieve a more evidence-based practice (Ingvarsson et al., 2022).

DOI: 10.4324/9781003318125-9

Social-cognitive theories

Cognitivism emerged in the 1950s in response to behaviourism. Cognitivists believed behaviourism neglected the importance of cognitions, that is, the mental processes involved in gaining knowledge and comprehension. Individual cognitions are considered processes that intervene between observable stimuli and responses in real-world situations (Luszczynska and Schwarzer, 2005). Social cognitivism recognizes that individuals also learn by observing others in social situations and through the influence of their social environment (Bandura, 1977). The cognitive process is viewed as a deliberative and rational process, involving evaluation of a behaviour based on some combination of utility, risk, capabilities and social influences, before developing hypotheses about the consequences of different actions (e.g. "What would happen if I deny this patient this test for which there is no evidence?") and finally acting (or not) on the intention (Norman and Conner, 2015). Social-cognitive theories have their roots in expectancy value theories from the 1950s that assume that individuals aim to maximize utility and prefer behaviours that are associated with the highest expected utility (Conner and Norman, 2015).

Implementation strategies in the form of courses on improving knowledge or skills, as well as strategies such as disseminating information and guidelines, can be said to be based on assumptions aligned with social-cognitive theories. Social-cognitive theories such as the Theory of Reasoned Action (Fishbein and Ajzen, 1975), the Social Cognitive Theory (Bandura, 1977), the Theory of Interpersonal Behaviour (Triandis, 1980) and the Theory of Planned Behaviour (Ajzen and Madden, 1986) have been applied in implementation science to identify variables that underlie healthcare practitioners' behaviours and to predict their behaviour change. A systematic review by Godin et al. (2008) identified 76 implementation studies that used social-cognitive theories. Since then, the use of social-cognitive theories in implementation science has been simplified through the development of the Theoretical Domains Framework, which is a determinant framework that synthesizes 33 social-cognitive theories into a framework consisting of 14 domains of behavioural influences (Michie et al., 2005; Cane et al., 2012).

Dual-process theories and habit theory

Despite their proven utility in explaining many behaviours, social-cognitive theories have been critiqued for not accounting sufficiently for the impact of non-reflective processes on behaviour (Norman and Conner, 2015). The assumption that human behaviour is largely under conscious control has taken a "theoretical battering" in the 2000s (Greenwald and Krieger, 2006, p. 945). The development of dual-process theories has drawn attention to the role of intuitive thinking on behaviours, providing a broader explanation of cognitive processes (Kahneman, 2011). Theories/models such as Dual-Process Theory (Evans and Over, 1996), Dual-System Theory (Sloman, 1996) and Two-System Theory (Stanovich and West, 2000) characterize two different cognitive processes or systems that work in parallel to influence behaviours. The two systems serve separate functions: System I is intuitive, automatic, fast, experiential and affect-based; System II is analytical, slow, verbal, deliberate and logical. System I is always active and can save time, energy and free up mental capacity for other purposes, whereas System II may be engaged or disengaged depending on the circumstances (Kahneman, 2011). Research has confirmed the relevance of both systems (Djulbegovic et al., 2012).

Studies have revealed that humans are susceptible to a range of cognitive biases that suggest that humans are "boundedly rational". Behavioural economics takes advantage of dual-process theories to provide input for behaviour change strategies, for example, using nudges that involve altering the way decisional options are presented to enable individuals to select the best option more easily (Last et al., 2021). However, these theories or strategies have scarcely been used in implementation science (Rendle and Beidas, 2021). Rather, theories applied in implementation science to analyse practitioners' behaviours have predominantly focused on the reflective processes (System II) that influence behaviours (Potthoff et al., 2022). In terms of implementation strategies, different types of reminders that prompt practitioners to perform a certain action can serve to disrupt habits and thus change habitual behaviours. There have been calls for increased use of dual-process and habit theories in implementation science (Sladek et al., 2006; Godin et al. 2008; Rochette et al. 2009; Nilsen et al., 2012; Rendle and Beidas, 2021; Nilsen et al., 2022; Potthoff et al., 2022).

Habit theory is consistent with dual-process theories because it posits that behaviours that are repeated in the same context (e.g. the same situation and place) become increasingly automated and reliant on System I (Lally et al., 2010; Potthoff et al., 2022). Habit is defined as a process whereby internal and contextual cues trigger automatic reactions based on a learned cue-response association (Gardner, 2015). Habit theory explains why specific tasks or practices are maintained due to repetition of a behaviour in a specific context. Once an action has become habitual, it becomes regulated by non-reflective processes (i.e. System I). Habit is a memory-based cognitive structure, and habitual behaviour is the potential consequence of this structure (Potthoff et al., 2022). Although there are definitional and measurement challenges, it has been estimated that 45% of people's everyday behaviours are repeated in the same location every day (Neal et al., 2006) and that between 40% and 95% of all human behaviours are habitual (Walesh, 2017).

Learning theories

Behaviour change can be seen as a subset of the broader concept of learning, which is typically defined in terms of change so that an individual is in some sense different than before this learning took place. The change in question can be anything from changes in understanding, attitudes and knowledge to changes in skills and behaviours. To be considered learning, the change should be relatively permanent and not the result of a maturation of the individual's existing potential (Illeris, 2009).

There are numerous ways to categorize different forms of learning and knowledge. First-order (or single-loop) learning takes place within given circumstances of an established practice. The result may be improvement of existing routines and working methods. Second-order (or double-loop) learning involves questioning of current circumstances, which creates favourable conditions for development and innovation; for example, new ways of providing patient consultations (Nilsen et al., 2017). The two concepts correspond to adaptive learning and developmental learning, respectively. Adaptive learning involves a gradual shift from slower, deliberate behaviours to faster, smoother and more efficient behaviours, yielding increasingly efficient, effective and reliable task performances. Developmental learning is conceptualized as a process in the opposite direction, whereby more or less automatically enacted behaviours are disrupted so that they become deliberate and conscious (Ellström, 2001).

Although behaviour change has been an important focus of research in implementation science, outcomes are also often considered in broader learning terms; for example, increased knowledge, more positive attitudes and improved motivation after taking part in a course intended to facilitate the use of an evidence-based guideline. Implementation of new evidence-based interventions typically requires both first-order and second-order learning: second-order learning to disrupt a current practice that needs to be changed to accommodate a new intervention and first-order learning to learn the new intervention and provide it to patients as part of regular practice (Nilsen et al., 2017). Despite the potential relevance of learning to understand and explain the changes involved in implementation, learning perspectives are not so common in implementation science.

Social group-level theories and concepts

Numerous theories and concepts relate to relationships between individuals in groups of varying size, from small units such as a work team to larger units such as professions, organizations or nations. Human beings are infinitely social creatures who need support and recognition provided by their peers. Hence, the relevance of the group level can be explained with regard to the importance of belonging to social groups. Substantial evidence suggests that social relationships are critical to our well-being because they fulfil a sense of belonging, which is a psychological need for survival (Allen, 2020). There is a reciprocal relationship between individuals and groups of people, which in essence is the study of sociology. Seven theories and concepts that have a group-level unit of analysis are described here: leadership; culture; social networks; homophily; social capital; community of practice; and routinization theory.

Leadership

Leadership is usually defined in terms of a process of influence to achieve certain goals; that is, guiding a group to accomplish a task (Yukl, 2006). The concept is not to be confused with management (although this often happens); leadership can be considered a social process or a relationship, whereas management is a position, which means that a manager does not have to be a leader and a leader does not have to hold a managerial position. For example, physicians are often described as leaders in many healthcare contexts, and their involvement in various change and improvement initiatives is often important for achieving desired goals (Danielsson et al., 2018).

The view of leadership has evolved from an early focus on leadership in the form of inherited traits to an increasingly multifaceted view that considers leadership as a complex interaction between the leader and the environment (Gill, 2011). Trait studies have been part of leadership research since the 1940s. Findings suggest that some traits are essential for effective leadership when other factors are present. Contingency-based leadership theories from the 1960s and 1970s recognized that different situations required different leadership styles. Hence, leaders should select a style that best fits with the situation at a given time. The 1980s saw changes in leadership theories as globalization demanded partially different skills from leaders. Contemporary leadership theories place greater emphasis on how leadership work affects employee motivation (Dinibutun, 2020).

The concepts of transformative and transactive leadership were introduced by Burns (1978) and have proved to be popular concepts in leadership research. Whereas transformative leadership means that leaders and employees increase each other's mo-tivation so that they see beyond their own needs, transactive leadership is a form of transaction between leaders and employees, where the leader offers rewards in ex-change for the employees' efforts and compliance with the leader's wishes and goals. Bass (1985) and Bass and Avolio (1997) further developed Burns' theory in their *Full Range Leadership*.

Despite extensive research and theory development on leadership, Gill (2011, p. 98) argues that "no theory or model of leadership so far has created a full or satisfactory explanation of leadership". Ellström et al. (2009) maintain that much leadership re-search tends to be overconfident about the possibility of identifying clear causal relation-ships between the leader and different outcomes. Implementation science has increasingly drawn attention to the role of leadership for implementation. Leadership is featured in several of the models and frameworks used in the field. However, research on the impor-tance of leadership in implementation is still fairly undeveloped and several researchers (e.g. Wensing et al., 2006; Yano, 2008; French et al., 2009; Reichenpfader et al., 2015) have called for an increased focus on leadership and management issues in implementa-tion science.

Culture

Many definitions of culture exist, but most convey that culture is something that indi-viduals learn based on experiences of dealing with social situations. This learning can become so ingrained that it is difficult to know how it influences our thoughts and be-haviours. Culture is often viewed in terms of one or more of four core elements: shared values (goals, ideals and priorities), norms (behaviours that are expected, accepted and supported), assumptions and perceptions of reality that develop in a social group when members interact with each other and the outside world (Bang, 1999). Culture is a group phenomenon because it is shared with people who interact within the social group in which it was learned (Hofstede et al., 2010). Culture in implementation science is usually considered in terms of organizational culture, but culture develops in any social group, from a family, work unit and community to an organization, ethnic group or a country. Culture can also be created in geographically dispersed organizations such as virtual internet communities.

Culture is linked with leadership because leaders are important "culture creators" because a leader has the power to influence the group members with his or her values, norms and descriptions of reality. At the same time, the culture influences who is ap-pointed a leader (Alvesson, 2009; Schein, 2008). An important question is whether it is possible to influence organizational culture and, if so, how. It is common to distinguish between two perspectives on culture: one that assumes that organizations "have" cul-ture and the other that builds on the organization "being" culture (Smircich, 1983). Many organizational culture researchers find themselves somewhere between the two perspectives on culture, viewing culture as something that develops in an organization and can be influenced even if it is often more difficult than suggested by the popular literature.

Cultural studies emerged in England in the late 1950s and subsequently spread inter-nationally. Research on organizational culture took off in the late 1970s and expanded greatly during the 1980s although the term organizational culture was first introduced by Elliott Jacques in his book *The Changing Culture of a Factory* (Jaques, 1951). Edgar

Schein is considered "the father" of organizational culture and has shown its importance in the management of organizational change. Schein emphasized the important role of culture in many types of social groups, claiming that as much as 90% of human behaviour is driven by culture (Culture University, 2019).

The importance of an organization's culture in implementation science is obvious because common values, norms, assumptions and perceptions of reality can influence the behaviours of individuals and groups in an organization. Organizational culture is included in many of the determinant frameworks used in implementation science; for example, Active Implementation Frameworks, Consolidated Framework for Implementation Research (CFIR) and Promoting Action on Research Implementation in Health Services (PARIHS) (Nilsen and Bernhardsson, 2019). The importance of professional cultures for implementation has not been recognized to the same extent as organizational culture, but there is research (e.g. Callen et al. 2009; Martinussen and Magnussen 2011) which shows that professional cultures in healthcare affect the success of the implementation of various practices and policies. There is also research that shows that specific healthcare settings (e.g. emergency departments) can have a particular culture that affects the behaviours of all professions working there (Kirk and Nilsen, 2016).

Social networks

Social networks is a concept that emerged in sociology in the 1960s. The concept refers to the relationship between individuals or other social actors (e.g. organizations and states). It was first put forward by the anthropologist Radcliffe Brown who believed that the informal connection between individuals is the essence of the meaning of social networks. A social network is a form of social organization based on a "network", that is the inter-connection between nodes (Li et al., 2021). Networks in terms of nodes and connections between them have been studied in many disciplines aside from sociology, including physics, biology and psychology. In sociological research on social networks, nodes are individuals and connections are relationships or flows of information between individuals (Cunningham et al., 2011).

Research on social networks is limited in implementation science, but several aspects of networking have been shown to be relevant for the dissemination of information and knowledge in healthcare. The density of the network is important for opportunities to implement changes in clinical practice. Research shows that physicians who are managers usually are part of networks with a higher density (i.e. "tighter") than the networks of nurses who are managers, suggesting that physicians who are managers have greater opportunities to support or counteract changes in clinical practice (West et al., 1999; West and Barron, 2005). The hierarchy of the network also affects the transfer of information. Nurses' networks tend to be more hierarchical than those of physicians (West et al., 1999; Creswick and Westbrook, 2007). Nurses who are managers have been shown to have more central roles in their networks than physicians who are managers (Creswick and Westbrook, 2007; Creswick et al., 2009).

Homophily

The concept of homophily provides an explanation for why individuals (e.g. healthcare practitioners) seek out and establish relationships with people who are in various respects reminiscent of themselves with regard to characteristics such as age, gender, education and profession. Similarity reduces the risk for conflict because partners who share goals and characteristics are more apt to agree than those who do not. Peer groups maintain cohesion and minimize internal strife through a de-selection process, wherein dissimilar individuals are excluded (Hafen et al., 2011). The realization that people tend to socialize with like-minded people is by no means new. Aristotle noted in his day that people "love those who are similar to themselves", and Plato observed that "similarity breeds friendship".

The concept has been applied in health services research although not in implementation science studies. Sociological research shows that homophily restricts individuals' social worlds by strongly influencing what information they receive, what attitudes and perceptions they develop, and which people they interact with (McPherson et al., 2001). Research focusing on healthcare has shown that homophily affects communication, so that healthcare practitioners predominantly seek advice from and discuss work-related issues with people from the same profession (Thunborg, 2004).

Social capital

Social capital is a complex multi-dimensional concept that has been studied in sociology, economics, political science and public health. The concept assumes that social relations are valuable resources, that is, social capital. In sociological research, social capital is used to understand how individuals can ensure access to information, knowledge and various abilities considered to be part of social capital (Frane and Roncevic, 2003). The origins of the concept can be traced to classical economists such as Adam Smith and John Stuart Mill, and sociologists such as Max Weber, who provided cultural explanations for economic phenomena. The concept came into the spotlight in the 1980s through sociologists Pierre Bourdieu, James Coleman and Robert Putman, and it has attracted a great deal of research since then (Bhandari and Yasunobu, 2009).

Healthcare research has shown the importance of social capital in the form of professional relationships that enable discussion and exchange of views with colleagues (Fattore et al., 2009; Mascia and Cicchetti, 2011). For example, research has pointed to the importance of trustworthy and experienced colleagues for social workers because many of their decisions are based on incomplete knowledge and less than clear-cut evidence even though the information may exist codified in research-based guidelines (Avby et al., 2015).

Community of practice

Community of practice is a social learning theory developed by Lave and Wenger (1991) that refers to learning at the group level. The theory has its roots in the psychology of socialization. Fundamental to the understanding of communities of practice is the social dimension of human development and learning, with pioneering work by psychologists Albert Bandura and Lev Vygotsky. The theory posits that learning is not primarily an individualistic process, but rather a process that takes place in social settings within a community of apprentices and more experienced workers (Phillips and Soltis, 2009). Participation in informal communities to solve problems can generate collective learning if there is a common purpose ("joint enterprise") and a common way of doing things ("shared repertoire"), which presupposes a shared commitment ("mutual engagement") to interact (Wenger, 1998).

The theory of community of practice has been applied in a wide range of fields, including health services, industry, business and education although not in implementation science. Healthcare is characterized by profession-led communities that usually have a strong internal cohesion but a more limited exchange with other groups or professions. These characteristics can make effective dissemination of information and knowledge in healthcare organizations more difficult (Fitzgerald and Dopson, 2005).

Routinization theory

Routines are collective phenomena, the repetitive, recognizable patterns of inter-dependent actions involving multiple participants, for example, a multi-professional team in a healthcare setting (Feldman, 2003). Routines enable coordination, solidify knowledge, reduce uncertainty and increase stability (Becker et al., 2005). Although often studied in organizational research as organizational routines, the concept does not necessarily belong to the organizational level because routines may exist with regard to particular tasks and apply to smaller groups or departments of an organization. Routines can be disrupted when participants in a routine start acting in a manner that is more individual than collective (Becker, 2004). There is some debate whether routines are predominantly habitual, characterized by nonconscious cognitive processes, or if they are the result of effortful, conscious processes (Becker, 2004). Rytterström et al. (2010) argue that nursing practice is guided largely by unquestioned routines that are rarely reflected upon. Potthoff et al. (2022) also maintain that organizational routines are predominantly nonconscious; that is, a form of a collective habitual behaviour.

From an implementation perspective, routinization theory suggests the importance of investigating existing healthcare routines that will be affected when a new evidence-based intervention is implemented. The degree to which a new intervention fits in with existing ingrained routines may be an important factor in explaining implementation success or failure. Most research on routines has been done in the commercial and manufacturing sectors. However, Greenhalgh (2008) argues that wider use of routinization theory would improve our understanding of the complexity of healthcare systems by focusing attention on what healthcare practitioners actually do rather than what they say they do.

Organizational-level theories and concepts

There is a wealth of theories and concepts that concern various organizational aspects, based on the premise that organizations influence the behaviours of individuals in these organizations, which makes the organization a relevant unit of analysis. The case has been made that these theories and concepts offer a highly relevant but largely untapped resource for implementation science (Birken et al., 2017; Leeman et al., 2019). This overview describes seven theories and concepts: organizational climate; organizational learning; learning organization; contingency theory; socio-technical theory; complexity theory; and institutional theory.

Organizational climate

Organizational culture is not to be confused with organizational climate (although this is very common). Research on organizational climate has a socio-psychological origin, which is also reflected in the methods used to study the phenomenon (i.e. mainly quantitative methods). In contrast, organizational culture is based on an anthropological research tradition, with a greater focus on qualitative methods. Organizational climate is usually described as a narrower and shallower concept than organizational culture (Bang, 1999). The term "organizational climate" was coined in 1939 by psychologist Kurt Lewin and his colleagues following a study of children's school clubs (Lewin, 1964). The concept came into use in the 1950s, but it was not until the 1970s that this research took off.

Organizational climate is the aggregate of the perceptions of individuals about their work environment, which makes it an important concept to understand work-related behaviours (James et al., 2008). Factors such as job satisfaction, organizational commitment and employee and organizational performance have been found to correspond with perceived organizational climate (Barth, 1974).

The concept of organizational climate has relevance for implementation science. Drawing on the concept, an implementation theory by Klein and Sorra (1996, p. 1060) defines implementation climate as "targeted employees' shared summary perceptions of the extent to which their use of a specific innovation is rewarded, supported and expected within an organization". The concept of organizational climate is also featured in some determinant frameworks, including CFIR (as implementation climate). However, organizational culture seems to be a slightly more common feature of these frameworks (Nilsen and Bernhardsson, 2019).

Organizational learning

Learning theories are mainly concerned with how individuals learn. The concept of organizational learning was first described in the 1960s by Cyert and March (1963), but it was not until the 1980s that the concept began to attract greater interest with the recognition that an organization is more than a collection of individuals. Thus, organizational learning is not simply the "sum" of individuals' learning. Employees in an organization may come and go, but an organization lives on because accumulated knowledge remains in the form of policies, work routines, rules, norms and values (Engeström, 2009). Definitions of organizational learning tend to emphasize that this learning leads to a change in organizational capacity in a broad sense (Kim, 1993).

The concept of organizational learning is given a slightly different meaning depending on the theoretical perspective. In behaviourism, this learning is considered a process that leaves formal traces in the organization; for example, revised guidelines, policies or rules. According to the cognitive tradition, organizational learning is seen as a process associated with changes in individuals' perception of their tasks and functions in the organization (Crossan et al., 1999). Viewed from a sociocultural perspective, organizational learning is qualitatively different from individual learning. According to this perspective, organizational learning is seen as "embedded in collective assumptions and systems of interpretation, routines, technologies and cultural practices" (Ellström, 2010, p. 48).

Organizational learning has not been studied much in implementation science. It is notable that organizational learning is not mentioned in any of the common process models or determinant frameworks in the field. Despite this, it seems obvious that achieving an evidence-based practice requires organizational learning to ascertain that the desirable behaviours are not restricted to just a few individuals in an organization. A study by

Dannapfel et al. (2014) explored how physiotherapists' learning through participation in a research project was transferred to colleagues for organizational learning.

Learning organization

Organizational learning is not to be confused with learning organization, a concept that became widespread in the 1990s, stimulated by Peter Senge's *The Fifth Discipline* (Senge, 1990). A learning organization is made up of employees skilled at creating, acquiring and transferring knowledge, and therefore able to adapt to unpredictable events or circumstances. Definitions of a learning organization reflect that this can be seen as a kind of ideal or goal, something organizations should strive to become. In this type of organization, employee learning is supported, enabling a continuous organizational renewal process (Ellström, 2010).

Informed by the learning organization concept, a learning health system was defined by the Institute of Medicine in 2007 as an organization with a culture of health system improvement where internal data are integrated with existing evidence and rapidly analysed, and thus transformed into knowledge and put into practice, and its effectiveness at closing practice gaps is evaluated (Nash et al., 2021). There has been increasing interest in the topic, but "implementation on a broad scale remains limited" (Menear et al., 2019).

Contingency theory

Contingency theory claims that there is no "best way" to structure work or an organization, to lead a company or to make decisions. Rather, the optimal course of action is contingent (i.e. dependent) on the internal and external situation. For example, the optimal way of structuring work will be contingent on characteristics of both the work being performed and the environment where the work is performed (Golembiewski, 1983; Otley, 2016). The theory posits that when uncertainty about a task is higher, unprogrammed means of coordination (e.g. transferring decision-making authority to frontline workers) will be a more effective way to carry out a task and when uncertainty is low, programmed means of coordination (e.g. rules, protocols, guidelines) will be more effective. Higher levels of inter-dependence (both within and between parts of an organization) will require greater investment in coordination. The greater the differentiation between departments, the more difficult it will be to coordinate (Schoonhoven, 1981). The theory was made popular by Fred Fiedler in his article "A contingency model of leadership effectiveness", which paved the way for further research on the topic (Fiedler, 1964).

The contingency theory has not been used in implementation science but its relevance has been pointed out by Birken et al. (2017), Leeman et al. (2019) and Birken et al. (2022). The theory suggests that implementation strategies should include assessment of uncertainty and inter-dependence related to the task and uncertainty in the task environment. For example, if the tasks involved in a new evidence-based intervention require inter-dependent interactions between departments in an organization, implementation strategies should strengthen coordination between departments, for example, by using implementation teams and local consensus discussions. The theory suggests the importance of using tailored implementation strategies adapted to both the characteristics of the work and the environment in which this work is carried out.

Socio-technical theory

Socio-technical theory takes a holistic system view of organizations, viewing social and technical subsystems as inter-related parts of one system. The theory posits that there are dynamic and mutual influences among two subsystems that are present in all organizations: the technical and the social (or human) subsystems (Mumford, 2006). These subsystems operate within a given environmental subsystem, which influences their function and interaction (Abbas and Michael, 2022). The socio-technical perspective originates from industry-based action research at the Tavistock Institute in London in the 1950s, led by Emery and Marek (1962) and Trist and Bamforth (1951). Their work deviated from the dominant technological paradigm at the time, favouring an approach that perceived people as a resource and encouraging a work environment that facilitated collaboration, commitment and risk-taking (Mumford, 2006). The theory is described with different labels, including socio-technical perspective and socio-technical analysis.

In terms of implementation science, the theory suggests that multi-level strategies targeting the three subsystems and their interaction and inter-dependency are required for successful implementation. The theory seems applicable in implementation science although it is not dissimilar to existing multi-level determinant frameworks such as CFIR and i-PARIHS. The use of socio-technical theory in implementation science has been promoted by Leeman et al. (2019) and others.

Complexity theory

Complexity theory focuses on understanding how change occurs in complex adaptive systems, which are systems that are made up of many inter-dependent, heterogeneous parts that interact in a nonlinear fashion. The system may be conceptualized as a unit within an organization, the organization as a whole and/or the wider inter-organizational system of which the organization is a part. Complexity theory emphasizes interactions and the accompanying feedback loops that constantly change systems (Waldrop, 1993; Plsek and Wilson, 2001).

Complexity theory and its associated concepts emerged in the 1990s across multiple disciplines, including physical, biological and social sciences. However, there is no one identifiable complexity theory, but rather several theories concerned with complex systems gathered under the banner of complexity science (Schneider and Somers, 2006). Complexity is an especially important concept in the study of organizations, organizational change and leadership; it can offer insights into how organizations adapt to their environments and cope with uncertainty (Lanham et al., 2013; Miller et al., 2019).

The relevance of complexity theory for implementation science was addressed by Braithwaite et al. (2018). Construing healthcare as a complex adaptive system, they argued that it is difficult to get evidence-based interventions into routine practice through a linear step-by-step implementation process. Rather, complexity science suggests that "the translation of evidence into new clinical or organizational practices does not unfold in a static and controlled environment awaiting the attention of top-down change agents; it takes place in settings comprised of diverse actors with varying levels of interest, capacity, and time, interacting in ways that are culturally deeply sedimented, and have often solidified" (Braithwaite et al., 2018, p. 7). The potential utility of harnessing complexity theory for implementation science has been suggested by Braithwaite et al. (2018), Leeman et al. (2019) and Birken et al. (2022). Complexity theory has been used in health services research to investigate the management, safety and organization of clinical services (e.g. McDaniel and Driebe, 2001; Bar-Yam et al., 2013).

Institutional theory

Institutional theory was introduced in the late 1970s by John Meyer and Brian Rowan to explore how organizations fit with, are related to and are shaped by their environments. The theory provides an answer to the question: why do organizations in a particular sector tend to look so similar? (Bill and Hardgrave, 1981). The theory has been applied in sociology and organizational research to investigate how structures in the form of (formal and informal) rules, norms, routines and schemes become established as authoritative guidelines for social behaviour, that is, individuals' behaviours that influence, or are influenced by, other individuals' behaviours (Scott, 2001; Hunt, 2007). An institution is an organization, establishment, foundation, society, or the like, devoted to the promotion of a particular cause, typically one of a public, educational or charitable character (Peters, 2000; Thornton et al., 2012).

The institutional environment can strongly influence the development of structures in an organization. Three types of pressures on the structures are described in institutional theory: coercive, mimetic and normative pressures. Coercive pressures are various influences from other organizations upon which an organization is dependent and expectations in the society within which the organization functions. Mimetic pressures are influences encouraging organizations to model their behaviour on other organizations in their field. Normative pressures are influences derived from members of an occupation or profession (e.g. physicians) defining the conditions of work (DiMaggio and Powell, 1983; Jensen et al., 2009; Novotná et al., 2012).

Institutional theory has not been applied in implementation science research, but its potential importance for the field has been proposed by Nilsen et al. (2013), Birken et al. (2017) and Leeman et al. (2019). The theory could be used for planning implementation strategies that account for existing or potential coercive, mimetic and normative pressures on the organization in which the implementation will be carried out. For example, coercive pressures may be augmented by specifying how an evidence-based intervention can assist an organization in meeting regulatory, reimbursing or accrediting body requirements. Mimetic pressures could be utilized by partnering with opinion-leading organizations to become early adopters and serve as models for other organizations in the field. Normative pressures may be taken into account by partnering with professional associations to support implementation.

Concluding remarks

This chapter provides an overview of theories and concepts that might be useful in implementation science, but does not claim to present a complete list. Rather, the purpose is to present a wide selection of theories and concepts to show different possibilities for researchers in implementation science. Less commonly used approaches in implementation science as well as approaches that have been used more frequently in the field are featured.

The theories and concepts presented in the chapter convey a systems perspective, meaning that implementation problems and solutions exist on several levels and that a holistic perspective is necessary for comprehending the entire phenomenon (Holmes et al., 2012).

This perspective is relevant in implementation science because there is broad agreement that an evidence-based intervention requires behaviours and behaviour changes that are influenced by multi-level determinants (Nilsen, 2020). Multi-level influences are evident in many determinant frameworks applied in the field although the relative emphasis on individual- versus collective-level determinants differs considerably among these theoretical approaches. For example, the individual-level constructs in the Theoretical Domains Framework are arguably its primary focus (12 of 14 domains, including motivation, goals and memory), although it also includes two domains at collective levels (environmental context and resources; social influences) (D'Lima et al., 2020). In contrast, CFIR features many more domains related to the inner and outer setting than domains representing the individual level (Damschroder et al., 2020).

Various group- and organizational-level concepts, such as culture, climate and leadership, are part of many determinant frameworks (Nilsen, 2015). However, empirical studies in the field are usually focused on individuals (e.g. clinicians) and their behaviours and/or behaviour changes. Moore and Evans (2017, p. 133) argue that collective-level theories and concepts are crucial because they address "deeper influences on behaviour" than individual-level theories and concepts, which focus more on "proximal surface influences" on behaviour. Arguably, implementation science has been more influenced by psychology than organizational theory or other disciplines that take a more collective approach to understanding practice change. There are also methodological challenges of conducting studies to capture the importance of collective levels. For example, professional or organizational culture depend partially on non-conscious cognitive processes and are largely "invisible" and difficult to grasp. Similar challenges likely exist with regard to studying abstract collective-level concepts such as institutional logics and routines to explain their influence on individuals' behaviours (Nilsen et al., 2022). Thus, despite the recognized importance of collective influences on implementation processes and outcomes, the field struggles somewhat to fully grasp and capture this in implementation science research and develop knowledge of use in achieving an evidence-based practice.

References

Abbas, R., Michael, K. (2022) Socio-technical theory: a review. In: Papagiannidis, S. (Ed.), *TheoryHub Book*. Pp. 64–80. Retrieved from https://open.ncl.ac.uk/theoryhub-book/ (accessed 28 July 2022).

Ajzen, I., Madden, T.J. (1986) Prediction of goal directed behaviour: attitudes, intentions and perceived behavioural control. *Journal of Experimental Social Psychology* 22, 453–474. https://doi.org/10.1016/0022-1031(86)90045-4.

Allen, K.-A. (2020) *The Psychology of Belonging*. Melbourne: Routledge. https://doi.org/10.4324/9780429327681

Alvesson, M. (2009) *Organisationskultur och ledning*. Malmö: Liber.

Avby, G., Nilsen, P., Ellström, P.-E. (2015) Knowledge use and learning in everyday social work practice: a study in child investigation work. *Child & Family Social Work* 22, 51–61. https://doi.org/10.1111/cfs.12227

Bandura, A. (1977). Self-efficacy: towards a unifying theory of behavioural change. *Psychological Review* 84, 191–215. https://doi.org/10.1037/0033-295X.84.2.191

Bang, H. (1999) *Organisationskultur*. Lund: Studentlitteratur.

Barth, R.T. (1974) Organizational commitment and identification of engineers as a function of organizational climate. *Relations Industrielles* 29, 185–199. https://doi.org/10.7202/028484ar

Bar-Yam Y, Bar-Yam S, Bertrand KZ, Cohen N, Gard-Murray AS, Harte HP, et al. (2013) A complexity science approach to healthcare costs and quality. In: Sturmberg, J., Martin, C. (Eds.),

Handbook of Systems and Complexity in Health. New York: Springer, pp. 855–877. https://doi.org/10.1007/978-1-4614-4998-0_48

Bass, B.M. (1985) *Leadership and Performance Beyond Expectations*. New York: Free Press.

Bass, B.M., Avolio, B.J. (1997) *Full Range Leadership Development Manual for the Multifactor Leadership Questionnaire*. Palo Alto, CA: Mindgarden.

Becker, M.C. (2004) Organizational routines: a review of the literature. *Industrial and Corporate Change* 13, 643–677. https://doi.org/10.1093/icc/dth026

Becker, M.C., Lazaric, N., Nelson, R.R., Winter, S.G. (2005) Applying organizational routines in understanding organizational change. *Industrial and Corporate Change* 14, 775–791. https://doi.org/10.1093/icc/dth071

Bhandari, H., Yasunobu, K. (2009) What is social capital? A comprehensive review of the concept. *Asian Journal of Social Science* 37, 480–510. https://doi.org/10.1163/156853109X436847

Bill, J.A., Hardgrave Jr., R.L. (1981) *Comparative Politics: The Quest for Theory*. Washington, DC: Bell & Howell, University Press of America.

Birken, S.A., Bunger, A.C., Powell, B.J., Turner, K., Clary, A.S., Klaman, S.L., et al. (2017) Organizational theory for dissemination and implementation research. *Implementation Science* 12, 62. https://doi.org/10.1186/s13012-017-0592-x

Birken, S.A., Ko, L.K., Wangen, M., Wagi, C.R., Bender, M., Nilsen, P., et al. (2022) Increasing access to organization theories for implementation science. *Frontiers in Health Services* 2, 891507. https://doi.org/10.3389/frhs.2022.891507

Braithwaite, J., Churruca, K., Long, J.C., Ellis, L.A., Herkes, J. (2018) When complexity science meets implementation science: a theoretical and empirical analysis of systems change. *BMC Medicine* 16, 63. https://doi.org/10.1186/s12916-018-1057-z

Burns, J.M. (1978) *Leadership*. New York: Harper and Row.

Callen, J., Braithwaite, J., Westbrook, J. (2009) The importance of medical and nursing sub-cultures in the implementation of clinical information systems. *Methods of Information in Medicine* 48, 196. https://doi.org/10.3414/ME9212

Cane, J., O'Connor, D., Michie, S. (2012) Validation of the theoretical domains framework for use in behaviour change and implementation research. *Implementation Science* 7, 37. https://doi.org/10.1186/1748-5908-7-37

Conner, M., Norman, P. (2015) Predicting and changing health behaviour: a social cognition approach. In: Conner, M., Norman, P. (Eds.), *Predicting and Changing Health Behaviour*. Maidenhead: McGraw-Hill Education, pp. 1–29.

Creswick, N., Westbrook, J.I. (2007) The medication advice-seeking network of staff in an Australian hospital renal ward. *Studies in Health Technology and Informatics* 130, 217–231.

Creswick, N., Westbrook, J.I., Braithwaite, J. (2009) Understanding communication networks in the emergency department. *BMC Health Services Research* 9, 247. https://doi.org/10.1186/1472-6963-9-247

Crossan, M.M., Lane, H.W., White, R.E. (1999) An organizational learning framework: from intuition to institution. *Academy of Management Review* 24, 522–537. https://doi.org/10.2307/259140

Culture University (2019) *Leadership, Humble Inquiry & the State of Culture Work – Edgar Schein*. Retrieved from www.humansynergistics.com/resources/culture-university/2014/03/10/leadership-humble-inquiry-the-state-of-culture-work---edgar-schein (accessed 15 April 2023).

Cunningham, T.R., Geller, S. (2012) A comprehensive approach to identifying intervention targets for patient-safety improvement in a hospital setting. *Journal of Organizational Behavior Management* 32, 194–220. https://doi.org/10.1080/01608061.2012.698114

Cunningham, F.C., Ranmuthugala, G., Plumb, J., Georgiou, A., Westbrook, J.I., Braithwaite, J. (2011) Health professional networks as a vector for improving healthcare quality and safety: a systematic review. *BMJ Quality and Safety* 21, 239–249. https://doi.org/10.1136/bmjqs-2011-000187

Cyert, R.M., March, J.G. (1963) *A Behavioural Theory of the Firm*. Englewood Cliffs, NJ: Prentice-Hall.

Damschroder, L.J., Reardon, C.M., Lowery, J.C. (2020) The consolidated framework for implementation research (CFIR). In: Nilsen, P., Birken, S.A. (Eds.), *Handbook on Implementation Science*. Cheltenham: Edward Elgar, pp. 88–113. https://doi.org/10.4337/9781788975995.00011

Danielsson, M., Nilsen, P., Rutberg, H., Carlfjord, S. (2018) The professional culture among physicians in Sweden: potential implications for patient safety. *BMC Health Services Research* 18: 543. https://doi.org/10.1186/s12913-018-3328-y

Dannapfel, P., Peolsson, A., Nilsen, P. (2014) A qualitative study of individual and organizational learning through physiotherapists' participation in a research project. *International Journal of Clinical Medicine* 5, 514–524. https://doi.org/10.4236/ijcm.2014.59071

Diener, L.H., McGee, H.M., Miguel, C.F. (2009) An integrated approach for conducting a behavioral systems analysis. *Journal of Organizational Behavior Management* 29, 108–135. https://doi.org/10.1080/01608060902874534

DiMaggio, P.J., Powell, W.W. (1983) The iron cage revisited: institutional isomorphism and collective rationality in organizational fields. *American Sociological Review* 48, 147–160. https://doi.org/10.2307/2095101

Dinibutun, S.R. (2020) Leadership: a comprehensive review of literature, research and theoretical framework. *Journal of Economics and Business* 3(1): 44–64. https://doi.org/10.31014/aior.1992.03.01.177

Djulbegovic, B., Hozo, I., Beckstead, J., Tsalatsanis, A., Pauker, S.G. (2012) Dual processing model of medical decision-making. *BMC Medical Informatics and Decision Making* 12, 94. https://doi.org/10.1186/1472-6947-12-94

D'Lima, D., Lorencatto, F., Michie, S. (2020) The behaviour change wheel approach. In: Nilsen, P., Birken, S.A. (Eds.), *Handbook on Implementation Science*. Cheltenham: Edward Elgar, pp. 168–214. https://doi.org/10.4337/9781788975995.00014

Ellström, P.E. (2001) Integrating learning and work: conceptual issues and critical conditions. *Human Resource Development Quarterly* 12, 421–435. https://doi.org/10.1002/hrdq.1006

Ellström, P.E. (2010) Organizational learning. *International Encyclopedia of Education* 1, 47–52. https://doi.org/10.1016/B978-0-08-044894-7.00006-3

Ellström, P.E., Fogelberg Eriksson, A., Kock, H. (2009) Traditioner inom ledarskapsforskningen. In: Ellström, P.E., Kock, H. (Eds.), *Mot ett förändrat ledarskap*. Lund: Studentlitteratur, pp. 17–46.

Emery, F.E., Marek, J. (1962) Some socio-technical aspects of automation. *Human Relations* 51, 17–25. https://doi.org/10.1177/001872676201500102

Engeström, Y. (2009) Expansive learning toward an activity-theoretical reconceptualization. In: Illeris, K. (Ed.), *Contemporary Theories of Learning*. Abingdon: Routledge, pp. 53–73.

Evans, J.S.B.T., Over, D.E. (1996) *Rationality and Reasoning*. Hove: Psychology Press.

Fattore, G., Frosini, F., Salvatore, D., Tozzi, V. (2009) Social network analysis in primary care: the impact of interactions on prescribing behaviour. *Health Policy* 92, 141–148. https://doi.org/10.1016/j.healthpol.2009.03.005

Feldman, M. (2003) A performative perspective on stability and change in organizational routines. *Industrial and Corporate Change* 12, 727–752. https://doi.org/10.1093/icc/12.4.727

Fiedler, F.E. (1964) A contingency model of leadership effectiveness. *Advances in Experimental Social Psychology* 1, 149–190. https://doi.org/10.1016/S0065-2601(08)60051-9

Fishbein, M., Ajzen, I. (1975) *Belief, Attitude, Intention, and Behaviour*. New York: John Wiley.

Fitzgerald, L., Dopson, S. (2005) Professional boundaries and the diffusion of innovation. In: Dopson, S., Fitzgerald, L. (Eds.), *Knowledge to Action?* pp. 104–131. Oxford: Oxford University Press. https://doi.org/10.1093/acprof:oso/9780199259014.003.0006

Frane, A., Roncevic, B. (2003) Social capital: recent debates and research trends. *Social Science Information* 42, 155–183. https://doi.org/10.1177/0539018403042002001

French, B., Thomas, L.H., Baker, P., Burton, C.R., Pennington, L., Roddam, H. (2009) What can management theories offer evidence-based practice? A comparative analysis of measurement tools for organizational context. *Implementation Science* 4, 28. https://doi.org/10.1186/1748-5908-4-28

Gardner, B. (2015) A review and analysis of the use of 'habit' in understanding, predicting and influencing health-related behaviour. *Health Psychology Review* 9, 277–295. https://doi.org/10.1080/17437199.2013.876238

Gill, R. (2011) *Theory and Practice of Leadership*. London: Sage Publications.

Godin, G., Bélanger-Gravel, A., Eccles, M., Grimshaw, J. (2008) Healthcare professionals' intentions and behaviours: A systematic review of studies based on social cognitive theories. *Implementation Science* 3, 36. https://doi.org/10.1186/1748-5908-3-36

Golembiewski, R.T. (1983) Professionalization, performance, and protectionism: a contingency view. *Public Productivity Review* 7, 251–268. https://doi.org/10.2307/3380328

Greenhalgh, T. (2008) Role of routines in collaborative work in healthcare organizations. *BMJ* 337, 1269–1271. https://doi.org/10.1136/bmj.a2448

Greenwald, A.G., Krieger, L.H. (2006) Implicit bias: scientific foundations. *California Law Review* 94, 945. https://doi.org/10.2307/20439056

Hafen, C.A., Laursen, B., Burk, W.J., Kerr, M., Stattin, H. (2011) Homophily in stable and unstable adolescent friendships: similarity breeds constancy. *Personality and Individual Differences* 51, 607–612. https://doi.org/10.1016/j.paid.2011.05.027

Hofstede, G, Hofstede, G.J., Minkov, M. (2010) *Cultures and Organizations*. New York: McGraw-Hill.

Holmes, B.J., Finegood, D.T., Riley, B.L., Best, A. (2012) Systems thinking in dissemination and implementation research. In: Brownson, R.C., Colditz, G.A., Proctor, E.K. (Eds.), *Dissemination and Implementation Research in Health*. New York: Oxford University Press, pp. 192–212. https://doi.org/10.1093/acprof:oso/9780199751877.003.0009

Hunt, M. (2007) *The Story of Psychology*. New York: Anchor Books.

Illeris, K. (2009) A comprehensive understanding of human learning. In: Illeris, K. (Ed.), *Contemporary Theories on Learning*. Abingdon: Routledge, pp. 7–20. https://doi.org/10.4324/9780203870426

Ingvarsson, S., Hasson, H., Augustsson, H., Nilsen, P., von Thiele Schwarz, U., Sandaker, I. (2022) Management strategies to de-implement low-value care – an applied behavior analysis. *Implementation Science Communications* 3, 69. https://doi.org/10.1186/s43058-022-00320-3

James, L.R., Choi, C.C., Ko, C.H.E., McNeil, P.K., Minton, M.K., Wright, M.A., et al. (2008) Organizational and psychological climate: a review of theory and research. *European Journal of Work and Organizational Psychology* 17, 5–32. https://doi.org/10.1080/13594320701662550

Jaques, E. (1951) *The Changing Culture of a Factory*. London: Tavistock Publications.

Jensen, T.B., Kjærgaard, A., Svejvig, P. (2009) Using institutional theory with sensemaking theory: a case study of information system implementation in healthcare. *Journal of Information Technology* 24, 343–353. https://doi.org/10.1057/jit.2009.11

Kahneman, D. (2011) *Thinking, Fast and Slow*. New York: Macmillan.

Kim, D.H. (1993) The link between individual and organizational learning. *Sloan Management Review* Fall, 37–50.

Kirk, J.W., Nilsen, P. (2016) Implementing evidence-based practices in an emergency department: contradictions exposed when prioritising a flow culture. *Journal of Clinical Nursing* 25, 555–565. https://doi.org/10.1111/jocn.13092

Klein, K.J., Sorra, J.S. (1996). The challenge of innovation implementation. *Academy of Management Review* 21, 1055–1080. https://doi.org/10.2307/259164

Lally, P., Van Jaarsveld, C.H.M., Potts, H.W.W., Wardle J. (2010). How are habits formed: modelling habit formation in the real world. *European Journal of Social Psychology* 40, 998–1009. https://doi.org/10.1002/ejsp.674

Lanham, H.J., Leykum, L.K., Taylor, B.S., McCannon, C.J., Lindberg, C., Lester, R.T. (2013) How complexity science can inform scale-up and spread in health care: understanding the role of self organization in variation across local contexts. *Social Science & Medicine* 93, 194–202. https://doi.org/10.1016/j.socscimed.2012.05.040

Last, B.S., Buttenheim, A.M., Timon, C.E., Mitra, N., Beidas, R.S. (2021) Systematic review of clinician-directed nudges in healthcare contexts. *BMJ Open* 11, e048801. https://doi.org/10.1136/bmjopen-2021-048801

Lave, J.C., Wenger, E. (1991) *Situated Learning: Legitimate Peripheral Participation*. New York: Cambridge University Press. https://doi.org/10.1017/CBO9780511815355

Leeman, J., Baquero, B., Bender, M., Choy-Brown, M., Ko, L.K., Nilsen, P., et al. (2019) Advancing the use of organization theory in implementation science. *Preventive Medicine* 139, 105832. https://doi.org/10.1016/j.ypmed.2019.105832

Lewin, K. (1964). *Field Theory in Social Change*. New York. Harper Torchbooks.

Li, N., Huang, Q., Ge, X., He, M., Cui, S., Huang, P., et al. (2021) A review of the research progress of social network structure. *Complexity* 2021, 6692210. https://doi.org/10.1155/2021/6692210

Luszczynska, A., Schwarzer, R. (2005) Social cognitive theory. In: Conner, M., Norman, P. (Eds.), *Predicting Health Behaviour*. Maidenhead: Open University Press, pp. 127–169.

Martinussen, P.E., Magnussen, J, (2011) Resisting market-inspired reform in healthcare: the role of professional subcultures in medicine. *Social Science & Medicine* 73, 193–200. https://doi.org/10.1016/j.socscimed.2011.04.025

Mascia, D., Cicchetti, A. (2011) Physician social capital and the reported adoption of evidence-based medicine: exploring the role of structural holes. *Social Science & Medicine* 72, 798–805. https://doi.org/10.1016/j.socscimed.2010.12.011

McDaniel, R.R., Driebe, D.J. (2001) Complexity science and health care management. In: Friedman, L.H., Goes, J., Savage, G.T. (Eds.), *Advances in Health Care Management*. Volume 2. Bingley: Emerald Group Publishing, pp. 11–36. https://doi.org/10.1016/S1474-8231(01)02021-3

McPherson, M., Smith-Lovin, L., Cook, J.M. (2001) Birds of a feather: homophily in social networks. *Annual Review of Sociology* 27, 415–444. https://doi.org/10.1146/annurev.soc.27.1.415

Menear, M., Blanchette, M.-A., Demers-Payette, O., Roy, D. (2019) A framework for value-creating learning health systems. *Health Research Policy and Systems* 17, 79. https://doi.org/10.1186/s12961-019-0477-3

Michie, S., Johnston, M., Abraham, C., Lawton, R., Parker, D., Walker, A., et al. (2005). Making psychological theory useful for implementing evidence based practice: a consensus approach. *Quality & Safety in Health Care* 14, 26–33. https://doi.org/10.1136/qshc.2004.011155

Miller, W.L., Rubinstein, E.B., Howard, J., Crabtree, B.F. (2019) Shifting implementation science theory to empower primary care practices. *Annals of Family Medicine* 17, 250–256. https://doi.org/10.1370/afm.2353

Moore, G.F., Evans, R.E. (2017) What theory, for whom and in which context? Reflections on the application of theory in the development and evaluation of complex population health interventions. *SSM – Population Health* 3, 132–135. https://doi.org/10.1016/j.ssmph.2016.12.005

Mumford, E. (2006) The story of socio-technical design: reflections on its successes, failures and potential. *Information Systems Journal* 164, 317–342. https://doi.org/10.1111/j.1365-2575.2006.00221.x

Nash, D.M., Bhimani, Z., Rayner, J., Zwarenstein, M. (2021) Learning health systems in primary care: a systematic scoping review. *BMC Family Practice* 22, 126. https://doi.org/10.1186/s12875-021-01483-z

Neal, D.T., Wood, W., Quinn, J.M. (2006) Habits – a repeat performance. *Current Directions in Psychological Science* 15, 198–202. https://doi.org/10.1111/j.1467-8721.2006.00435.x

Nilsen, P. (2015) Making sense of implementation theories, models and frameworks. *Implementation Science* 10, 53. https://doi.org/10.1186/s13012-015-0242-0

Nilsen, P. (2020) Overview of theories, models and frameworks in implementation science. In: Nilsen, P., Birken, S.A. (Eds.), *Handbook on Implementation Science*. Cheltenham: Edward Elgar, pp. 8–31. https://doi.org/10.4337/9781788975995.00008

Nilsen, P., Bernhardsson, S. (2019) Context matters in implementation science: a scoping review of determinant frameworks that describe contextual determinants for implementation outcomes. *BMC Health Services Research* 19, 189. https://doi.org/10.1186/s12913-019-4015-3

Nilsen, P., Roback, K., Broström, A., Ellström, P.E. (2012) Creatures of habit: accounting for the role of habit in implementation research on clinical behaviour change. *Implementation Science* 7, 53. https://doi.org/10.1186/1748-5908-7-53

Nilsen, P., Ståhl, C., Roback, K., Cairney, P. (2013) Never the twain shall meet? -a comparison of implementation science and policy implementation research. Implementation *Science* 8, 63. https://doi.org/10.1186/1748-5908-8-63

Nilsen, P., Neher, M., Ellström, P.E., Gardner, B. (2017). Implementation of evidence-based practice from a learning perspective, *Worldviews on Evidence-Based Nursing* 14, 192–199. https://doi.org/10.1111/wvn.12212

Nilsen, P., Birken, S.A., Potthoff, S. (2022) Conceptualizing four categories of behaviours: implications for implementation strategies to achieve behaviour change. *Frontiers in Health Services* 1, 795144. https://doi.org/10.3389/frhs.2021.795144

Norman, P., Conner, M. (2015) Predicting and changing health behaviour: future directions. In: Conner, M., Norman, P. (Eds.), *Predicting and Changing Health Behaviour*. Maidenhead: McGraw-Hill Education, pp. 390–430.

Novotná, G., Dobbins, M., Henderson, J. (2012) Institutionalization of evidence-informed practices in healthcare settings. *Implementation Science* 7, 112. https://doi.org/10.1186/1748-5908-7-112

Otley, D. (2016) The contingency theory of management accounting and control: 1980–2014. *Management Accounting Research* 31, 45–62. https://doi.org/10.1016/j.mar.2016.02.001

Peters, B.G. (2000) *Institutional Theory: Problems and Prospects*. Vienna: Institut für Höhere Studien (IHS). Retrieved from www.ssoar.info/ssoar/bitstream/handle/document/24657/ssoar-2000-peters-institutional_theory.pdf?sequence=1 (accessed 27 July 2022).

Phillips, D.C., Soltis, J.F. (2009) *Perspectives on Learning*. New York: Teachers College Press.

Plsek, P.E., Wilson, T. (2001) Complexity science: complexity, leadership, and management in healthcare organisations. *BMJ* 323, 746–749. https://doi.org/10.1136/bmj.323.7315.746

Potthoff, S., Kwasnicka, D., Avery, L., Finch, T., Gardner, B., Hankonen, N., et al. (2022) Changing health professionals' non-reflective processes to improve the quality of care. *Social Science & Medicine* 298, 114840. https://doi.org/10.1016/j.socscimed.2022.114840

Reichenpfader, U., Carlfjord, S., Nilsen, P. (2015) Leadership in evidence-based practice: a systematic review. *Leadership in Health Services* 28, 298–316. https://doi.org/10.1108/LHS-08-2014-0061

Rendle, K.A., Beidas, R.S. (2021) Four strategic areas to advance equitable implementation of evidence-based practices in cancer care. *Translational Behavioral Medicine* 11, 1980–1988. https://doi.org/10.1093/tbm/ibab105

Rochette, A., Korner-Bitensky, N., Thomas, A. (2009) Changing clinicians' habits: is this the hidden challenge to increasing best practices? *Disability and Rehabilitation* 31, 1790–1794. https://doi.org/10.1080/09638280902803773

Rytterström, P., Unosson, M., Arman, M. (2010) The significance of routines in nursing practice. *Journal of Clinical Nursing* 20, 3513–3522. https://doi.org/10.1111/j.1365-2702.2010.03522.x

Schein, E.H. (2008). *Organizational Culture and Leadership*. 3rd edition. San Francisco, CA: Jossey-Bass.

Schneider, M., Somers, M. (2006) Organizations as complex adaptive systems: Implications of Complexity Theory for leadership research. *Leadership Quarterly* 17, 351–365. https://doi.org/10.1016/j.leaqua.2006.04.006

Schoonhoven, C.B. (1981) Problems with contingency theory: testing assumptions hidden within the language of contingency "theory". *Administrative Science Quarterly* 26, 349–377. https://doi.org/10.2307/2392512

Scott, W.R. (2001) *Institutions and Organizations*. Thousand Oaks, CA: Sage.

Senge, P.M. (1990) *The Fifth Discipline: The Art and Practice of the Learning Organization*. London: Century Business.

Sladek, R.M., Phillips, P.A., Bond, M.J. (2006) Implementation science: a role for parallel dual processing models of reasoning? *Implementation Science* 1, 12. https://doi.org/10.1186/1748-5908-1-12

Sloman, SA (1996) The empirical case for two systems of reasoning. *Psychological Bulletin* 119, 3–22. https://doi.org/10.1037/0033-2909.119.1.3

Smircich, L. (1983) Concepts of culture and organizational analysis. *Administrative Science Quarterly* 28, 339–358. https://doi.org/10.2307/2392246

Stanovich, K.E., West, R.F. (2000) Individual differences in reasoning: implications for the rationality debate? *Behavioral and Brain Sciences* 23, 645–665. https://doi.org/10.1017/S0140525X00003435

Thornton, P.H., Ocasio, W., Lounsbury, M. (2012) *The Institutional Logics Perspective: A New Approach to Culture, Structure and Process*. Oxford: Oxford University Press. https://doi.org/10.1093/acprof:oso/9780199601936.001.0001

Thunborg, C. (2004) Yrkesidentiteter i rörelse. In: Ellström, P.-E., Hultman, G. (Eds.), *Lärande och förändring i organisationer*. Lund: Studentlitteratur, pp. 117–136.

Triandis, H.C. (1980) Values, attitudes, and interpersonal behaviour. In: Howe, H.E., Page, M.M. (Eds.), *Nebraska Symposium on Motivation, 1979: Attitudes, Values and Beliefs*. Lincoln, NB: University of Nebraska Press, pp. 195–259.

Trist, E.L., Bamforth, K.W. (1951) Some social and psychological consequences of the longwall method of coal-getting. *Human Relations* 41, 3–38. https://doi.org/10.1177/001872675100400101

Waldrop, M.M. (1993) *Complexity: The Emerging Science at the Edge of Order and Chaos*. New York: Simon and Schuster.

Walesh, S.G. (2017) *Introduction to Creativity and Innovation for Engineers*. London: Pearson Education.

Wenger, E. (1998) *Communities of Practice*. Cambridge: Cambridge University Press.

Wensing, M., Wollersheim, H., Grol, R. (2006) Organizational interventions to implement improvements in patient care: a structured review of reviews. *Implementation Science*, 1, 2. https://doi.org/10.1186/1748-5908-1-2

West, E., Barron, D.N. (2005) Social and geographical boundaries around senior nurse and physician leaders: an application of social network analysis. *Canadian Journal of Nursing Research* 37, 132–148.

West, E., Barron, D.N., Dowsett, J., Newton, J.N. (1999) Hierarchies and cliques in the social networks of health care professionals: Implications for the design of dissemination strategies. *Social Science & Medicine* 48, 633–646. https://doi.org/10.1016/S0277-9536(98)00361-X

Wilder, D.A., Austin, J., Casella, S. (2009) Applying behavior analysis in organizations: organizational behavior management. *Psychological Services* 6, 202–211. https://doi.org/10.1037/a0015393

Yano, E.M. (2008) The role of organizational research in implementing evidence-based practice: QUERI Series. *Implementation Science* 3, 29. https://doi.org/10.1186/1748-5908-3-29

Yukl, G. (2006) *Leadership in Organizations*. 6th edition. Upper Saddle River, NJ: Prentice Hall.

9 Implementation strategies and outcomes

Per Nilsen and Hanna Augustsson

Taxonomies of implementation strategies

Implementation strategies constitute the "how to" of integrating evidence-based interventions, programmes and other practices into routine use in healthcare and other settings. Implementation strategies have been defined as "methods or techniques used to enhance the adoption, implementation and sustainability of a clinical programme or practice" (Proctor et al., 2013). Another definition posits that an implementation strategy is "a systematic intervention process to adopt and integrate" evidence-based practices into usual care (Powell et al., 2012). Definitions of implementation strategies are typically analogous with those of interventions; in other words, they involve some sort of concerted effort, action or process to achieve desired outcomes.

The implementation science literature describes many different implementation strategies, from mailing printed material to healthcare professionals to complex, multi-faceted strategies targeting different levels of a healthcare organization. Strategies vary in their scale, their targets, the settings in which they are applied and the nature of the evidence-based practices they are intended to support. Multiple taxonomies exist that classify the different types of implementation strategies. Such taxonomies can facilitate understanding of the nature of specific strategies and enable synthesis and comparison of the evidence of the effectiveness of different strategies (Mazza et al., 2013).

Early taxonomies

Early taxonomies focused on strategies for changing physician behaviour. For example, a taxonomy by Davies et al. (1992) included education, reminder systems and audit and feedback, among other strategies intended to increase physicians' adherence to evidence-based guidelines. Oxman et al. (1995) broadened the scope to all healthcare professions and included ten categories of strategies:

- Educational materials: distribution of published or printed recommendations for clinical care, including clinical practice guidelines, audio-visual materials and electronic publications.
- Conferences: participation of healthcare providers in conferences, lectures, workshops or traineeships outside their practice settings.
- Outreach visits: use of a trained person who meets with providers in their practice setting to provide information.
- Local opinion leaders: use of providers explicitly nominated by their colleagues to be "educationally influential".

DOI: 10.4324/9781003318125-10

- Patient-mediated interventions: interventions aimed at changing the performance of healthcare providers for which information was sought from or given directly to patients by others, for example, direct mailings to patients, patient counselling delivered by others, or clinical information collected directly from patients and given to the provider.
- Audit and feedback: summaries of clinical performance of healthcare over a specified period, with or without recommendations for clinical action.
- Reminders: interventions (manual or computerized) that prompt the healthcare provider to perform a clinical action, for example, concurrent or inter-visit reminders to professionals about desired actions such as screening or other preventive services, enhanced laboratory reports or administrative support.
- Marketing: use of personal interviewing, group discussion or a survey of targeted providers to identify barriers to change and the subsequent design of an intervention.
- Local consensus processes: inclusion of participating providers in discussions to ensure agreement that the chosen clinical problem is important and the approach to managing it is appropriate.
- Multi-faceted interventions: any intervention that includes two or more of the last six interventions described here.

Effective Practice and Organisation of Care

Based on the Oxman et al. (1995) taxonomy, groups within the Cochrane Collaborative have proposed taxonomies that have moved beyond behaviour change to include strategies that target the levels of the healthcare setting and system and the wider regulatory environment. In 2011, Cochrane's Effective Practice and Organisation of Care (EPOC) review group developed a taxonomy that included four domains: professional strategies (e.g. educational meetings, reminders, audit and feedback); financial strategies (e.g. financial incentives); organizational strategies (e.g. multi-disciplinary teams, interventions to boost morale); and regulatory strategies (e.g. peer review, management of patient complaints) (EPOC, 2011).

The EPOC taxonomy was subsequently revised between 2013 and 2015 to address gaps identified in the taxonomy and to align the taxonomy with other taxonomies that were being used to classify "health systems interventions" in online databases. The 2015 EPOC taxonomy includes four overarching categories of health system interventions (EPOC, 2015):

- Delivery arrangements: changes in how, when and where healthcare is organized and delivered, and who delivers healthcare.
- Financial arrangements: changes in how funds are collected, insurance schemes, how services are purchased, and the use of targeted financial incentives or disincentives.
- Governance arrangements: rules or processes that affect how power is exercised, particularly with regard to authority, accountability, openness, participation, and coherence.
- Implementation strategies: interventions designed to bring about changes in healthcare organizations, the behaviour of healthcare professionals or the use of health services by healthcare recipients; they are divided into interventions targeted at healthcare organizations and/or healthcare workers and specific types of practice, conditions or settings.

Research Unit for Research Utilisation

In 2003, the Research Unit for Research Utilisation (RURU) in Scotland took a theory-informed approach by distinguishing between different strategy categories based on their underlying assumptions and hypothesized mechanisms of change (Walter et al., 2007). The RURU taxonomy was further developed by Nutley et al. (2007), who presented a taxonomy consisting of five categories of strategies:

- Dissemination: circulating or presenting research findings to potential users in formats that may be more or less tailored to their target audience.
- Interaction: developing stronger links and collaborations between the research and policy or practice communities.
- Social influence: relying on influential others, such as experts and peers, to inform individuals about research and to persuade them of its value.
- Facilitation: enabling the use of research through technical, financial, organizational and emotional support.
- Incentives and reinforcement: using rewards and other forms of control to reinforce appropriate behaviour.

Expert Recommendations for Implementing Change

Powell et al. (2012) reviewed the literature and proposed a consolidated list of 68 implementation strategies, which was then refined by the Expert Recommendations for Implementing Change (ERIC) project. ERIC drew on the initial review by generating expert consensus on a common nomenclature for implementation strategy terms, definitions and categories (Waltz et al., 2014). The ERIC project yielded a list of 73 discrete implementation strategies with the goal of providing a menu of implementation strategies that could be combined to target the multi-level determinants critical for integrating an intervention into routine practice (Powell et al., 2015). The strategies have been categorized into nine conceptually different groups (Waltz et al., 2015):

- Use evaluative and iterative strategies: assessing for readiness and identifying barriers and facilitators, auditing and providing feedback, and developing a formal implementation blueprint.
- Provide interactive assistance: facilitation, provision of local technical assistance and providing clinical supervision.
- Adapt and tailor to context: tailoring strategies, promoting adaptability and using data experts.
- Develop stakeholder inter-relationships: identifying and preparing champions, informing local opinion leaders and identifying early adopters.
- Train and educate stakeholders: conducting ongoing training, distribution of educational materials and creating a learning collaborative.
- Support clinicians and healthcare professionals: reminding clinicians, developing resource-sharing agreements and revising professional roles.
- Engage patients and service users: involving patients, consumers and family members and preparing patients and consumers to be active participants.
- Utilize financial strategies: altering incentive or allowance structures, using other payment schemes and developing disincentives.
- Change infrastructure: mandating change, creating or changing credentialing and/or licensure standards, and changing liability laws.

Tools for matching implementation determinants and strategies

Matching determinants with appropriate implementation strategies can be difficult. It is rarely obvious what strategies are appropriate for various determinants. If barriers to the implementation of a new intervention include a lack of knowledge and skills in using the intervention, it may be apparent that some form of training or education might be an appropriate strategy. But what strategies are relevant if the implementation of an intervention is hindered by management and leadership resistance to changes in current practice? Three tools have been proposed to facilitate this matching process:

- The Behaviour Change Wheel (BCW).
- Consolidated Framework for Implementation Research (CFIR)-Expert Recommendations for Implementing Change (ERIC) Strategy Matching Tool.
- The Integrated Theory-Based Framework for Intervention Tailoring Strategies (ItFits) Toolkit.

The Behaviour Change Wheel

The BCW is a tool for analysing determinants of behaviour change and matching them with potentially appropriate implementation strategies, referred to as intervention functions and policy categories. The tool provides "a systematic and theoretically guided method for identifying the types of interventions and supporting policies that would

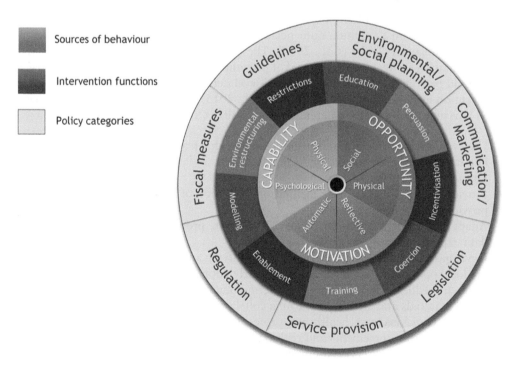

Figure 9.1 The Behaviour Change Wheel.

Source: Michie et al. (2014)

be expected to be effective for a given behaviour, context and target individual, group or population" (Michie et al., 2014, p. 110). BCW is premised on conducting a "behavioural diagnosis" of what needs to change using Capability Opportunity Motivation – Behaviour (COM-B) and/or the Theoretical Domains Framework (TDF). BCW is depicted as a wheel with the three components of COM-B at the hub encircled by intervention functions and policies to change behaviour (Figure 9.1) (Michie et al., 2011). A webpage provides information on the BCW, including COM-B and TDF (www.behaviourchangewheel.com).

After the behavioural diagnosis, the next step of BCW involves linking this diagnosis with intervention functions and policy categories (i.e. implementation strategies). Intervention functions are broad categories of ways in which interventions can change behaviour. Policy categories represent different types of decisions made by authorities that help to support and enact the strategies. BCW features nine intervention functions and seven policy categories. They were identified through a systematic literature review of 19 frameworks (Michie et al., 2011).

The BCW tool also provides information to facilitate the matching of determinants and interventions. A group of experts matched determinants (COM-B and/or TDF) and intervention functions in a consensus exercise. For each COM-B component or TDF domain, the intervention functions most likely to be effective in bringing about the desired change are described. BCW also provides information about what policy categories can support different intervention functions (Michie et al., 2011).

The next step in the BCW system is to identify which behaviour change techniques (BCTs) can deliver the identified intervention functions under the relevant policy options. It is important to identify precisely how the strategies will be delivered. Intervention functions are made up of smaller component BCTs, which are defined as active components of interventions designed to change behaviour. BCTs are observable, replicable and irreducible components of interventions designed to change behaviour. Examples of BCTs include "feedback on behaviour" and "instruction on how to perform the behaviour" (Michie et al., 2014).

Consolidated Framework for Implementation Research-Expert Recommendations for Implementing Change Strategy Matching Tool

The CFIR-ERIC Strategy Matching Tool (https://cfirguide.org/choosing-strategies/) is another tool that can match determinants and strategies. It matches implementation strategies from the ERIC compilation to contextual barriers from the CFIR. The tool consists of an Excel workbook that provides a list of strategies to consider based on the prioritized CFIR barriers that are entered.

The tool was developed based on rankings by 169 implementation experts regarding which implementation strategies they believed would best address each barrier. Participants were allowed to choose up to seven implementation strategies for each barrier. There was considerable heterogeneity in implementation strategies chosen by the participants, showing that there are few obvious relationships between CFIR-based barriers and ERIC implementation strategies (Waltz et al., 2019). Despite this, the tool provides a list of the highest-ranked strategies for each barrier and may help the process of considering which of the numerous implementation strategies could be most appropriate to address CFIR-based barriers.

The Integrated Theory-Based Framework for Intervention Tailoring Strategies toolkit

The Integrated Theory-Based Framework for Intervention Tailoring Strategies (ItFits) toolkit is an online tool to support tailored implementation (https://itfits-toolkit.com). It was developed as part of the ImpleMentAll study, which is a European collaboration to support effective implementation of eHealth interventions (ImpleMentAll, 2023). The ItFits toolkit is based on Normalization Process Theory and includes four modules:

- Identify: guidance on how to identify implementation goals and what the barriers are to achieve those goals and how to prioritize among goals and barriers.
- Match: guidance on how to match barriers with a range of potential implementation strategies that others have used previously to help overcome these barriers.
- Design: guidance on how to design the implementation strategies and how to adapt them to the needs of the people and organizations where the implementation takes place.
- Apply and review: guidance on how to apply the chosen implementation strategies and how to review their impact.

The ItFits toolkit has been evaluated in a stepped-wedge randomized trial where the effectiveness of implementation, measured as normalization, using the toolkit was compared with implementation-as-usual. Implementation guided by the ItFits toolkit showed higher normalization levels compared with usual implementation, but the effect was small (Vis et al., 2023).

Methods for matching implementation determinants and strategies

A few methods to map strategies to barriers and facilitators when implementing a particular evidence-based practice in a given setting have been described in the literature (Powell et al., 2017; Fernandez et al., 2019). Five methods are addressed here:

- Concept mapping.
- Group model building.
- Conjoint analysis.
- Intervention mapping.
- Implementation mapping.

Concept mapping

Concept mapping, also referred to as group concept mapping, is a mixed-methods participatory approach that aims to identify, organize and prioritize ideas or concepts related to a pre-defined problem or topic (Trochim and Kane, 2005). It is designed to be actionable, that is, the results can be used to guide action on the issue addressed by the concept mapping (Trochim and Kane, 2005). Concept mapping can help tailor implementation strategies, for example, by identifying important barriers to the implementation of a specific evidence-based practice in a given setting and by identifying implementation strategies that may be feasible and effective in addressing specific barriers (Powell et al., 2017).

The process of concept mapping typically involves engaging a group of stakeholders in a brainstorming session to generate a list of ideas or statements, which are individually sorted into categories and rated based on aspects such as their relative importance and feasibility. The brainstorming is centred around a focus prompt to which participants generate as many meaningful statements as possible. Examples of prompts related to tailoring implementation strategies could be "A potential barrier to implement this evidence-based intervention is . . ." or "A strategy to address this barrier to implementation of this evidence-based intervention is . . .". In the next step, stakeholders sort the statements into categories based on their similarities. This yields conceptually distinct categories of statements. Participants are asked to rank the statements based on different dimensions, for example, relative importance and feasibility. The data from the sorting are then analysed using multi-dimensional scaling and hierarchical cluster analysis. This results in maps that visually depict the views of the group and indicate the priorities of the group on the importance and feasibility of the categories.

An empirical example of the use of concept mapping to tailor implementation is presented in a study by Kwok et al. (2020). They used concept mapping to identify and choose strategies for improving the implementation of an evidence-based outcome measurement tool in paediatric speech-language pathology. The concept mapping yielded 14 prioritized implementation strategies to address identified barriers to implementation from the TDF.

Group model building

Group model building is a participatory method that involves stakeholders in identifying and proposing solutions to unstructured or wicked problems, that is, problems with many inter-dependent factors that make solving them seem impossible (Saryazdi et al., 2020). Group model building has developed to include a range of different formats. Powell et al. (2017) highlight one of the most used, the so-called reference group approach. This method involves a group of stakeholders with interest and expertise in the problem in a series of meetings. The discussions are led by a facilitator, but the process can also include other roles such as a gatekeeper, process coach, modelling coach and recorder (Saryazdi et al., 2020).

The reference group method features three steps. In the first step, the reference group articulates a problem statement. In relation to implementation, this may, for instance, be that an evidence-based intervention is not sufficiently integrated in practice. In the second step, model building is initiated. The reference group outlines factors that are relevant to the problem and the solution to the problem. For instance, important factors to include in the model may be training needs, resources, clinician confidence, time constraints and supervision. This information is then used to create a causal loop diagram (visualizes how different components of a system are causally inter-related) or a stock and flow diagram (visualizes a system's behaviour and how stocks and flows interact, where stocks are entities that can accumulate or be depleted and flows are entities that make stocks increase or decrease). In the third step, the group model-building team generates a mathematical formula to quantify specified parameters. The model is then used for simulation of the proposed solution (Powell et al., 2017).

Examples of how group model building can be used to match implementation determinants and strategies are scarce. Muttalib et al. (2021) used group model building to identify barriers and facilitators to acute care delivery in a resource-limited setting but did not map these to strategies. The results yielded causal maps that identified severe patient illness and a high volume of patients as strains on the system in several areas, including physical space, resource needs and utilization, staff capabilities and quality improvement. Stress in these areas resulted in worsening patient condition and negative reinforcing feedback loops.

Conjoint analysis

Conjoint analysis originates from marketing research and is a method to determine how consumers make decisions and what they value in products when making a purchase (Green et al., 2001). This method can also be used in implementation science research to assess stakeholders' preferences for a service, programme, implementation strategy, etc. The method is especially useful in situations where trade-offs must be made, for example, when implementation strategy X has more support than strategy Y, but strategy Y is less costly than strategy X (Powell et al., 2017).

There are different types of conjoint analysis (Orme, 2009) but all ask respondents to consider multiple attributes of a product and to rate, rank or select the products that they prefer. The first step is to define a set of attributes that are important; for example, factors that are important for the decisions to implement a specific evidence-based practice or strategies that can be used to implement a certain practice. The attributes can be determined using different methods such as literature reviews and interviews or focus groups with stakeholders involved in the issue (Bridges et al., 2011). Different combinations of attributes are presented to relevant stakeholders who are asked to rate their preference of each combination. For instance, stakeholders might be presented with multi-component implementation strategies with different sets of discrete strategies (e.g. educational materials, training, supervision, fidelity monitoring and reminders) and be asked to rate how likely they would be to use each strategy to implement a specific practice in a specified context. Next, a statistical analysis is conducted to quantify the impact score of each attribute in terms of its contribution to the stakeholder's decision.

Lewis et al. (2018) provide an example of how conjoint analysis can be carried out for matching implementation determinants and strategies. They used conjoint analysis to generate a strategy for implementing a cognitive behavioural therapy intervention in a youth residential centre. They prioritized identified barriers according to feasibility and importance, before selecting strategies from a published compilation and rating them for feasibility and likelihood of having an impact on the fidelity of the intervention. Another example of application is presented in a study by Cunningham et al. (2014) that used conjoint analysis to model factors influencing the decision of educators to adopt strategies for improving children's mental health outcomes. The results showed that educators preferred small-group workshops led by experts and strategies that focused on teaching skills applicable to all students (rather than only to students at risk).

Intervention mapping

Intervention mapping is a method to plan for the development, implementation and evaluation of interventions (Bartholomew et al., 2016). It was originally used for health promotion interventions, for example, concerning overweight and physical activity. The method involves identifying determinants for change and developing strategies to match those determinants. Intervention mapping consists of six steps (Bartholomew et al., 2016):

- Establish a comprehensive understanding of the health problem by means of a needs assessment or problem analysis.

- Create matrices of change objectives by combining performance objectives with determinants that should be targeted by the intervention to address the problem.
- Identify and select theory- and evidence-based interventions that can influence the determinants.
- Integrate the interventions into a coherent programme.
- Develop implementation strategies to support the adoption, implementation and sustainability of the programme.
- Plan process and outcome evaluations to assess the implementation and the efficacy or effectiveness of the intervention.

Although intervention mapping features a series of steps, the process is usually iterative rather than linear. Intervention mapping has been used in a few studies to develop implementation strategies. Examples include strategies for implementing clinical guidelines (Zwerver et al., 2011) and an intervention to increase adherence to mammography (Highfield et al., 2018).

Implementation mapping

Implementation mapping is a further development of the intervention mapping method (Fernandez et al., 2019). It expands on the fifth step of intervention mapping with the aim of guiding a systematic process for developing strategies for the adoption, implementation and maintenance of evidence-based practices. Thus, implementation mapping can be used instead of intervention mapping when an evidence-based practice already exists and should be implemented. Implementation mapping involves five steps (Fernandez et al., 2019):

- Conduct an implementation needs assessment and identify programme adopters and implementers.
- State adoption and implementation outcomes and performance objectives, identify determinants and create matrices of change objectives.
- Choose or design theory-based strategies to influence individual- and organization-level determinants.
- Produce implementation protocols, activities and/or materials.
- Evaluate implementation outcomes.

The five steps are iterative to ensure that all adopters, implementers, outcomes, determinants and objectives are addressed. Empirical examples of the application of implementation mapping are scarce so far.

Taxonomies of implementation outcomes

Implementation science distinguishes between the effectiveness of an implemented practice (e.g. an evidence-based treatment or programme) and the effectiveness of the implementation of this practice. An implemented practice will not be effective if it is not implemented well. Thus, favourable implementation outcomes constitute necessary preconditions for attaining the desired benefits of a treatment, programme or other evidence-based practice (Proctor et al., 2011). Implementation outcomes have been defined by Proctor et al. (2011) as "the effects of deliberate and purposive actions to implement new treatments, practices, and services". Two widely used taxonomies of implementation outcomes are described here.

Reach, Effectiveness, Adoption, Implementation and Maintenance

First described in 1999, the Reach, Effectiveness, Adoption, Implementation and Maintenance (RE-AIM) framework was developed for use in public health to enable broader evaluations of interventions that might be delivered to large numbers of people over longer periods (Glasgow et al., 1999). The framework was developed "to address the issue that the translation of scientific advances into practice, and especially into public health impact and policy, have been slow and inequitable" (Glasgow et al., 2019, p. 1).

The ultimate impact of an intervention is conceptualized as the combined effects of the five dimensions of RE-AIM (Figure 9.2). These dimensions operate at both the individual level and multiple ecological levels, most frequently at staff and setting levels in health systems although RE-AIM has also been applied at community and national levels (Holtrop et al., 2021):

- Reach (individual level): the absolute number, proportion and representativeness of individuals who are willing to participate in a given initiative, intervention or programme.
- Effectiveness (individual level): the impact of an intervention on important outcomes, including potential negative effects, quality of life and economic outcomes.
- Adoption (staff, setting, system, policy or other levels): the absolute number, proportion and representativeness of settings and intervention agents (people who deliver the programme) who are willing to initiate a programme.
- Implementation (staff, setting, system, policy or other levels): the intervention agents' fidelity to the various elements of an intervention's protocol, including consistency of delivery as intended and the time and cost of the intervention.
- Maintenance (both individual level and staff, setting, system, policy or other levels): at the individual level, maintenance is the long-term effects of a programme on outcomes after 6 or more months after the most recent intervention contact; at collective levels, maintenance is the extent to which a programme or policy becomes institutionalized or part of the routine organizational practices and policies.

RE-AIM has become a popular and broadly used framework. Holtrop et al. (2021) stated that it has been used in over 700 publications. It has proven to be flexible, having been used in a broad range of settings, populations and health issues across diverse clinical, community and corporate contexts, including policy and environmental change. The framework has evolved over time. It is not used just for evaluation purposes but also for planning implementation endeavours (Holtrop et al., 2021).

Proctor et al.'s (2011) taxonomy

The taxonomy by Proctor et al. (2011) was developed by a multi-disciplinary workgroup, which conducted a narrative review of implementation science research to identify concepts for labelling and assessing implementation outcomes. Through recurring meetings,

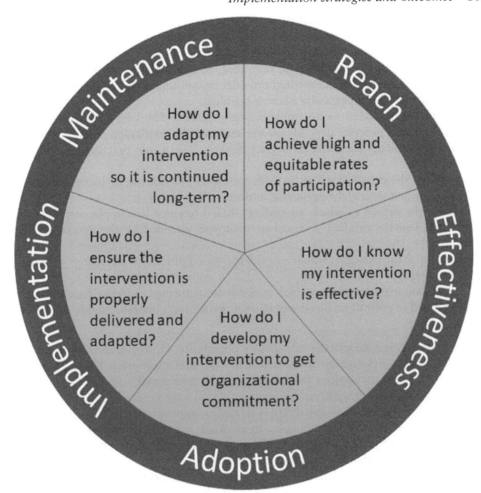

Figure 9.2 Reach, Effectiveness, Adoption, Implementation and Maintenance (RE-AIM).
Source: Glasgow et al. (1999, 2019)

team members engaged in discussions on the similarities and distinctions reflected in uses of the term "implementation outcomes". Identified constructs were assembled in a proposed heuristic taxonomy to portray the current state of vocabulary and conceptualization of terms used to assess implementation outcomes.

The resultant taxonomy includes eight constructs:

- Acceptability: the perception among implementation stakeholders that a given evidence-based practice (i.e. treatment, service, practice or innovation) is agreeable, palatable or satisfactory. The referent of acceptability (or the "what" is acceptable) may be a specific intervention, practice, technology or service within a particular setting of care. Acceptability should be viewed as a dynamic construct, subject to change with experience with the practice or implementation process.

- Adoption: the intention, initial decision, or action to use an evidence-based practice. Adoption also may be referred to as "uptake". Adoption may be studied from the perspective of individual providers or the organization.
- Appropriateness: the perceived fit, relevance, or compatibility of the evidence-based practice for a given practice setting, provider or consumer; and/or perceived fit of the practice to address a particular issue or problem.
- Cost: the cost related to an implementation effort. The cost of implementing an evidence-based practice depends on the costs of the particular practice, the implementation strategy used and the service delivery (e.g. a solo practitioner's office or a hospital).
- Feasibility: the extent to which an evidence-based practice can be successfully used or carried out within a given agency or setting.
- Fidelity: the degree to which an evidence-based practice was implemented as it was prescribed in the original protocol or as it was intended by the developers of the practice.
- Penetration: the extent to which an evidence-based practice is integrated within a service setting and its subsystems.
- Sustainability: the extent to which a newly implemented evidence-based practice is maintained or institutionalized within a service setting's ongoing, stable operations.

Appropriateness is conceptually similar to acceptability. However, the two concepts are distinguishable: a given intervention may be perceived as appropriate but not acceptable, and vice versa. For example, a treatment might be considered a good fit for treating a given condition, but its features (e.g. rigid protocol) may render it unacceptable to the provider. Similarly, although feasibility is related to appropriateness, the two constructs are conceptually distinct. For example, an evidence-based practice may be appropriate for a service setting in that it is compatible with the setting's mission but may not be feasible due to unmet resource or training requirements.

A systematic review by Khadjesari et al. (2020) of implementation outcome instruments to measure outcomes in accordance with the "Proctor taxonomy" identified 55 methodologically and psychometrically appraised instruments for evaluating the implementation of evidence-based practices in healthcare settings. Most of the included studies reported instruments that assessed acceptability ($n = 33$), followed by appropriateness ($n = 7$), adoption ($n = 4$), feasibility ($n = 4$), penetration ($n = 4$) and sustainability of evidence-based practice ($n = 3$). No studies of instruments measuring implementation cost were identified.

Concluding remarks

This chapter has described several taxonomies for categorizing different types of implementation strategies. Despite the smorgasbord of implementation strategies to choose from, evidence for the effectiveness of implementation strategies is weak. Reviews have consistently found that implementation strategies have modest effects overall, with substantial variations across studies (Grimshaw et al., 2012). Evidence to date suggests that passive dissemination has limited effects, and more active implementation strategies have, at best, small effects on adoption and implementation (Grol and Grimshaw, 2003). Oxman et al. (1995) noted that there are no "magic bullets" for the successful implementation of evidence-based practices into routine use; this conclusion is also valid today, 30 years later.

A common notion is that combining multiple strategies is more effective than a single strategy because more barriers can be addressed if several strategies are used. However, reviews have shown mixed effects of such strategies. Multi-faceted strategies are likely to be more resource-consuming and complex to deliver and sustain and may not lead to better outcomes than discrete implementation strategies or less complex multi-faceted strategies (Squires et al., 2014). It is possible that the effect of a multi-faceted strategy is attributed to one or a few of the included strategies and other components are not providing added effects. Furthermore, previous studies have provided limited guidance on the specific combinations of strategies that are most effective under which circumstances (Powell et al., 2019).

It is generally assumed that tailored implementation, that is, using implementation strategies that are specifically adapted to address specific determinants for implementation, has a higher chance of being effective. However, tailored implementation has shown variable effectiveness, and effects tend to be small to moderate (Baker et al., 2015). Some of the limitations concerning the lack of convincing effectiveness of implementation strategies may be due to poor matching of determinants and appropriate strategies. The results of a diagnostic analysis of barriers and facilitators should ideally "correspond as closely as possible" to the strategies that are chosen and enacted (Grol and Wensing, 2005, p. 123). However, this matching is often complex because there is "no reproducible, algorithmically operationalised process" for achieving this (Bhattacharyya et al., 2006). The matching process will likely be influenced by human judgement and numerous biases. However, it is important to conduct research concerning the matching tools and methods described in this chapter for improved understanding of how matching can be carried out for best possible results.

References

Baker, R., Camosso-Stefinovic, J., Gillies, C., Shaw, E.J., Cheater, F., Flottorp, S., et al. (2015) Tailored interventions to address determinants of practice. *Cochrane Database of Systematic Reviews* 29(4), CD005470. https://doi.org/10.1002/14651858.CD005470.pub3

Bartholomew, E.L.K., Markham, C.M., Ruiter, R.A.C., Fernandez, M.E., Kok, G., Parcel, G.S. (2016) *Planning Health Promotion Programs: An Intervention Mapping Approach*. San Francisco, CA: Jossey-Bass.

Bhattacharyya, O., Reeves, S., Garfinkel, S., Zwarenstein, M. (2006) Designing theoretically-informed implementation interventions: Fine in theory, but evidence of effectiveness in practice is needed. *Implementation Science* 1, 5. https://doi.org/10.1186/1748-5908-1-5

Bridges, J.F., Hauber, A.B., Marshall, D., Lloyd, A., Prosser, L.A., Regier, D.A., et al. (2011) Conjoint analysis applications in health—a checklist: a report of the ISPOR Good Research Practices for Conjoint Analysis Task Force. *Value Health* 14, 403–413. https://doi.org/10.1016/j.jval.2010.11.013

Cunningham, C.E., Barwick, M., Short, K., Chen, Y., Rimas, H., Ratcliffe, J., et al. (2014) Modeling the mental health practice change preferences of educators: a discrete-choice conjoint experiment. *School Mental Health* 6, 1–14. https://doi.org/10.1007/s12310-013-9110-8

Davies, D.A., Thomson, M.A., Oxman, A.D., Haynes, R.B. (1992) Evidence for the effectiveness of CME: a review of 50 randomized controlled trials. *Journal of the American Medical Association* 268, 1111–1117. https://doi.org/10.1001/jama.1992.03490090053014

EPOC (2011) *Data Collection Checklist*. Ontario: Institute of Population Health, University of Ottawa.

EPOC (2015). EPOC Taxonomy. Available from https://epoc.cochrane.org/epoc-taxonomy (accessed 15 July 2023).

Fernandez, M.E., Ten Hoor, G.A., van Lieshout, S., Rodriguez, S.A., Beidas, R.S., Parcel, G., et al. (2019) Implementation mapping: using intervention mapping to develop implementation strategies. *Frontiers in Public Health* 7, 158. https://doi.org/10.3389/fpubh.2019.00158

Glasgow, R.E., Vogt, T.M., Boles, S.M. (1999) Evaluating the public health impact of health promotion interventions: the RE-AIM framework. *American Journal of Public Health* 89, 1322–1327. https://doi.org/10.2105/AJPH.89.9.1322

Glasgow, R.E., Harden, S.M., Gaglio, B., Rabin, B., Smith, M.L., Porter, G.C., et al. (2019) RE-AIM planning and evaluation framework: adapting to new science and practice with a 20-year review. *Frontiers in Public Health* 7, 64. https://doi.org/10.3389/fpubh.2019.00064

Green, P.E., Krieger, A.M., Wind, Y. (2001) Thirty years of conjoint analysis: reflections and prospects. *Interfaces* 31, S56–S73. https://doi.org/10.1287/inte.31.4.56.9676

Grimshaw, J.M., Eccles, M.P., Lavis, J.N., Hill, S.J., Squires, J.E. (2012) Knowledge translation of research findings. *Implementation Science* 7, 50. https://doi.org/10.1186/1748-5908-7-50

Grol, R., Grimshaw, J. (2003) From best evidence to best practice: effective implementation of change in patients' care. *Lancet* 362, 1225–1230. https://doi.org/10.1016/S0140-6736(03)14546-1

Grol, R., Wensing, M. (2005) Selection of strategies. In: Grol, R., Wensing, M., Eccles, M. (Eds.), *Improving Patient Care: The Implementation of Change in Clinical Practice*. Edinburgh: Elsevier, pp. 122–134.

Highfield, L., Valerio, M.A., Fernandez, M.E., Eldridge-Bartholomew, L.K. (2018) Development of an implementation intervention using intervention mapping to increase mammography among low income women. *Frontiers in Public Health* 6, 300. https://doi.org/10.3389/fpubh.2018.00300

Holtrop, J.S., Estabrooks, P.A., Gaglio, B., Harden, S.M., Kessler, R.S., King, D.K., et al. (2021) Understanding and applying the RE-AIM framework: clarifications and resources. *Journal of Clinical and Translational Science* 5, e126. https://doi.org/10.1017/cts.2021.789

ImpleMentAll (2023). Getting eHealth implementation right. Retrieved from www.implementall.eu/ (accessed 4 July 2023).

Khadjesari, Z., Boufkhed, S., Vitoratou, S., Schatte, L., Ziemann, A., Daskalopoulou, C., et al. (2020) Implementation outcome instruments for use in physical healthcare settings: a systematic review. *Implementation Science* 15, 66. https://doi.org/10.1186/s13012-020-01027-6

Kwok, E.Y.L., Moodie, S.T.F., Cunningham, B.J., Oram Cardy, J.E. (2020) Selecting and tailoring implementation interventions: a concept mapping approach. *BMC Health Services Research* 20, 385. https://doi.org/10.1186/s12913-020-05270-x

Lewis, C.C., Scott, K., Marriott, B.R. (2018) A methodology for generating a tailored implementation blueprint: an exemplar from a youth residential setting. *Implementation Science* 13, 68. https://doi.org/10.1186/s13012-018-0761-6

Mazza, D., Bairstow, P., Buchan, H., Chakraborty, S.P., Van Hecke, O., Grech, C., et al. (2013) Refining a taxonomy for guideline implementation: results of an exercise in abstract classification. *Implementation Science* 8, 32. https://doi.org/10.1186/1748-5908-8-32

Michie, S., van Stralen, M.M., West, R. (2011) The behaviour change wheel: a new method for characterising and designing behaviour change interventions. *Implementation Science* 6, 42. https://doi.org/10.1186/1748-5908-6-42

Michie, S., Atkins, L., West, R. (2014) *The Behaviour Change Wheel: A Guide to Designing Interventions*. London: Silverback Publishing.

Muttalib, F., Ballard, E., Langton, J., Malone, S., Fonseca, Y., Hansmann, A., et al. (2021) Application of systems dynamics and group model building to identify barriers and facilitators to acute care delivery in a resource limited setting. *BMC Health Services Research* 21, 26. https://doi.org/10.1186/s12913-020-06014-7

Nutley, S.M., Walter, I., Davies, H.T.O. (2007) *Using Evidence: How Research Can Inform Public Services*. Bristol: The Policy Press. https://doi.org/10.56687/9781847422323

Orme, B.K. (2009) Which Conjoint Method Should I Use? Washington: Sawtooth Software, pp. 1–7.

Oxman, A.D., Thomson, M.A., Davis, D.A., Haynes, R.B. (1995) No magic bullets: a systematic review of 102 trials of interventions to improve professional practice. *Canadian Medical Association Journal* 153, 1423–1431.

Powell, B.J., McMillen, J.C., Proctor, E.K., Carpenter, C.R., Griffey, R.T., Bunger, A.C., et al. (2012) A compilation of strategies for implementing clinical innovations in health and mental health. *Medical Care Research and Review* 69, 123–157. https://doi.org/10.1177/1077558711430690

Powell, B.J., Waltz, T.J., Chinman, M.J., Damschroder, L.J., Smith, J.L., Matthieu, M.M., et al. (2015) A refined compilation of implementation strategies: results from the Expert Recommendations for Implementing Change (ERIC) project. *Implementation Science* 10, 21. https://doi.org/10.1186/s13012-015-0209-1

Powell, B.J., Beidas, R.S., Lewis, C.C., Aarons, G.A., McMillen, J.C., Proctor, E.K., et al. (2017) Methods to improve the selection and tailoring of implementation strategies. *Journal of Behavioral Health Services & Research* 44, 177–194. https://doi.org/10.1007/s11414-015-9475-6

Powell, B.J., Fernandez, M.E., Williams, N.J., Aarons, G.A., Beidas, R.S., Lewis, C.C., et al. (2019) Enhancing the impact of implementation strategies in healthcare: a research agenda. *Frontiers in Public Health* 7, 3. https://doi.org/10.3389/fpubh.2019.00003

Proctor, E., Silmere, H., Raghavan, R., Hovmand, P., Aarons, G., Bunger, A., et al. (2011) Outcomes for implementation research: conceptual distinctions, measurement challenges, and research agenda. *Administration and Policy in Mental Health* 38, 65–76. https://doi.org/10.1007/s10488-010-0319-7

Proctor, E.K., Powell, B.J., McMillen, J.C. (2013) Implementation strategies: recommendations for specifying and reporting. *Implementation Science* 8, 139. https://doi.org/10.1186/1748-5908-8-139

Saryazdi, A.H.G., Ghatari, A.R., Mashayekhi, A.N., Hassanzadeh, A. (2020) Group model building: a systematic review of the literature. *Journal of Business School* 3, 98–136. https://doi.org/10.26677/TR1010.2021.631

Squires, J.E., Sullivan, K., Eccles, M.P., Worswick, J., Grimshaw, J.M. (2014) Are multifaceted interventions more effective than single-component interventions in changing health-care professionals' behaviours? An overview of systematic reviews. *Implementation Science* 9, 152. https://doi.org/10.1186/s13012-014-0152-6

Trochim, W., Kane, M. (2005) Concept mapping: an introduction to structured conceptualization in health care. *International Journal for Quality in Health Care* 17, 187–191. https://doi.org/10.1093/intqhc/mzi038

Vis, C., Schuurmans, J., Aouizerate, B., Atipei Craggs, M., Batterham, P., Bührmann, L., et al. (2023) Effectiveness of self-guided tailored implementation strategies in integrating and embedding internet-based cognitive behavioral therapy in routine mental health care: results of a multi-center stepped-wedge cluster randomized trial. *Journal of Medical Internet Research* 25, e41532. https://doi.org/10.2196/41532

Walter, I., Nutley, S.M., Davies, H.T.O. (2007) *Using Evidence: How Research Can Inform Public Services*. Bristol: Policy Press. https://doi.org/10.56687/9781847422323

Waltz, T.J., Powell, B.J., Chinman, M.J., Smith, J.L., Matthieu, M.M., Proctor, E.K., et al. (2014) Expert recommendations for implementing change (ERIC): protocol for a mixed methods study. *Implementation Science* 9, 39. https://doi.org/10.1186/1748-5908-9-39

Waltz, T.J., Powell, B.J., Matthieu, M.M., Damschroder, L.J., Chinman, M.J., Smith, J.L., et al. (2015) Use of concept mapping to characterize relationships among implementation strategies and assess their feasibility and importance: results from the Expert Recommendations for Implementing Change (ERIC) study. *Implementation Science*, 10, 109. https://doi.org/10.1186/s13012-015-0295-0

Waltz, T.J., Powell, B.J., Fernández, M.E., Abadie, B., Damschroder, L.J. (2019) Choosing implementation strategies to address contextual barriers: diversity in recommendations and future directions. *Implementation Science* 14, 42. https://doi.org/10.1186/s13012-019-0892-4

Zwerver, F., Schellart, A.J., Anema, J.R., Rammeloo, K.C., van der Beek, A.J. (2011) Intervention mapping for the development of a strategy to implement the insurance medicine guidelines for depression. *BMC Public Health* 11, 9. https://doi.org/10.1186/1471-2458-11-9

10 Causal pathway diagrams to understand how implementation strategies work

Rosemary D. Meza, Predrag Klasnja, Cara C. Lewis, Michael D. Pullmann, Kayne D. Mettert, Rene Hawkes, Lorella Palazzo and Bryan J. Weiner

Introduction

Over the past two decades, numerous implementation strategies have been developed to target the determinants of implementation. There has been progress in consolidating, defining and organizing these implementation strategies (Powell et al., 2012, 2015; Waltz et al., 2015); however, little concerted effort has been made to articulate and evaluate how implementation strategies work (Williams, 2016). Consequently, the field lacks the precision in knowledge to answer questions such as "Which implementation strategies are equipped to address which determinants?" or "Under what conditions will this implementation strategy work?" By establishing causal accounts of implementation strategy functioning, the field can accumulate practical knowledge to guide evidence-based selection of implementation strategies equipped to address influential determinants that can be successful in the contexts in which they are deployed. Answering these questions will require exploration of the causal processes through which implementation strategies operate (specifically, their mechanisms of action) and the factors that influence how well a strategy works in different contexts. What is needed, in other words, is that we develop and test theories of strategy operation. Yet, theorizing about implementation strategy functioning occurs infrequently.

Theories and frameworks bring clarity to complex systems within which implementation occurs (Damschroder, 2020) and provide a testable way of explaining phenomena by specifying relationships among variables and enabling prediction of outcomes (Glanz and Bishop, 2010). Thus, they support efficiency in generalizing knowledge across contexts (Foy et al., 2011). By specifying the causal relationships between variables, researchers can evaluate whether implementation strategies operate according to expected mechanisms, how contextual factors affect the causal processes involved in implementation strategies, and how much variation in outcomes is accounted for by those mechanisms. Over time, utilizing causal models can serve a dual purpose of contributing to the development of more robust theories of implementation processes and improving implementation practice by tackling practical implementation issues. For instance, the use of causal models can (1) help create improved implementation strategies, (2) enhance the effectiveness of existing strategies, and (3) prioritize which strategies to use in which contexts. Causal pathway diagrams (CPDs) are a tool for structuring the process of theorizing about the causal mechanisms behind implementation strategies.

Causal pathway diagrams as a tool for theorizing

CPDs are box-and-arrow graphical representations that provide a structure for articulating the causal theory of how implementation strategies are hypothesized to work. They

DOI: 10.4324/9781003318125-11

are based on the statistical literature on path analysis (Stage et al., 2004), structural equation modelling (Hoyle, 1995; Bowen and Guo, 2011) and causal inference (Pearl, 1998, 2009), which use path diagrams and directed acyclic graphs to depict and estimate causal relationships that underpin observable phenomena and measurements. CPDs expand upon existing visualization tools by making the role that each element plays in the causal chain represented in the diagram explicit. In implementation science, CPDs provide a structure through which researchers can articulate, based on existing theory and empirical evidence, the chain of events through which an implementation strategy is expected to have an impact on an implementation outcome and the factors (effect modifiers) that can impede or facilitate the strategy's operation.

CPDs can be created with varying degrees of abstraction, which has implications for their generalizability and their utility for different audiences. At lower levels of abstraction, implementers can use CPDs to articulate how a concretely operationalized implementation strategy is expected to work under well-defined conditions in which it is being implemented. A CPD of this type might describe how clinical supervision, involving case review, symptom and fidelity monitoring, and role play, provided for 1 hour per week to mental health clinicians working in community mental health clinics would influence clinicians' fidelity to delivering cognitive behavioural therapy. The product of this kind of application of a CPD is more akin to a programme theory, or "small theory", that articulates a concrete theory of change that is practical and highly embedded within a particular context (Davidoff et al., 2015). This type of CPD may draw on existing theory (e.g. implementers may draw on the tandem model of supervision to articulate putative mechanisms of supervision) (Milne and Dunkerley, 2010) and empirical evidence, but might also draw heavily on the personal experience of stakeholders in the setting (Dixon-Woods, 2014). Their limited abstraction and high degree of contextual embeddedness make them practical but limit their generalizability to other contexts and different operationalizations of an implementation strategy.

At higher levels of abstraction, CPDs can be used to develop middle-range theories, which offer explanations that are both practical and applicable to various contexts, and provide focused propositions that can be tested and used to guide empirical investigations (Merton, 1968; Weick, 1989). In such theorizing using CPDs, implementation strategies may be broadly defined to capture their core activities without concretely operationalizing their deployment, the implementation object (e.g. clinical intervention) may be undefined and the context only loosely defined to provide a more generalizable account of how implementation strategies operate. Although benefiting from a higher degree of generalizability, theories developed in this way require further contextualization when applying them to a specific deployment of an implementation strategy. Both programme and middle-range theories can contribute to advancing implementation science (Kislov et al., 2019). This chapter focuses on the application of CPDs to developing middle-range theories that can produce testable propositions about how implementation strategies work in their general form.

Elements of causal pathway diagrams

A basic CPD consists of two parts: (1) the "stem" (the central part of Figure 10.1), describing the main causal process through which an implementation strategy operates, and

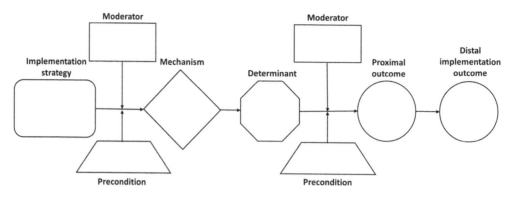

Figure 10.1 Causal pathway diagram.

(2) "leaves" (top and bottom boxes of Figure 10.1), which represent "effect modifiers", that is, factors that influence whether, and to what extent, the process represented by the stem unfolds successfully. Specification of elements in a CPD for a middle-range theory should prioritize existing relevant theory and empirical evidence that spans contexts and implementation objects. Because of the limited theoretical and empirical literature focused on how implementation strategies work, the development of such CPDs will also require scientists to engage in novel theorizing. As with all theories, but especially when engaging in novel theorizing, the resulting propositions will need to be treated as tentative and refined with the accumulation of evidence.

CPD stem

The stem visually represents the intended sequence of the impacts of an implementation strategy. It begins, on the left, with the name of the strategy, and ends, on the right, with the distal implementation outcome that the strategy is intended to achieve. The stem will typically consist of the following elements (Table 10.1).

Table 10.1 Causal pathway diagram: terms and definitions.

Term	Definition
Implementation strategy component	Methods used to improve the adoption, fidelity, or sustained use of an evidence-based treatment, practice or service
Mechanism	The process through which an implementation strategy operates to affect an implementation outcome
Determinant	Commonly referred to as barriers or facilitators, a factor that has an enabling or hindering influence on an implementation outcome; determinants are often the targets that implementation strategies are intended to affect
Proximal outcome	The most immediate, observable outcome of an implementation strategy
Distal implementation outcome	The downstream implementation outcome that the implementation strategy is ultimately intended to achieve
Precondition	A factor that is necessary for an implementation strategy to exert its influence on an implementation outcome
Moderator	A factor that can strengthen or weaken the influence of an implementation strategy

Implementation strategy: CPDs can describe the functioning of a discrete implementation strategy, such as distributing educational materials, or a complex multifaceted implementation strategy, such as a learning collaborative. In the development of a theory, the implementation strategy should be defined in terms of its core components. Those components may not be immediately clear due to the lack of empirical evidence of which components are core to an implementation strategy's effectiveness. In the absence of evidence, a key part of theorizing will involve identifying components that are both common (i.e., those commonly found across different operationalizations of a strategy) and that are believed to be responsible for the strategy's function. Aspects of a strategy that appear to be present to address circumstances specific to a particular context (i.e., the adaptable periphery) should not be included in a general theory of the strategy.

Mechanism: This is the process through which a strategy is thought to impact the determinant it is intended to address. It describes how and why a strategy works. Rather than simply reflecting a construct, mechanisms should describe a process that may consist of multiple steps that explain the causal process. Implementation strategies may work through a single or multiple mechanisms. Determining potential mechanisms through which a strategy works is *the* central task of theory development we are describing in this chapter.

Determinant: This is a barrier that impedes the desired implementation outcome or facilitator that enables successful implementation. While an implementation strategy may be poised to address multiple determinants, theories should include those that are most directly and plausibly addressed by the strategy. If a strategy is poised to resolve multiple determinants, CPDs can represent the causal paths through which each of those determinants might be addressed by that strategy, as each process may involve a different mechanism and contain distinct preconditions or moderators.

Proximal outcomes: These represent measurable impacts that, if the strategy is operating as intended, will occur before a more distal implementation outcome. Proximal outcomes (Brenner, Curbow and Legro, 1995; Javdani and Allen, 2011) are a sequence of observable effects through which the strategy impacts implementation outcomes, meaning they mediate the impact of the strategy on the distal implementation outcome. Articulating proximal outcomes can support the field's understanding of early indicators of implementation strategy success and the development of measurement approaches that can facilitate early diagnosis of strategy success.

Distal implementation outcome: This refers to the global intended effect of an implementation strategy. While implementation strategies are intended to have downstream effects on health outcomes, implementation strategies in and of themselves are not sufficient to bring about change in health outcomes and therefore are not centered in the causal pathway. Instead, CPDs typically end with implementation outcomes (e.g., fidelity or adoption) that can more directly be achieved by the implementation strategy being theorized. Similarly, CPDs only include implementation outcomes that the implementation strategy can plausibly bring about without the necessity of additional implementation strategies. For instance, while training can exert influence on adoption, it is unlikely to ensure the sustained use of a practice without additional implementation strategies.

CPD leaves

The CPD leaves represent contextual factors that facilitate or impede a strategy's operation. We describe two types of effect modifiers: preconditions and moderators. The positioning of preconditions and moderators is not fixed. That is, both preconditions and moderators may exert their influence on the relationship between any two elements in the stem. For instance, a moderator may strengthen or weaken the relationship between an implementation strategy and its mechanism or a proximal and distal outcome.

Preconditions: These are factors that must be present for a part of the strategy's causal process to take place but might not be (Mackie, 1965). Similar to the all-or-nothing effect of flipping a light switch, if preconditions are not present (i.e. the light switch is off), preconditions block the strategy from having any effect. When present (i.e. the light switch is on), they allow for the strategy to function unimpeded. Although any given implementation strategy may have many preconditions, only those that plausibly might not be present should be included.

Moderators: Moderators refer to factors that can either facilitate or impede the functioning of an implementation strategy. In contrast to preconditions, moderators function like a dimmer switch, which can produce brighter or dimmer light, depending on the position of the dimmer. For instance, if trust positively moderates the relationship between providing clinical supervision (implementation strategy) and experiential learning (mechanism), then as trust increases (i.e. the position of the dimmer is turned up), the effect of clinical supervision on experiential learning will also increase and vice versa. The identification of moderators points to conditions under which strategies will work better or worse.

Using causal pathway diagrams to develop theories of implementation strategy functioning

To advance the field's ability to understand how and under what conditions implementation strategies work, our team is developing middle-range theories for 30 of the most used implementation strategies (Lewis et al., 2022). Here, we describe the process and products for two of those implementation strategies: practice facilitation and innovation championing.

To develop the CPDs, we reviewed conceptual articles, systematic reviews and empirical articles for statements about (a) the purpose or goal of the strategy, useful for identifying the distal outcome that could be attained; (b) the rationale for the strategy, useful for identifying the determinant (barrier) the strategy could be deployed to overcome; (c) the contextual factors that influence whether or not, or how well, the strategy works; and (d) any clues about the strategy's plausible mechanism(s) and proximal outcomes. In addition, we noted variations in how the strategies were defined and operationalized, common strategy activities that might constitute core components, and any theories mentioned in relation to the strategy.

In the process of developing these CPDs, we sought to:

- Balance the specificity and generality of the descriptions of the strategy, mechanism(s), and barrier(s).
- Clarify the causal logic of the proposed mechanism(s) and consider any theoretical support for that logic.
- Differentiate the proposed mechanism(s) from both the barrier(s) the strategy addresses and the strategy's core components to eliminate tautologies.
- Identify the boundary conditions governing the appropriateness and feasibility of strategy deployment.
- Consider the length of the causal chain to ascertain whether the strategy, in isolation, could realistically produce an implementation outcome as a distal outcome.

A theory of how practice facilitation operates to influence implementation

Practice facilitation refers to "a process of interactive problem solving and support that occurs in a context of a recognized need for improvement and a supportive inter-personal relationship". Practice facilitators engage in various activities to help primary care practices implement the best evidence to improve the quality of care and develop quality improvement capacity. The core activity of practice facilitation, in our view, is quality improvement (QI). Informed by the literature on practice facilitation, we have developed an initial theory of how practice facilitation functions, depicted in the CPD shown in Figure 10.2.

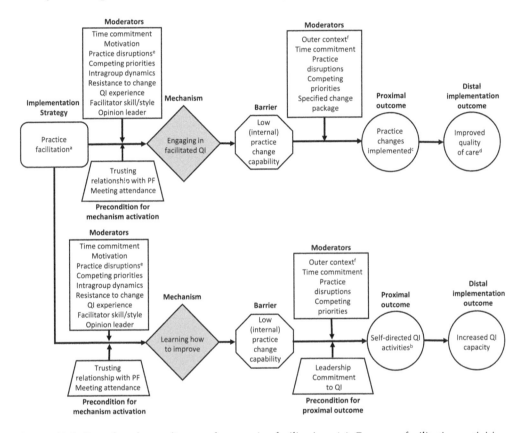

Figure 10.2 Causal pathway diagram for practice facilitation. (a) Common facilitation activities: assess performance/barriers/readiness, support development of a QI plan, help the practice establish a QI team, help practices map and redesign the workflow, train practices in QI methods, assist practices in using methods such as PDSA cycles, help practices develop performance monitoring systems. (b) QI activities are those mentioned as common facilitation activities. This is not circular because the facilitator trains, guides, encourages, etc. ("helps them do it"). (c) Practice changes refer to substantive organizational and behavioural changes that support improved quality (e.g. use of ASCVD calculators, ask-advise-refer, changes to EHR, group visits, collaborative care model, etc.). (d) Improved quality of care can be conceptualized/measured as service penetration (percentage of eligible patients receiving EBIs). (e) Practice disruptions include staff/clinician turnover, new IT systems, ownership changes, etc. (f) Outer context: supportive payment systems, quality initiatives/reporting. ASCVD, atherosclerotic cardiovascular disease; EBI, evidence-based intervention; EHR, electronic health record; PDSA, plan-do-study-act; PF, practice facilitation; QI, quality improvement.

We propose that practice facilitation targets the barrier of low practice change capability by activating two mechanisms: engaging in facilitated QI and learning to improve. That is, we hypothesize that practice facilitation "works" to improve the quality of care (distal outcome) by engaging practice members in facilitated QI. Engaging in facilitated QI involves practice members actively participating in QI activities initiated and supported by the practice facilitator. However, engaging practice members in facilitated QI is insufficient to increase a practice's QI capacity (distal outcome). For that to occur, another mechanism, learning to improve, must be activated.

A theory of how innovation champions operate to influence implementation

A champion is an individual who "dedicates themselves to supporting, marketing, and driving an implementation, overcoming indifference or resistance that the intervention may provoke in an organization" (Powell et al., 2012). Informed by the work of Shea (2021), Miech et al. (2018) and early writings about innovation champions, we developed an initial theory of innovation championing depicted in the CPD shown in Figure 10.3. Innovation championing involves various actions to positively influence targeted organizational members' perceptions of the innovation or change initiative, the implementation context, and the implementers or users themselves. We propose that innovation championing targets the barrier of organizational inertia, indifference and resistance by activating three mechanisms: organizational members' buying into the vision, experiencing a positive implementation climate and feeling greater collective efficacy. This, in turn, brings about practice participation in implementation activities, initial use of an evidence-based intervention (EBI), improvement in skill in delivering the EBI, and ultimately promotes EBI penetration and fidelity.

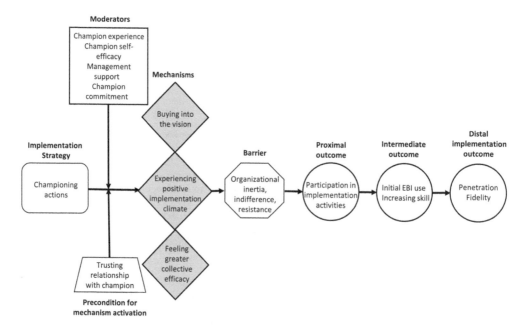

Figure 10.3 Causal pathway diagram for innovation champions.

Challenges in developing theories of implementation strategy functioning

There are several challenges that the field must grapple with when approaching the task of articulating how implementation strategies work. Implementation strategies are often poorly defined (Michie et al., 2009) or are complex, multi-faceted strategies, with flexibility in what activities constitute the strategy (Alexander and Hearld, 2012). Without clearly defined strategies, it is challenging to articulate how those strategies work. However, these challenges are not unique to theory articulation. Ambiguities in what constitutes a particular strategy have long posed challenges for deploying, testing, replicating and scaling strategies (Proctor et al., 2013). Attempting to define core activities of implementation strategies through theorizing can help unify approaches to deploying strategies and measuring their impact.

There is limited theoretical and empirical literature that describes how strategies work, beyond proposing and testing links between implementation strategies and implementation outcomes. A systematic review found limited studies in implementation science that examined mechanisms of change in implementation outcomes and, among those, even fewer explored mechanisms of how an implementation strategy exerts an influence on an implementation outcome (Lewis et al., 2020). The utility of theories lies in their ability to both predict and explain, but often theories fail to provide explanations (Bacharach, 1989). The limited source of empirical and theoretical material for informing mechanistic explanations of how strategies work will require significant novel theorizing about mechanisms. Through engaging in theorizing and supporting researchers using CPDs in their own theorizing, our team has identified challenges to articulating explanatory mechanisms.

First, mechanisms are commonly conflated with components of an implementation strategy. For instance, supervisor modelling, a clinical supervision component, might be described as a mechanism through which clinical supervision works to influence fidelity. Rather than describing the process by which supervision works, this is equivalent to saying that supervision works by providing supervision. Instead, mechanisms should be described in terms of the process of change that occurs within the recipient of the implementation strategy. In our example, the mechanism could be re-articulated as clinician learning through observation. This describes the process of change (learning through observation) that occurs within the recipient of supervision (the clinician).

Second, other forms of non-explanatory mechanisms that are common when engaging in theorizing are those that rely on circular reasoning. For instance, conducting educational meetings (strategy) improves low leader support (determinant) by improving leader support (mechanism). This circular reasoning is equivalent to saying that a strategy works by resolving the determinant, and therefore adds no explanation to the theory. An explanatory mechanism might suggest that conducting educational visits works by enhancing leaders' perceived value of the intervention, thereby improving their support for the intervention.

Third, determining the appropriate level of granularity when articulating a mechanism is challenging. Unlike in engineering where mechanisms align with physical pieces of machinery, mechanisms in implementation science serve as a metaphor for capturing a causal process. Thus, choosing the appropriate explanatory label for a mechanism will depend on the function of articulating the mechanism. In our view, the purpose of a mechanism is to improve clarity on which strategy to use based on how it works, to understand the outcomes a strategy is likely and unlikely to bring about based on how it works, and to provide a means for measuring whether a strategy's causal process has been activated. Our team has found it useful to provide mechanistic accounts that are descriptive, capture an active process, are abstract enough to encompass a series of steps, and are measurable.

Using theories of implementation strategies to guide theoretically informative research

The development of theories of implementation strategies is intended to stimulate a body of research that can advance the precision of implementation science and practice to bring about meaningful change in public health. This research should be informed by and inform theories of implementation strategy functioning, such that theories are being revised and improved in light of the accumulation of empirical evidence (Kislov et al., 2019). Theorizing about the mechanisms of implementation strategies has the potential to organize research that can answer three important questions.

1 How do implementation strategies work? It is unlikely that each implementation strategy produces change through unique processes. Instead, we may discover that common mechanisms (e.g. learning, garnering commitment, creating accountability) are shared across several strategies. This has implications for selecting and designing implementation strategies. By understanding how strategies work, we can narrow the field of potential strategies to select from. Moreover, when we understand mechanistic processes that address determinants, these can guide the design of new strategies that are intended to activate those mechanisms.
2 How do we optimize the impact of implementation strategies? Understanding the processes that account for change in implementation outcomes provides a path for optimizing that change. When the core components of strategies and how they operate are understood, we can focus on maximizing the impact of those components. For instance, within clinical supervision, should we focus more on case reviews, role plays, or modelling to maximize the impact on clinician fidelity? Understanding how these components work allows for tailored design of strategies to maximize the components that are most critical to address a given determinant.
3 Under what conditions do implementation strategies work as planned? Knowing the process through which a strategy can work does not guarantee that the process will be activated. Clinical supervision may work, in part, by activating observational learning. But whether, or the extent to which, the process of observational learning is activated might depend on the supervisor's competence or a clinician's existing knowledge. Research that explores the conditions under which implementation strategies activate their mechanisms can help to explain inconsistencies in implementation strategy effectiveness and can clarify whether there are certain conditions (e.g. organizational or innovation characteristics) for which implementation strategies are best suited based on their moderators or preconditions.

For research informed by implementation strategy theories to also be theoretically informative, findings should also be leveraged to (in)validate the propositions proposed in theories (Kislov et al., 2019). The field must conduct research that facilitates the assessment of the congruence between theoretical assertions and empirical evidence (Fawcett,

2005). If empirical evidence does not support or suggests modifications to the theoretical postulates, researchers should participate in the process of theorizing by suggesting refinements or modifications to the theory in light of the accumulation of empirical evidence. Such a process will support the evolution of theory that is empirically supported and practically meaningful.

Concluding remarks

Understanding how implementation strategies function is an important next step in implementation science (Powell et al., 2019). The ultimate purpose of this chapter is to promote advances in our understanding of how implementation strategies work to produce downstream improvements in the precision with which we design, select, and deploy implementation strategies. The intellectual exercise of theorizing about how implementation strategies work is intended to have practical implications for how implementation science is practised. That process begins with advancing the clarity of the field's thinking about how implementation strategies work. To fully realize the impact of a strong unifying theory, these theories will need to be followed by a body of research that tests and refines their propositions.

References

Alexander, J.A., Hearld, L.R. (2012) Methods and metrics challenges of delivery-system research. *Implementation Science* 7, 15. https://doi.org/10.1186/1748-5908-7-15

Bacharach, S.B. (1989) Organizational theories: some criteria for evaluation. *Academy of Management Review* 14, 496–515. https://doi.org/10.2307/258555

Bowen, N.K., Guo, S. (2011) *Structural Equation Modeling*. New York: Oxford University Press. https://doi.org/10.1093/acprof:oso/9780195367621.001.0001

Damschroder, L.J. (2020) Clarity out of chaos: use of theory in implementation research. *Psychiatry Research* 283, 1–8. https://doi.org/10.1016/j.psychres.2019.06.036

Davidoff, F., Dixon-Woods, M., Leviton, L., Michie, S. (2015) Demystifying theory and its use in improvement. *BMJ Quality & Safety* 24, 228–238. https://doi.org/10.1136/bmjqs-2014-003627

Dixon-Woods, M. (2014) The problem of context in quality improvement, *Perspectives on Context*, pp. 87–101. Retrieved from www.health.org.uk/publications/perspectives-on-context/.

Fawcett, J. (2005) Criteria for evaluation of theory, *Nursing Science Quarterly* 18, 131–135. https://doi.org/10.1177/0894318405274823

Foy, R., Ovretveit, J., Shekelle, P.G., Pronovost, P.J., Taylor, S.L., Dy, S., et al. (2011) The role of theory in research to develop and evaluate the implementation of patient safety practices. *BMJ Quality and Safety* 20, 453–459. https://doi.org/10.1136/bmjqs.2010.047993

Glanz, K., Bishop, D.B. (2010) The role of behavioral science theory in development and implementation of public health interventions. *Annual Review of Public Health* 31, 399–418. https://doi.org/10.1146/annurev.publhealth.012809.103604

Hoyle, R.H. (Ed.) (1995) *Structural Equation Modeling: Concepts, Issues, and Applications*. Thousand Oaks, CA: Sage Publications.

Kislov, R., Pope, C., Martin, G.P., Wilson, P.M. (2019) Harnessing the power of theorising in *implementation science*. Implementation Science 11, 103. https://doi.org/10.1186/s13012-019-0957-4.

Lewis, C.C., Boyd, M.R., Walsh-Bailey, C., Lyon, A.R., Beidas, R., Mittman, B., et al. (2020) A systematic review of empirical studies examining mechanisms of implementation in health. *Implementation Science* 15, 21. https://doi.org/10.1186/s13012-020-00983-3

Lewis, C.C., Klasnja, P., Lyon, A.R., Powell, B.J., Lengnick-Hall, R., Buchanan, G., et al. (2022) The mechanics of implementation strategies and measures: advancing the study of implementation mechanisms. *Implementation Science Communications* 3, 114. https://doi.org/10.1186/s43058-022-00358-3

Mackie, J.L. (1965) Causes and conditions. *American Philosophical Quarterly* 2, 245–264.

Merton, R.K. (1968) *Social Theory and Social Structure*. New York: Free Press.

Michie, S., Fixsen, D., Grimshaw, J.M., Eccles, M.P. (2009) Specifying and reporting complex behaviour change interventions: the need for a scientific method., *Implementation science* 4, 40. https://doi.org/10.1186/1748-5908-4-40.

Miech, E.J., Rattray, N.A., Flanagan, M.E., Damschroder, L., Schmid, A.A., Damush, T.M. (2018) Inside help: an integrative review of champions in healthcare-related implementation. *SAGE Open Medicine* 6, 2050312118773261. https://doi.org/10.1177/2050312118773261

Milne, D., Dunkerley, C. (2010) Towards evidence-based clinical supervision: the development and evaluation of four CBT guidelines. *Cognitive Behaviour Therapist* 3, 43–57. https://doi.org/10.1017/S1754470X10000048

Pearl, J. (1998) Graphs, causality, and structural equation models. *Sociological Methods & Research* 27, 226–284.

Pearl, J. (2009) *Causality*. New York: Cambridge University Press.

Powell, B.J., McMillen, J.C., Proctor, E.K., Carpenter, C.R., Griffey, R.T., Bunger, A.C., et al. (2012) A compilation of strategies for implementing clinical innovations in health and mental health. *Medical Care Research and Review* 69, 123–157. https://doi.org/10.1177/1077558711430690

Powell, B.J., Waltz, T.J., Chinman, M.J., Damschroder, L.J., Smith, J.L., Matthieu, M., et al. (2015) A refined compilation of implementation strategies: results from the expert recommendations for implementing change (ERIC) project. *Implementation Science* 10, 21. https://doi.org/10.1186/s13012-015-0209-1

Powell, B.J., Fernandez, M.E., Williams, N.J., Aarons, G.A., Beidas, R.S., Lewis, C.C., et al. (2019) Enhancing the impact of implementation strategies in healthcare: a research agenda. *Frontiers in Public Health* 7, 3. https://doi.org/10.3389/fpubh.2019.00003

Proctor, E.K., Powell, B.J., McMillen, J.C. (2013) Implementation strategies: recommendations for specifying and reporting. *Implementation Science* 8, 139. https://doi.org/10.1186/1748-5908-8-139

Shea, C.M. (2021) A conceptual model to guide research on the activities and effects of innovation champions. *Implementation Research and Practice* 2, 2633489521990443. https://doi.org/10.1177/2633489521990443

Stage, F.K., Carter, H.C., Nora, A. (2004) Path analysis: an introduction and analysis of a decade of research. *Journal of Educational Research* 98, 5–12. https://doi.org/10.3200/JOER.98.1.5-13

Waltz, T.J., Powell, B.J., Matthieu, M.M., Damschroder, L.J., Chinman, M.J., Smith, J., et al. (2015) Use of concept mapping to characterize relationships among implementation strategies and assess their feasibility and importance: results from the expert recommendations for implementing change (ERIC) study. *Implementation Science* 10, 109. https://doi.org/10.1186/s13012-015-0295-0

Weick, K.E. (1989) Theory construction as disciplined imagination. *Academy of Management Review*, 14, 516–531. https://doi.org/10.5465/amr.1989.4308376

Williams, N.J. (2016) Multilevel mechanisms of implementation strategies in mental health: integrating theory, research, and practice. *Administration and Policy in Mental Health and Mental Health Services Research* 43, 783–798. https://doi.org/10.1007/s10488-015-0693-2

Part II

Application

11 Implementation science research methods

Soohyun Hwang, Sarah A. Birken and Per Nilsen

Studies to identify barriers and facilitators

Studies aimed at identifying and/or assessing barriers and facilitators, also referred to as diagnostic or problem analysis (Grol et al., 2013), can use quantitative, qualitative and mixed methods to analyse various determinants. Fundamentally, quantitative and qualitative methods differ on whether the data are numeric or non-numeric. Some also assert that they differ epistemologically, with quantitative methods deriving from positivist traditions and qualitative from constructivist traditions (Grbich, 2007).

Qualitative methods

Qualitative methods refer to approaches to collecting and analysing non-numeric data. Data produced from these sources are nuanced in the sense that they are not restricted to predetermined values. Thus, qualitative methods can achieve in-depth understanding of issues, develop detailed stories to describe phenomena and generate new theories or hypotheses (Trochim and Donnelly, 2008). The methodological focus is on people and their experiences, opinions and behaviours. Qualitative methods seek to answer questions of "how" and "why" (Patton, 2015; Gill and Baillie, 2018).

These characteristics make qualitative methods valuable for implementation science research. Qualitative methods are used to elicit the perspectives of different stakeholders (e.g. healthcare providers and managers) and to gather information about barriers and facilitators to implementing an evidence-based practice. Given that implementation is not a simple switch-on/-off process, qualitative methods are well appreciated by researchers to understand the process, the people involved and the context regarding the implementation of an evidence-based intervention or programme.

Individual interviews and focus group interviews are two widely used qualitative methods in implementation science. Interviewing involves asking individuals or small groups questions about a topic. Focus groups are a specific form of group interview, where interaction between participants is encouraged. Focus groups range in size from 6 to 12 individuals. The researcher conducting a focus group interview plays the role of a facilitator encouraging discussion, rather than an interviewer asking questions. The interactive nature of focus group interviews can reveal information that might not be gathered from a single person (Miles and Huberman, 1994; Gillham, 2005; Patton, 2015). It has been suggested that focus group interviews generate a wider range of views than could be captured in individual interviews. On the other hand, individual interviews tend to produce more detail and offer more insight into an informant's personal thoughts, feelings and perspectives (Guest et al., 2017).

DOI: 10.4324/9781003318125-13

Interviews can be affected by social desirability, meaning that informants say what they think the researcher wants to hear rather than what they actually believe or do. Observational studies conducted in practice settings allow a first-hand account of behaviours and interactions, thus allowing a picture of practices from the perspective of the researcher rather than the participant. Observing researchers can adopt a detached role (non-participant observation) or participate in the activities being observed (participant observation). Several positions in between these two stances are possible. The knowledge of being observed tends to make people self-conscious, which may affect their behaviours (i.e. the Hawthorne effect). However, research has shown that as participants become accustomed to the observer's presence, their behaviours will more closely resemble normal, everyday behaviours (Patton, 2015; Twycross and Shorten, 2016).

There are several approaches to analysing the qualitative data. Content analysis is the systematic analysis of text with the major purpose of identifying patterns in the text. With ample data to work with, the researcher(s) divides each text into segments that will be treated as separate units of analysis in the study. The next step is to apply one or more codes to each unitized text segment, which is also called coding (Trochim and Donnelly, 2008). The researcher(s) then analyses the coded data to determine themes and contexts and how they might be correlated.

The grounded theory approach involves a constant comparison of coding and analysing data through three stages: open coding; axial coding; and selective coding. Each interview or observation is coded before the next is conducted so that new information obtained from the process can be incorporated into subsequent encounters (for more details, see Corbin and Strauss, 2014). Unlike the prescriptive requirements for grounded theory, template analysis is considered a more flexible technique with fewer specified procedures, allowing the researchers to tailor it to match their own requirements (King, 1998). The template analysis approach uses a priori codes and focuses on the balance between within and across case analysis. This is particularly useful when the aim is to compare the perspectives of different groups of staff within a specific context (King, 1998).

Quantitative methods

Quantitative methods use numerical data. Quantitative data are often derived from non-quantitative data, such as knowledge, beliefs, and costs that were transformed into quantitative form. The main strength of quantitative data is their potential for generalizability given their standardized form.

Analysing quantitative data requires several processes. The data must be prepared, which involves checking or logging in the data, checking the data for accuracy, entering and transforming the data, and developing a database structure that integrates various measures (Trochim and Donnelly, 2008). Researchers may use descriptive statistics to describe the basic features of the data. To address a research question or hypothesis, inferential statistics should be considered; this involves using the data as the basis for drawing broader inferences rather than simply describing the data. To understand inferential statistics, familiarity with the general linear model is required; this is the basic structure of the t test, analysis of variance, regression analysis, and many of the multi-variate methods used for analysing quantitative data (for details, see Wooldridge, 2019).

Quantitative methods may be useful in implementation science research for understanding phenomena across organizations or stakeholders, given that one premise of implementation is that patterns are likely to exist across units of analysis. For example, barriers to the implementation of a particular intervention in one setting may be at least somewhat consistent across providers or practices. Quantitative methods and data collection approaches could also be beneficial in answering implementation questions related to the context, actors, depth and breadth of implementation across subunits.

Mixed methods

Mixed methods use both quantitative and qualitative data, integrating the two to varying degrees, and then drawing interpretations based on the combined strengths of both sets of data to understand research problems (Creswell, 2015). Using mixed methods requires a clear rationale (i.e. neither quantitative nor qualitative data alone are sufficient to gain an understanding of the research question) and an approach to mixing methods that are relevant for answering the research question. Basic mixed methods include convergent, explanatory sequential, and exploratory sequential designs.

The convergent design involves the separate collection and analysis of the quantitative and qualitative data (Creswell, 2015). Merging the data follows as the results of the analyses of quantitative and qualitative data are brought together and compared. After the separate results have been merged, researchers examine to what extent the quantitative results are confirmed by the qualitative results and vice versa. A popular way to represent the merging is through a discussion in which the quantitative and qualitative results are arrayed one after the other, in parallel fashion. Researchers could also develop a table or graph that illustrates the results from both databases; this is often referred to as a joint display (Creswell, 2015).

The explanatory sequential design begins with quantitative methods and adds qualitative methods to explain the quantitative results (Creswell, 2015). This design is useful to further explore the results found through quantitative data that are often limited to statistical significance, confidence intervals, and effect sizes due to the nature of the data.

The exploratory sequential design first explores a problem through qualitative data, develops an instrument or intervention based on qualitative findings, and finally tests the instrument or intervention using quantitative data (Creswell, 2015). This is helpful when researchers lack sufficient knowledge of the subject matter to generate quantitative data collection instruments for distribution to a large number of prospective study participants or to develop and design an intervention; in-depth understanding based on the qualitative data collection and analysis generates the knowledge necessary to do so.

Studies to evaluate the effectiveness of implementation strategies

There are broadly two types of study designs for investigating the effectiveness of implementation strategies: experimental and observational studies. The basic difference between them is that the experimental design includes an intervention to achieve desired outcomes, whereas observational studies do not include this. There is also quasi-experimental design, which has some of the characteristics of experimental design. Both quantitative and qualitative methods may be used in experimental, quasi-experimental and observational designs.

Experimental design

To show causal relationships (e.g. between an evidence-based intervention, treatment, programme, etc. and desired outcomes), experimental design is often regarded as the most rigorous approach and is often labelled as the gold standard in research design with respect to internal validity (Trochim and Donnelly, 2008). Experimental design relies on the idea of random assignment of study subjects to the intervention of interest; random assignment is intended to uphold the assumption that groups (usually intervention versus control) are probabilistically equivalent, allowing us to isolate the effect of the intervention on the outcome of interest. Interventions in implementation science are usually referred to as strategies.

Brown et al. (2017) have examined three broad categories of designs for comparisons of implementation strategies:

- Within-site comparisons.
- Between-site comparisons.
- Within- and between-site comparisons.

The basic type of study in the between-site design category is a head-to-head comparison of two implementation strategies that target different outcomes with no site receiving both (Brown et al., 2017). This is effective in that it allows processes and output to be compared among sites that have different exposures. Brown et al. (2017) also emphasize that randomization should be at the "level of implementation" in the between-site designs to avoid cross-contamination. When sample size is insufficient, researchers may consider matched-pair randomized designs that improve power with fewer units of randomization or may consider other adaptive designs for randomized trials (Brown et al., 2009). The Sequential Multiple Assignment Randomized Trial (SMART) design allows for building time-varying adaptive interventions (or stepped-care strategies) that take into account the order in which components are presented (Collins et al., 2007).

Ayieko et al. (2019) conducted a cluster randomized trial examining the effect of enhanced audit and feedback (an implementation strategy) on the uptake of the new pneumonia guidelines by clinical teams within county hospitals in Kenya. The investigators performed restricted randomization, which involved retaining balance on key covariates to ensure balance in terms of geographic location and monthly pneumonia admissions between treatment and control arms. The study also used random intercept multi-level models to account for any residual imbalances in performance at baseline so that the findings could be attributed to the intervention.

Finch et al. (2019) examined the effectiveness of two implementation strategies, performance review and facilitated feedback, in increasing the implementation of healthy eating and physical activity-promoting policies and practices in childcare services in a parallel group randomized controlled trial design. Finch et al. delivered the implementation strategies to control arm childcare services after the intervention period (i.e. waitlist control; Trochim and Donnelly, 2008), a common approach in randomized trials.

Quasi-experimental design

Quasi-experimental design shares experimental design's goal of assessing the effect of an intervention on outcomes of interest. Unlike experiments, however, quasi-experiments do not randomly assign participants to intervention and usual care groups. This key distinction from experiments limits the internal validity of quasi-experiments; differences between groups cannot be attributed exclusively to the intervention; however, when randomization is not possible or desirable for assessing an intervention's effectiveness, quasi-experimental designs are appealing. Quasi-experimental study designs use techniques of varying strength to bolster internal validity in lieu of randomization, including before and after designs, interrupted time series, non-equivalent group designs, propensity score matching, synthetic control, and regression-discontinuity designs (Newcomer et al., 2015).

Quasi-experiments have the advantage that they are typically cheaper to carry out than experiments that require substantial investment in the trial process (Yapa and Barnighausen, 2018). Thus, quasi-experiments have been popular to establish causal impacts of interventions in resource-poor settings. Myriad other quasi-experimental designs with various combinations of sampling, measurement, or analytic approach exist. For additional detail on these methods, see *The Research Methods Knowledge Base* (Trochim and Donnelly, 2008) or the *Handbook of Practical Program Evaluation* (Newcomer et al., 2015).

Martens et al. (2007) conducted a quasi-experimental study to assess the initial effects of a behaviour independent financial incentive on the volume of drug prescribing by general practitioners (GPs). This study also used a quasi-experimental design, a controlled before-after study with a concurrent control group. The intervention group consisted of 119 GPs in a region in the south of the Netherlands that was known for over-prescription of certain drug categories and medications. Martens et al. (2007) searched for a control region in another part of the country that was as comparable as possible consisting of 118 GPs. The differences between the two groups were receipt of the financial incentive and awareness of the performance being checked. The study indicated that there were no differences in the age and gender of the GPs between the regions, however, there could have been additional elements (e.g. years of experience) that they could also have controlled for to make a compelling control group that was similar to the intervention group.

Observational design

In observational studies, the investigator is not acting on study participants but instead is observing the natural relationship between an implementation strategy (e.g. a course in delivering an evidence-based treatment) and outcomes of interest (Thiese, 2014). Quasi-experiments apply statistical methods to observational data to approximate what, from a scientific perspective, would ideally be achieved with random assignment. In contrast to quasi-experiments, which attempt to predict relationships among constructs, observational studies seek to describe phenomena. Thus, observational studies may be particularly useful for evaluating the real-world applicability of evidence. These descriptive, observational studies may use approaches to data collection and analysis that are quantitative, qualitative, or both.

Concluding remarks

This chapter has reviewed several commonly used study designs and methods in the social sciences that are relevant to implementation science research. There are other types of study design that researchers could explore and consider, such as case studies, cohort studies, etc., that are not covered in this chapter. Given the nascent stage of the field, researchers must actively seek opportunities to discover emerging methods and refinements to traditional methods to optimize understanding of implementation.

Implementation science research involves several methodological challenges. An acknowledged difficulty is to capture the importance of collective-level concepts, such as culture, climate and leadership. Most empirical studies in implementation science are premised on collecting data from individuals. The challenge of capturing collective-level influences is articulated in a study by Jacobs et al. (2014) on implementation climate. Results were mixed with respect to the validity of using survey questionnaires to measure implementation climate based on aggregated individual responses (e.g. "I am rewarded for implementing the evidence-based practice") versus collective-referenced responses (e.g. "We are rewarded for implementing the evidence-based practice"). Fundamentally, aggregating responses may amount to reductionist fallacy, that is, making inferences about group or other collective-level processes drawn from individual-level data (Trochim, 2020). Avoiding this fallacy requires modes of data collection that do not focus on individuals. Observational studies in various practice settings (Kirk and Haines, 2020) may be a route to investigating collective-level influences, but such studies are uncommon in implementation science.

Diagnostic analyses of barriers and facilitators present some challenges. There is the issue of whether the barriers that are identified are the actual barriers. The perceived importance of particular barriers may not necessarily correspond with actual importance. It may also be difficult to account for synergistic effects such that two seemingly minor barriers constitute an important obstacle to implementing an evidence-based practice if they interact. Johns (2006) has talked about "deadly combinations" of otherwise facilitating factors that can yield unfavourable outcomes. Changes in specific barriers may affect other barriers, suggesting that there are no simple cause-and-effect relationships between individual factors and the extent to which desired outcomes are attained. Rather, it is reasonable to assume that many factors are associated and interrelated in various ways that are not always predictable (or measurable using surveys). Studying various barriers and facilitators in isolation makes research more manageable, but it may hinder in-depth understanding of how an evidence-based practice can be attained (Nilsen and Bernhardsson, 2019).

Another issue is whether all relevant barriers are identified in diagnostic studies. Studies using quantitative survey questionnaires usually consist of a number of barriers (e.g. "the research is not reported clearly and readably" and "the amount of research information is overwhelming"), which the respondents are requested to rank on a Likert scale (e.g. Iles and Davidson, 2006) or in terms of selecting "your three greatest barriers to the use of evidence-based practice in your clinical practice" (e.g. Jette et al., 2003). The studies also incorporate questions regarding attitudes to achieving an evidence-based practice (e.g. "Evidence-based practice is an essential component of physiotherapy practice") and skills/self-efficacy in working in accordance with an evidence-based practice (e.g. "I do not feel capable of evaluating the quality of the research"). Although these studies can cover many factors influencing the implementation of an evidence-based practice, they probably do not encompass all potentially relevant barriers and facilitators. Surveying the perceived importance of a finite set of predetermined barriers and facilitators can yield insights into the relative importance of these particular factors, but may fail to identify factors that independently affect desired outcomes (Nilsen and Bernhardsson, 2019).

References

Ayieko, P., Irimu, G., Ogero, M., Mwaniki, P., Malla, L., Julius, T., et al. (2019) Effect of enhancing audit and feedback on uptake of childhood pneumonia treatment policy in hospitals that are part of a clinical network: a cluster randomized trial. *Implementation Science* 14, 20. https://doi.org/10.1186/s13012-019-0868-4

Brown, C.H., Ten Have, T.R., Jo, B., Dagne, G., Wyman, P.A., Muthen, B., et al. (2009) Adaptive designs for randomized trials in public health. *Annual Reviews of Public Health* 30, 1–25. https://doi.org/10.1146/annurev.publhealth.031308.100223

Brown, C.H., Curran, G., Palinkas, L.A., Aarons, G.A., Wells, K.B., Jones, L., et al. (2017) An overview of research and evaluation designs for dissemination and implementation. *Annual Reviews of Public Health* 38, 1–22. https://doi.org/10.1146/annurev-publhealth-031816-044215

Collins, L.M., Murphy, S.A., Strecher, V. (2007) The multiphase optimization strategy (MOST) and the sequential multiple assignment randomized trial (SMART): new methods for more potent eHealth interventions. *American Journal of Preventive Medicine* 32, S112–S118. https://doi.org/10.1016/j.amepre.2007.01.022

Corbin, J., Strauss, A. (2014) *Basics of Qualitative Research. Techniques and Procedures for Developing Grounded Theory*. 4th edition. Thousand Oaks, CA: Sage Publications.

Creswell, J.W. (2015) *A Concise Introduction to Mixed Methods Research*. Thousand Oaks, CA: Sage Publications.

Finch, M., Stacey, F., Jones, J., Yoong, S.L., Grady, A., Wolfenden, L. (2019) A randomised controlled trial of performance review and facilitated feedback to increase implementation of healthy eating and physical activity-promoting policies and practices in centre-based childcare. *Implementation Science* 14, 17. https://doi.org/10.1186/s13012-019-0865-7

Gill, P., Baillie, J. (2018) Interviews and focus groups in qualitative research: an update for the digital age. *British Dental Journal* 225, 668–672. https://doi.org/10.1038/sj.bdj.2018.815

Gillham, B. (2005) *Research Interviewing - The Range of Techniques*. Maidenhead: Open University Press.

Grbich, C. (2007) *Qualitative Data Analysis: An Introduction*. Thousand Oaks, CA: Sage Publications.

Grol, R., Wensing, M., Eccles, M., Davis, D. (2013) *Improving Patient Care: The Implementation of Change in Health Care*. Chichester: John Wiley. https://doi.org/10.1002/9781118525975

Guest, G., Namey, E., Taylor, J., Eley, N., McKenna, K. (2017) Comparing focus groups and individual interviews: findings from a randomized study. *International Journal of Social Research Methodology* 20, 693–708. https://doi.org/10.1080/13645579.2017.1281601

Iles, R., Davidson, M. (2006) Evidence based practice: a survey of physiotherapists' current practice. *Physiotherapy Research International* 11, 93–103. https://doi.org/10.1002/pri.328

Jacobs, S.R., Weiner, B.J., Bunger, A.C. (2014) Context matters: measuring implementation climate among individuals and groups. *Implementation Science* 9, 46. https://doi.org/10.1186/1748-5908-9-46

Jette, D.U., Bacon, K., Batty, C., Carlson, M., Ferland, A., Hemingway, R.D., et al. (2003) Evidence-based practice: beliefs, attitudes, knowledge, and behaviors of physical therapists. *Physical Therapy* 83, 786–805. https://doi.org/10.1093/ptj/83.9.786

Johns, G. (2006) The essential impact of context on organizational behavior. *Academy of Management Review* 31, 386–408. https://doi.org/10.5465/amr.2006.20208687

King, N. (1998) Template analysis. In: Symon, G., Cassell, C. (Eds.), *Qualitative Methods and Analysis in Organizational Research*. London: Sage.

Kirk, J.W., Haines, E.R. (2020) Ethnography. In: Nilsen, P., Birken, S.A. (Eds.), *Handbook on Implementation Science*. Cheltenham: Edward Elgar, pp. 480–486. https://doi.org/10.4337/9781788975995.00032

Martens, J.D., Werkhoven, M.J., Severens, J.L., Winkens, R.A. (2007) Effects of a behaviour independent financial incentive on prescribing behaviour of general practitioners. *Journal of Evaluation in Clinical Practice* 13, 369–373. https://doi.org/10.1111/j.1365-2753.2006.00707.x

Miles, M.B., Huberman, A.M. (1994) *Qualitative Data Analysis*. Thousand Oaks, CA: Sage Publications.

Newcomer, K.E., Hatry, H.P., Wholey, J.S. (2015) *Handbook of Practical Program Evaluation*. Hoboken, NJ: John Wiley. https://doi.org/10.1002/9781119171386

Nilsen, P., Bernhardsson, S. (2019) Context matters in implementation science: a scoping review of determinant frameworks that describe contextual determinants for implementation outcomes. *BMC Health Services Research* 19, 189. https://doi.org/10.1186/s12913-019-4015-3

Patton, M.Q. (2015) *Qualitative Research & Evaluation Methods*. Thousand Oaks, CA: Sage Publications.

Thiese, M.S. (2014) Observational and interventional study design types; an overview. *Biochemica Medica (Zagreb)* 24, 199–210. https://doi.org/10.11613/BM.2014.022

Trochim, W.M.K., Donnelly, J.P. (2008) *The Research Methods Knowledge Base*. Mason, OH: Cengage Learning.

Trochim, W.M.K. (2020) The Research Methods Knowledge Base. Retrieved from conjointly.com/kb (accessed 27 April 2020).

Twycross, A., Shorten, A. (2016). Using observational research to obtain a picture of nursing practice. *Evidence-Based Nursing* 19, 66–67. https://doi.org/10.1136/eb-2016-102393

Wooldridge, J. (2019) *Introductory Econometrics: A Modern Approach*. Mason, OH: Cengage Learning.

Yapa, H.M., Barnighausen, T. (2018) Implementation science in resource-poor countries and communities. *Implementation Science* 13, 154. https://doi.org/10.1186/s13012-018-0847-1

12 Selecting theories, models and frameworks

Margit Neher and Sarah A. Birken

Use of theories, models and frameworks in implementation science

Despite their potential benefits, theories, models and frameworks (collectively referred to as TMFs) are often underused, used superficially or misused in implementation science; this represents a challenge to moving the field of implementation science forward (Grol et al., 2007; Colquhoun et al., 2010; Davies et al., 2010; Tinkle et al., 2013; Powell et al., 2014; Liang et al., 2017). Tinkle et al. (2013) highlighted the underuse of TMFs (i.e. not using a TMF at all), revealing that most projects funded by the United States National Institutes of Health that they reviewed did not use a TMF. Similarly, Davies et al. (2010) reviewed evaluations of guideline dissemination and implementation strategies from 1966 to 1998 and found that only 23% used a TMF.

Although the use of TMFs may be increasing, it is often done superficially. For example, in a systematic review of studies citing the Consolidated Framework for Implementation Research (CFIR), Kirk et al. (2016) found that few studies applied the framework in a meaningful way. Many articles only cited the CFIR in the background or discussion sections and did not apply the CFIR to data collection, analysis or organization of the results. Another review of articles citing the Promoting Action on Research Implementation in Health Services (PARIHS) framework echoed the pervasive superficial use of the framework (Helfrich et al., 2010). TMF misuse is another issue. Gaglio et al. (2013) found that studies often misused the "reach" domain of the Reach, Effectiveness, Adoption, Implementation and Maintenance (RE-AIM) framework, which should compare intervention participants (numerator) with non-participants (denominator). Examples of misuse include comparisons of participants with each other as opposed to non-participants (e.g. Haas et al., 2010).

Which TMFs do implementation science researchers most commonly select and what do they use them for?

A survey of an international group of implementation science researchers (Birken et al., 2017a) was conducted to investigate their use of TMFs. Survey respondents reported using more than 100 TMFs across disciplines (e.g. implementation science, health behaviour, organizational studies, sociology and business). The most commonly used TMFs included CFIR (Damschroder et al., 2009), RE-AIM (Glasgow et al., 1999), Diffusion of Innovations (Rogers, 2010), Theoretical Domains Framework (TDF) (Michie et al., 2005) and Exploration, Preparation, Implementation, Sustainment (EPIS) framework (Aarons et al., 2011). Many implementation science researchers reported combining TMFs or developing them in-house.

DOI: 10.4324/9781003318125-14

In their implementation work, implementation science researchers ($n = 223$) reported applying the most frequently used TMFs to identify key constructs that may act as implementation barriers and facilitators (80%), to inform data collection (77%), to enhance conceptual clarity (66%) and to guide implementation planning (66%). They also used TMFs to inform data analysis, drive hypotheses about relationships among constructs, clarify terminology, frame an evaluation, specify implementation processes and/or outcomes, convey the larger context of the study and guide the selection of implementation strategies.

In their qualitative study, Strifler et al. (2020) noted that implementation science researchers and practitioners perceived that TMFs were a good starting point for implementation, provided a systematic or pragmatic approach, facilitated an overview of key categories or processes of implementation and increased methodological rigour. TMFs were used to inform the research question, to justify and organize an implementation project, to guide the selection and tailoring of implementation strategies, to help achieve intended outcomes and to analyse, interpret, generalize or apply the findings of an implementation project.

How do implementation science researchers select theoretical approaches?

Implementation science researchers ($n = 212$) reported using a large number of criteria to select TMFs, with little consensus on which are the most important (Birken et al., 2017a):

- Analytical level (e.g. individual, organizational, system): 58.02%.
- Logical consistency/plausibility (i.e. inclusion of meaningful, face-valid explanations of proposed relationships): 56.13%.
- Description of a change process (i.e. provides an explanation of how changes in process factors lead to changes in implementation-related outcomes): 53.77%.
- Empirical support (i.e. use in empirical studies with results relevant to the framework or theory, contributing to cumulative theory building): 52.83%.
- Generalizability (i.e. applicability to various disciplines, settings and populations): 47.17%.
- Application to a specific setting (e.g. hospitals, schools) or population (e.g. cancer): 44.34%.
- Inclusion of change strategies/techniques (i.e. provision of specific method(s) for promoting change in implementation-related processes and/or outcomes): 44.34%.
- Outcome of interest (i.e. conceptual centrality of the variable to which included constructs are thought to be related): 41.04%.
- Inclusion of a diagrammatic representation (i.e. elaboration in a clear and useful figure representing the concepts within and their inter-relations): 41.04%.
- Associated research method, for example, informs qualitative interviews, associated with a valid questionnaire or methodology for constructing one (i.e. recommended or implied method to be used in an empirical study that uses the framework or theory): 40.09%.
- Process guidance (i.e. provision of a step-by-step approach for application): 38.68%.
- Disciplinary approval (i.e. frequency of use, popularity, acceptability and perceptions of influence among a given group of scholars or reviewers, country, funding agencies, etc.; endorsement or recommendation by credible authorities in the field): 33.96%.

- Explanatory power/testability (i.e. the ability to provide explanations around variables and effects; generates hypotheses that can be empirically tested): 32.55%.
- Simplicity/parsimony (i.e. relatively few assumptions are used to explain effects): 32.08%.
- Specificity of causal relationships among constructs (i.e. summary, explanation, organization and description of relationships among constructs): 32.08%.
- Disciplinary origins (i.e. philosophical foundations): 18.40%.
- Falsifiability (i.e. verifiable; ability to be supported with empirical data): 15.09%.
- Uniqueness (i.e. the ability to be distinguished from other theories or frameworks): 12.74%.
- Fecundity (i.e. offers a rich source for generating hypotheses): 9.91%.
- None of the above: 0.00%.

This heterogeneity of selection criteria may contribute to the underuse, superficial use and misuse of TMFs. Moreover, qualitative results from the survey suggested that TMFs are often selected haphazardly or based on convenience or previous exposure. Strifler et al. (2020) reported that study participants did not usually follow an explicit process to identify a new theory, model or framework and that they "favoured one or more implementation theories, models or frameworks and used them repeatedly, stating that it was easy to use what was familiar".

What are the advantages of deliberate TMF selection?

Favouring one or more implementation TMFs and using them repeatedly may come at a cost. The unreflective selection of TMFs may inhibit the selection of TMFs that contribute with real quality to users' objectives. The tendency to use convenient or familiar TMFs may create silos in implementation science, limiting our ability to generalize findings, promote shared understanding and advance the field. Being open to novel ways of potentially explaining determinants for implementation and developing implementation strategies may inform the TMF selection process and open the door to more effective solutions.

For example, implementation science has long identified changes in the behaviour of individuals and groups as key to implementation. The field has mainly strived to explain behaviour change by using well-developed theoretical support from the fields of sociology and psychology. There has been a relative research emphasis on individual-level determinants. Empirical studies about behaviour change have often been targeted at single levels of socioecological frameworks, as have the implementation strategies for behaviour change (Birken et al., 2017a). Empirical studies designed to elucidate the influence on behaviour at the collective level (such as culture, climate, leadership and resources) often draw inferences from scientific methods that involve collecting and aggregating data from individuals, which may, in effect, amount to a reductionist fallacy. Novel theoretical approaches and scientific methodology in implementation science could provide a deeper understanding of collective-level influences on behaviour change of individuals and groups (Nilsen et al., 2022). Similarly, organizational theory may contribute to implementation science (Birken et al., 2022).

Much-diffused TMFs have also one-sidedly focused on conscious thought processes as key for behaviour and behaviour change in clinical practice. However, as implementation science has repeatedly shown that changing healthcare professionals' behaviour can be difficult, other theoretical approaches may be of interest. Understanding healthcare professionals' behaviour in terms of non-reflective processes in the form of ingrained habits and routines could provide an alternative lens to the understanding of human behaviours and ways to change them (Potthoff et al., 2022).

Recent research shows that addressing factors at the individual level may have a limited effect, and more knowledge is being developed about the impact of collective influences on behaviour change. Nilsen et al. (2022) propose a 2 × 2 conceptual map that may be used to consider and reflect on the nature of the behaviours that need to be changed, thus providing guidance on the type of TMF that might be most relevant for understanding and facilitating behaviour change.

What are common problems in finding a suitable TMF for a project?

The perspectives of implementation researchers and practitioners working in healthcare were studied by Strifler et al. (2020) in an interview study. Although most participants perceived that the use of TMFs was important and self-evident for planning, developing and sustaining effective evidence-based practices and implementation strategies, they also highlighted that selecting a TMF was difficult.

The study showed that major barriers to selection included inadequate background or training in the implementation of TMFs and lack of training or expertise in implementation research methods or practice. The participants perceived that clear and concise language and terminology (including definitions of constructs) were key factors for identification and selection, especially to help differentiate the various TMFs, which they perceived as often overlapping and sometimes highly derivative of each other.

Participants identified a need for more information on the context in which the TMF was developed or had been applied to be able to assess the fit of a TMF within the context of their own implementation project. Relevant examples of applications of the TMF from the literature were perceived to facilitate comparisons concerning the research question, purpose or goal, health problem, setting, population and level of behaviour change (Strifler et al., 2020).

A tool for selecting TMF(s) for a project

TMFs in implementation science derive from a range of disciplines (e.g. sociology, health services research, psychology, management science) and, increasingly, have been developed within implementation science itself (Nilsen, 2015). Efforts to synthesize TMFs may help address potential overlap among them. However, given that TMFs have varying strengths, weaknesses and appropriateness for any given project, the question of how to select a relevant TMF remains (Birken et al., 2017b). Therefore, implementation science researchers would benefit from guidance in selecting a TMF for a specific project. Such guidance could promote meaningful use of TMFs and discourage underuse; this, in turn, could promote opportunities to test, report and enhance their utility and validity and provide evidence to support adaptation or replacement.

T-CaST (Theory Comparison and Selection Tool) was developed to facilitate implementation science researchers' selection of TMFs. As a first step towards the development of this tool, colleagues conducted an international survey of implementation researchers and practitioners to explore which TMF they used, how they used them and which criteria they used to select them (Birken et al., 2017a).

When developing T-CaST, the study team first engaged implementation scientists in concept mapping exercises to review the criteria for TMF selection identified in the survey and participate in sorting and rating activities that yielded conceptually distinct categories of selection criteria and ratings of their clarity and importance. Second, the study team used the concept mapping results to develop a tool to guide TMF selection. Third, the team assessed the tool's usefulness through expert consensus, cognitive interviews and semi-structured interviews with implementation science researchers. The tool and methods are described in detail in a publication in *Implementation Science* (Birken et al., 2018).

The instructions for using T-CaST are as follows:

1 Complete Table 12.1 with information about your implementation project.
2 Complete Table 12.2 to evaluate the fit of one or more TMFs to your project. The tool can be used to evaluate, assess gaps and/or identify opportunities to combine TMFs.

- Step 1: In column 1, select the characteristics that are relevant to your project.
- Step 2: Note potential TMFs at the top of the third and/or fifth columns.
- Step 3: For each selected characteristic, rate the fit of the potential theory to your project and include notes that explain your score.

    o 0 = Poor fit (TMF does not fit the project along this characteristic).
    o 1 = Moderate fit (TMF somewhat fits the project along this characteristic).
    o 2 = Good fit (TMF fits the project well along this characteristic).

- Step 4 (optional): Calculate the average score in the final row and use it to assess the fit of the TMF to the particular project. If multiple team members are completing the tool, consider averaging scores across team members.
- Step 5: Repeat as needed with alternative TMFs.
- Step 6: In the action section, describe how you will apply the information from the completed tool to your project.

Tables 12.1 and 12.2 show how researchers can make both the project information and the criteria the research group use for selecting TMFs explicit with the help of T-CaST and evaluate the TMFs' performance with respect to relevant criteria.

The tool is available online (https://impsci.tracs.unc.edu/tcast) and includes hyperlinks to descriptions of the purpose of T-CaST, how T-CaST was developed and where users can find TMFs to rate using T-CaST. The tool provides instructions for use, examples of

Table 12.1 Project information.

Project title:	
Research questions: Study design: Data collection:	Aims: Constructs: Analysis plan:

Table 12.2 Theories, models and frameworks (TMF) evaluation.

Select to include X	TMF characteristic	TMF 1:		TMF 2:	
		Score (0, 1, 2)	Notes	Score (0, 1, 2)	Notes
	1. Usability				
	a. TMF includes relevant constructs (e.g. self-efficacy, climate)				
	b. Key stakeholders (e.g. researchers, clinicians, funders) are able to understand, apply, and operationalize the TMF				
	c. TMF has a clear and useful figure depicting included constructs and relationships among them				
	d. TMF provides a step-by-step approach for applying it				
	e. TMF provides methods for promoting implementation in practice				
	f. TMF provides an explanation of how included constructs influence implementation and/or each other				
	2. Testability				
	a. TMF proposes testable hypotheses				
	b. TMF includes meaningful, face-valid explanations of proposed relationships				
	c. TMF contributes to an evidence base and/or theory development because it has been used in empirical studies				
	3. Applicability				
	a. TMF focuses on a relevant implementation outcome (e.g. fidelity, acceptability)				
	b. A particular research method (e.g. interviews, surveys, focus groups, chart review) can be used				
	c. TMF addresses a relevant analytic level (e.g. individual, team, organizational, community)				
	d. TMF has been used in a relevant population (e.g. children, adults) and/or conditions (e.g. attention deficit hyperactivity disorder, cancer)				
	e. TMF is generalizable to other disciplines (e.g. education, health services, social work), settings (e.g. schools, community-based organizations), and/or populations (e.g. children, adults with serious mental illness)				
	4. Acceptability				
	a. TMF is familiar to key stakeholders (e.g. researchers, scholars, clinicians, funders)				
	b. TMF comes from a particular discipline (e.g. education, health services, social work)				
	Scoring (optional)				
	Total score				
	Number of characteristics				
	Average score (total score/number of characteristics)				
	Average score among team				
	Action: How will you apply the information from this tool? (e.g. Which TMF(s) did you select? What is your rationale for selecting the TMF(s)? If applicable, how will you combine multiple TMFs?)				

its application in both research and practice, fields for project description and TMFs under consideration, and a table in which users may select criteria that are relevant to their project and rate candidate TMFs along relevant criteria. Additional useful information about TMFs in the field of implementation science, including key strategies on how to select, apply and assess TMFs is available online (https://dissemination-implementation.org/select).

T-CaST has several potential benefits. First, because it aids in TMF selection, T-CaST has the potential to reduce fragmentation in the literature and address the underuse of TMFs in implementation science. Second, T-CaST may limit the prevalent misuse of TMFs in implementation science. Participants in semi-structured interviews reported that T-CaST encouraged them to be explicit about the criteria that they used to select a TMF. In light of our previous finding that TMF selection is often driven by convenience or previous exposure, we recommend that T-CaST be used to facilitate transparent reporting of the criteria used to select TMFs whenever a TMF is used in an implementation-related study. Transparent reporting of the criteria used to select TMFs may limit the often superficial use of TMFs. Third, T-CaST has the potential to curb the proliferation of TMFs by prompting users to consider that an appropriate TMF (or multiple TMFs in combination) may already exist.

Recent contributions in the literature

The selection of TMFs may be facilitated by recent contributions to the literature. Smith et al. (2020) have proposed additional guidance for selecting optimal TMF(s) for a project. In the process of designing an Implementation Research Logic Model (IRLM) for an implementation process, the researcher or practitioner may explore the shared relationships among the resources, activities, outputs, outcomes and impact for the programme (Smith et al., 2020). This (simplified) "logical" overview of the different parts of a project may support the researchers in the design process and facilitate their choice of appropriate TMFs.

IRLMs may be simple or complex and can be used for different purposes and stages of research to plan, execute, report and synthesize research. In an exploratory process, researchers formulate a theory about the central processes or drivers by which change comes about (Theory of Change) and a Theory of Action describing how programme components are constructed to activate the Theory of Change. Ideally, an IRLM is co-created with stakeholders, iteratively reviewed and changed to accommodate new insights. One of the examples that Smith et al. (2020) provide on their website (https://cepim.northwestern.edu) illustrates the IRLM implementation of sustained regular exercise for people with Parkinson disease (Table 12.3).

Building a logic model involves linking mechanisms of action to implementation strategies and relevant outcomes. Although the authors do not mention any method for the selection of TMFs in their description of developing an IRLM, there are opportunities for using the T-CaST in parts of the process, for example, when weighing up different TMF alternatives. Using an evaluation model such as T-CaST may facilitate the selection of a TMF that supports this logic, for example, by comparing TMF characteristics such as "applicability" (3a: TMF focuses on a relevant implementation outcome (e.g. fidelity, acceptability)) and "testability" (2b: TMF includes meaningful, face-valid explanations of proposed relationships) (see Table 12.2).

Table 12.3 Explanation of the Implementation Research Logic Model for the implementation of sustained regular exercise for people with Parkinson disease.

Clinical outcomes	The "distal" clinical/patient outcome of sustained regular exercise is associated with a slower decline in mobility and quality of life in the Parkinson patient population. A more proximal and measurable outcome was the exercise performed by patients, both in duration and intensity.
Service outcomes	To be able to reach those clinical outcomes/client goals, the service would need to provide sustainable and effective access to physical therapy.
Implementation outcomes	To facilitate sustainable and effective access to physical therapy, the members of the healthcare organization would need to increase physician referrals to physical therapy, physiotherapists would need to deliver the exercise programme with high fidelity, and referrers, physical therapists and patients would need to commit to a more proactive approach to physical therapy over the long term.
Mechanisms of action	The developers of the logic model designed actions that could facilitate implementation outcomes related to the physicians, the physiotherapists and the patients using a theory of "mechanisms of action".
Implementation strategies	To facilitate those actions, the developers of the logic model devised several "key implementation strategies"; the strategies were informed by the intervention characteristics of the evidence-based clinical intervention itself and by their analysis of implementation barriers and facilitators.
Implementation determinants	A structure for the analysis of implementation barriers and facilitators was provided by the CFIR, detailing domains and subdomains in the inner and outer context of implementation, the implementation process and the characteristics of the people involved.

Future directions

Selecting TMFs for implementation science research projects is likely to remain somewhat of a challenge to both newcomers and veterans in the implementation science community and beyond, but as we have seen in recent contributions, steps are being taken in the research field to reduce the complexity. The future may see some developments to support practice implementers and researchers in their selection process. Some of the following issues could be addressed:

• Dissemination of TMFs with a more holistic perspective
• Exemplars of the use of TMFs
• Combining implementation science and contextual expertise in the selection of TMFs
• Refining the selection tool

Dissemination of TMFs with a more holistic perspective

In the future, the selection of TMFs may be enriched by the TMFs that contribute to a more holistic perspective on implementation. Although the underuse, superficial use and misuse of implementation TMFs are usually attributed to the challenge of selecting from among the (too) many existing TMFs in the field (Tabak et al., 2012; Flottorp et al., 2013), there are promising TMFs that have seldom been selected because they are relatively unknown by researchers in the field. Researchers who recognize the need for a more holistic view of implementation will integrate TMFs designed to focus on multilevel influences on implementation, collective-level and systems perspectives or conscious versus non-conscious thought processes at the individual level in their selection process.

Exemplars of the use of TMFs

An online list of TMFs and a selection tool will not always suffice for successfully identifying one or several suitable TMFs for a project. In an ideal world, the network resources would include both a list of TMF options, a history of their development and examples of applications in different contexts together with a summary of how useful they had been in these instances. An overview of settings where various TMFs have been used and shown to function well would be of great assistance to both novice and expert TMF users.

Combining implementation science and contextual expertise in the selection of TMFs

As pointed out by Strifler et al. (2020), the process of identifying and selecting suitable TMFs for a project involves not only navigating through large numbers of different TMFs with varied language and terminology but also making judicious project decisions based on knowledge and understanding of the specific logic inherent in implementation science and an understanding of how the selected TMFs fit within the project context. The implementation team selecting and using TMFs could benefit from having both these capacities available in the team involved in the TMF selection process. This could include one or more persons with knowledge of the project context and one or more individuals with either implementation training or knowledge (or with the resources, capacity and motivation to learn more) and someone or some persons willing to lead the design of an implementation plan.

Refining the selection tool

The developers of T-CaST will explore ways to refine the tool for more deliberate TMF selection. Online exemplars of the use of TMFs are provided on the site. Future versions of T-CaST could include examples of the use of less frequently selected TMFs that contribute to a more holistic perspective. In recognition of the need for combined implementation science training and contextual expertise in the selection of TMFs, the site in its current form provides templates for both practitioners and experts in separate versions. The future version of T-CaST may include an integrated approach to facilitate the work of combined theory-practice audiences.

T-CaST could be developed to support awareness in people selecting TMFs concerning the aims and goals of the project, and if relevant, which type of outcomes should be considered. Users of TMFs might find it useful to begin by defining the general objective of the implementation project and decide if the goal is to understand factors of importance for implementation (before or after an implementation process), to plan for an implementation process or to support the choice of implementation strategies. Having a clear idea of which of these three overarching aims can be identified in the project will facilitate the selection of relevant approaches (Nilsen, 2015).

Concluding remarks

The use of TMFs in implementation science practice and research has been largely accepted as desirable to generalize findings, promote shared understanding and advance the field. The multitude of TMFs in implementation science are a rich source of potentially inspiring ways to plan, conduct and evaluate implementation projects. However, more research is needed about the process of building an appreciation of which TMF(s) fit a specific project context. The selection should ideally be aligned with the research question as well as satisfy the needs of the implementation research project or the practical implementation project at hand. The discussion around the best way to select TMFs will likely continue for some time. The implementation science community will continue to focus on better ways to further the use of TMFs and facilitate access to and understanding of TMFs and their applications among novice and expert implementation researchers and practitioners.

References

Aarons, G. A., Hurlburt, M., Horwitz, S. M. (2011) Advancing a conceptual model of evidence-based practice implementation in public service sectors. *Administration and Policy in Mental Health* 38, 4–23. https://doi.org/10.1007/s10488-010-0327-7

Birken, S.A., Powell, B.J., Shea, C.M., Haines, E.R., Kirk, M.A., Leeman, J., et al. (2017a) Criteria for selecting implementation science theories and frameworks: results from an international survey. *Implementation Science* 12, 124. https://doi.org/10.1186/s13012-017-0656-y

Birken, S.A., Powell, B.J., Presseau, J., Kirk, M.A., Lorencatto, F., Gould, N.J., et al. (2017b) Combined use of the Consolidated Framework for Implementation Research (CFIR) and the Theoretical Domains Framework (TDF): a systematic review. *Implementation Science* 12, 2. https://doi.org/10.1186/s13012-016-0534-z

Birken, S.A., Rohweder, C.L., Powell, B.J., Shea, C.M., Scott, J., Leeman, J., et al. (2018) T-CaST: an implementation theory comparison and selection tool. *Implementation Science* 13, 143. https://doi.org/10.1186/s13012-018-0836-4

Birken, S.A., Ko, L.K., Wangen, M., Wagi, C.R., Bender, M., Nilsen, P., et al. (2022) Increasing access to organization theories for implementation science. *Frontiers in Health Services* 2, 891507. https://doi.org/10.3389/frhs.2022.891507

Colquhoun, H.L., Letts, L.J., Law, M.C., MacDermid, J.C., Missiuna, C.A. (2010) A scoping review of the use of theory in studies of knowledge translation. *Canadian Journal of Occupational Therapy* 77, 270–279. https://doi.org/10.2182/cjot.2010.77.5.3

Damschroder, L.J., Aron, D.C., Keith, R.E., Kirsh, S.R., Alexander, J.A., Lowery, J.C. (2009) Fostering implementation of health services research findings into practice: a consolidated framework for advancing implementation science. *Implementation Science* 4, 50. https://doi.org/10.1186/1748-5908-4-50

Davies, P., Walker, A.E., Grimshaw, J.M. (2010) A systematic review of the use of theory in the design of guideline dissemination and implementation strategies and interpretation of the results of rigorous evaluations. *Implementation Science* 5, 14. https://doi.org/10.1186/1748-5908-5-14

Flottorp, S.A., Oxman, A.D., Krause, J., Musila, N.R., Wensing, M., Godycki-Cwirko, M., et al. (2013) A checklist for identifying determinants of practice: A systematic review and synthesis of frameworks and taxonomies of factors that prevent or enable improvements in healthcare professional practice. *Implementation Science* 8, 35. https://doi.org/10.1186/1748-5908-8-35

Gaglio, B., Shoup, J.A., Glasgow, R.E. (2013) The RE-AIM framework: a systematic review of use over time. *American Journal of Public Health* 103, e38–e46. https://doi.org/10.2105/ajph.2013.301299

Glasgow, R.E., Vogt, T.M., Boles, S.M. (1999) Evaluating the public health impact of health promotion interventions: the RE-AIM framework. *American Journal of Public Health* 89, 1322–1327. https://doi.org/10.2105/ajph.89.9.1322

Grol, R.P., Bosch, M.C., Hulscher, M.E., Eccles, M.P., Wensing, M. (2007) Planning and studying improvement in patient care: the use of theoretical perspectives. *Milbank Quarterly* 85, 93–138. https://doi.org/10.1111/j.1468-0009.2007.00478.x

Haas, J.S., Iyer, A., Orav, E.J., Schiff, G.D., Bates, D.W. (2010) Participation in an ambulatory e-pharmacovigilance system. *Pharmacoepidemiology and Drug Safety* 19, 961–969. https://doi.org/10.1002/pds.2006

Helfrich, C.D., Damschroder, L.J., Hagedorn, H.J., Daggett, G.S., Sahay, A., Ritchie, M., et al. (2010) A critical synthesis of literature on the promoting action on research implementation in health services (PARIHS) framework. *Implementation Science* 5, 82. https://doi.org/10.1186/1748-5908-5-82

Kirk, M.A., Kelley, C., Yankey, N., Birken, S.A., Abadie, B., Damschroder, L. (2016) A systematic review of the use of the Consolidated Framework for Implementation Research. *Implementation Science* 11, 72. https://doi.org/10.1186/s13012-016-0437-z

Liang, L., Bernhardsson, S., Vernooij, R.W., Armstrong, M.J., Bussières, A., Brouwers, M.C., et al. (2017) Use of theory to plan or evaluate guideline implementation among physicians: a scoping review. *Implementation Science* 12, 26. https://doi.org/10.1186/s13012-017-0557-0

Michie, S., Johnston, M., Abraham, C., Lawton, R., Parker, D., Walker, A. (2005) Making psychological theory useful for implementing evidence based practice: a consensus approach. *BMJ Quality & Safety in Health Care* 14, 26–33. https://doi.org/10.1136/qshc.2004.011155

Nilsen, P. (2015) Making sense of implementation theories, models and frameworks. *Implementation Science* 10, 53. https://doi.org/10.1186/s13012-015-0242-0

Nilsen, P., Potthoff S., Birken S.A. (2022) Conceptualising four categories of behaviours: Implications for implementation strategies to achieve behaviour change. *Frontiers in Health Services* 1, 795144. https://doi.org/10.3389/frhs.2021.795144

Potthoff, S., Kwasnicka, D., Avery, L., Finch, T., Gardner, B., Hankonen, N., et al. (2022) Changing healthcare professionals' non-reflective processes to improve the quality of care. *Social Science & Medicine* 298, 114840. https://doi.org/10.1016/j.socscimed.2022.114840

Powell, B.J., Proctor, E.K., Glass, J.E. (2014) A systematic review of strategies for implementing empirically supported mental health interventions. *Research on Social Work Practice* 24, 192–212. https://doi.org/10.1177%2F1049731513505778

Rogers, E.M. (2010) *Diffusion of Innovations*. 4th edition. New York: Simon and Schuster.

Smith, J.D., Li, D.H., Rafferty, M.R. (2020) The Implementation Research Logic Model: a method for planning, executing, reporting, and synthesizing implementation projects. *Implementation Science* 15, 84. https://doi.org/10.1186/s13012-020-01041-8

Strifler, L., Barnsley, J.M., Hillmer, M., Straus, S.E. (2020) Identifying and selecting implementation theories, models and frameworks: a qualitative study to inform the development of a decision support tool. *BMC Medical Informatics and Decision Making* 20, 91. https://doi.org/10.1186/s12911-020-01128-8

Tabak, R.G., Khoong, E.C., Chambers, D.A., Brownson, R.C. (2012) Bridging research and practice: models for dissemination and implementation research. *American Journal of Preventive Medicine* 43, 337–350. https://doi.org/10.1016/j.amepre.2012.05.024

Tinkle, M., Kimball, R., Haozous, E.A., Shuster, G., Meize-Grochowski, R. (2013) Dissemination and implementation research funded by the US National Institutes of Health, 2005–2012. *Nursing Research and Practice* 2013, 909606. https://doi.org/10.1155/2013/909606

13 Applying the Exploration, Preparation, Implementation, Sustainment framework

*Erika L. Crable, Ryan G. Kenneally,
Theresa S. Betancourt and Gregory A. Aarons*

Introduction

The Exploration, Preparation, Implementation, and Sustainment (EPIS) framework is a widely applied dissemination and implementation science (D&I) framework (Skolarus et al., 2017). Its flexibility allows for examination of determinants and mechanisms influencing the implementation of evidence-based innovations (e.g. practices, programmes, policies) across socioecological levels, settings and populations. This chapter describes how EPIS was applied in three different projects (Table 13.1).

The goal of this chapter is to showcase EPIS' flexibility and utility for guiding implementation efforts of diverse innovations across service sectors and countries. Each case study is organized with a description of the healthcare access and quality gap that led to the implementation of an evidence-based innovation, the overall study approach, and discussion of how EPIS phases and constructs were investigated in and/or facilitated the implementation study. Ideas for future directions for EPIS-guided research and practice are also provided.

Table 13.1 Overview of case studies by Exploration, Preparation, Implementation, Sustainment (EPIS) phases and determinants.

	Case 1	Case 2	Case 3
EPIS phases			
Exploration	Systems leaders, community-based organizations, advocacy groups, and parent representatives examined the need for service delivery changes to prevent child maltreatment and assessed the costs/benefits of different practices before selecting SafeCare as the focal innovation	Medicaid programme leadership examined the unmet need for substance use treatment and decided which services would be added to create care continuums	Researchers identified an unmet need for youth mental health services that persisted during the Ebola epidemic. Non-governmental organizations received short-term behaviour-change funding to support the implementation of the Youth Readiness Intervention (YRI)

DOI: 10.4324/9781003318125-15

	Case 1	*Case 2*	*Case 3*
EPIS phases			
Preparation	Inter-agency collaborators developed strategies, processes and contracting plans to support implementation and sustainment activities	Medicaid programme leadership established funding and contracting arrangements to pay for new services and planned strategies to reduce implementation barriers	Non-governmental organizations and systems partners planned how to best integrate YRI into the ongoing entrepreneurship training programme and service delivery system
Implementation	Local seed teams provided ongoing support for continuous SafeCare training, coaching, and implementation. Inter-agency collaborative teams were trained to deliver SafeCare with fidelity	Healthcare providers received training on care continuum services and delivered new substance use treatment services to clients	Invested actors assessed the ideological fit between YRI and existing training efforts. A Collaborative Team Approach supported YRI implementation with local training and supervision
Sustainment	Inter-agency collaborative teams supported ongoing communication, information and workload sharing to embed SafeCare as a routine practice	Medicaid programme staff planned training and funding strategies to support continued service delivery over time	Local teams considered ways to integrate YRI with other education and entrepreneurial programmes for youth, pending government commitment and continued funding
EPIS determinants			
Outer setting	A countywide child welfare service system environment, partnering agencies and community-based organizations. Federal, state and county resources influencing implementation	Federal and state environments with multi-level leadership, resources, sociopolitical factors, and media attention around the opioid epidemic and healthcare spending	Sierra Leone's broad country-level context, executive leadership, service environment, historical traumas related to civil war and the Ebola epidemic, and external funding
Inner setting	Provider organizations tasked with delivering SafeCare	State-run Medicaid programmes that revised benefit arrays to adopt substance use treatment care continuums	A non-governmental organization responsible for integrating YRI into existing Youth FORWARD programming

(Continued)

Table 13.1 (Continued)

	Case 1	Case 2	Case 3
EPIS determinants			
Bridging factors	Local inter-agency collaborative seed teams facilitated training and implementation efforts	Training and educational efforts, revised provider contracts, and service delivery manuals embedded services, reimbursement rates incentivized service delivery	Funding and contracting arrangements supported YRI integration into local programming. Collaborative Team Approach teams facilitated training and implementation efforts
Innovation factors	The SafeCare curriculum and its fit with the structure, culture and needs of service populations and organizations	Substance use treatment care continuum services, their complexity, and fit with the available resources of state programmes and service providers, and client needs	YRI programme components and their fit with existing entrepreneurship programming and goals for human capital and support services to youth

Case 1: Inter-agency collaborative teams to scale up evidence-based practice

EPIS was used in framing and supporting the implementation of an evidence-based intervention for preventing child neglect in the child welfare system in the sixth largest county in the United States (Hurlburt et al., 2014). This case demonstrates the interplay between EPIS' multi-level contexts throughout the implementation phases.

Healthcare access and quality gap

A child welfare system typically provides a group of services intended to ensure the safety, health and well-being of children and youth. Child welfare systems in the United States are required to include evidence-based services to prevent child abuse and neglect. Neglected children can experience physical harms, cognitive difficulties and social, emotional and language skill deficits. Despite the importance of ensuring access to evidence-based services for preventing maltreatment, successful implementation of these practices across publicly funded child welfare programmes is hindered by limited policies to support evidence-based practices (EBPs), funding, and the shortage of dedicated staff for such services. Strategies to successfully implement, scale up, and sustain these EBPs are critical for effective prevention of child maltreatment.

Innovation

SafeCare is an EBP designed to prevent/reduce child neglect and abuse by engaging parents in structured behavioural skills training and education and supporting communication; it is provided in the home (Chaffin et al., 2012; Gershater-Molko et al., 2003).

SafeCare-certified home visitors are expected to deliver services with fidelity to the model, and fidelity is assessed and coached through in-vivo observation and feedback from certified trainers/coaches. The curriculum includes advancing parent communication and problem-solving skills and has three modules focused on child health: home safety, parent-child or parent-infant interactions; each module is administered via role-playing scenarios, hands-on demonstrations, training, follow-up assessments and feedback to facilitate parent progress towards module goals (Chaffin et al., 2012; Gershater-Molko et al., 2003).

Study approach

A mixed methods study examined the implementation process of SafeCare in the sixth largest county in the United States. Inter-agency collaborative teams (ICTs) composed of diverse stakeholders and staff from the philanthropic funding agency, the county child welfare system, advocates, and partnering service delivery organizations were formed. A local ICT "seed team" was created and contracted to provide local capacity for ongoing SafeCare training and coaching to home visitors, support model fidelity and provide a flexible, local resource for countywide scale-up, and to function as an ongoing resource to address staff turnover. The main hypothesis was that the ICT scale-up strategy would lead to SafeCare fidelity that was non-inferior between the seed team and subsequently trained service provider ICTs.

The EPIS framework was used to inform qualitative interview guides for individual and focus group discussions with policy makers and programme staff about system- and organizational-level factors influencing implementation and the overall fit of SafeCare with local populations and service delivery contexts (Hurlburt et al., 2014; Willging et al., 2018).

EPIS phases

ICT activities took place through phases in both outer and inner contexts. Implementation processes were designed to align with EPIS phases (Aarons et al., 2014; Hurlburt et al., 2014). During the Exploration phase, decision makers from the external start-up funder, the child welfare system and its partnering agencies, community-based organizations, advocacy groups and parent representatives examined the need for service delivery changes to prevent child maltreatment. This was the outer context ICT whose stakeholders convened to review information about the costs and benefits of specific EBPs informed by presentations from three EBP developers. Through these inter-agency discussions, stakeholders committed to investing in resources to implement and sustain SafeCare. Sustainment, rather than implementation, was the goal from the outset. Preparation activities began with inter-agency collaborators developing strategies and processes and contracting plans to support implementation and sustainment activities. During implementation, the inner context ICT seed team, consisting of employees from multiple local organizations, was convened, trained and certified as SafeCare trainers/coaches. During active implementation, the seed teams provided ongoing support for continuous SafeCare training, coaching and implementation over time. Seed teams trained ICTs consisting of practitioners and staff from local community-based organizations to deliver SafeCare with fidelity. The inter-agency nature of the ICTs promoted highly communicative, information- and workload-sharing networks of providers throughout the Implementation and Sustainment phases.

EPIS constructs

The use of EPIS to guide the scale-up of SafeCare demonstrates the engagement of diverse stakeholders within and across outer and inner contexts. The outer context represented the county service system environment, including government agencies and community-based organizations involved in the prevention of child maltreatment, and the families in the county involved in services. The inner context described the provider organizations, including the seed team agency and direct service provider agencies that delivered SafeCare.

Cross-level and cross-context leadership was critical for SafeCare implementation. Leadership from outer (philanthropy and service system) and inner (provider agencies) contexts engaged in initial discussions to identify SafeCare as the focal EBP, and then collaborated throughout the EPIS phases, although not without some degree of negotiation (Aarons et al., 2014). Policy makers from state and county government agencies were also identified as leaders who were critical for championing SafeCare implementation, fostering collaboration from cross-context stakeholders and navigating the transition from philanthropic start-up funding to child welfare system contracts to fund ongoing seed team activities and provision of SafeCare (Willging et al., 2015). Seed team members also held leadership roles because they were responsible for training, fidelity assessment and coaching SafeCare home visitors. Outer context funding/contracting described the federal, state and county funding available to support SafeCare as well as the contractual requirements of community-based organizations that provided SafeCare to clients. Research on the nature and utility of these formal arrangements in a larger study revealed that contracts served as EPIS bridging factors, allowing service systems and community-based organizations to have bi-directional influence (Lengnick-Hall et al., 2020). For example, the outer context child welfare system proposed contract arrangements that altered inner context community-based organization behaviour around funding and inter-organizational networking. In turn, community-based organizations influenced the child welfare system by negotiating contract requirements specific to their needs, altering system-level processes and prompting greater inter-organizational collaboration (Aarons et al., 2014).

Diverse practitioners and non-profit staff within the outer context of the inter-organizational environment and network interacted in ICTs to support SafeCare implementation. Qualitative research highlighted how dissimilar organizational cultures, strategies and approaches to collaboration across these outer context entities initially introduced conflict during implementation activities, but inter-agency communications led to a shared commitment to implementing SafeCare. Innovation factors describe SafeCare's overall curriculum (innovation characteristics). The ICT model and its seed teams enhanced the innovation fit of SafeCare with the structure, culture and local needs of service populations and organizations delivering the curriculum. With regard to long-term implementation outcomes, the ICT approach led to fidelity of the SafeCare model as it was scaled up across new service teams in the service system (Chaffin et al., 2016).

Case 2: Implementing US federal- and state-level policies to improve substance use treatment for publicly insured individuals

This case study demonstrates EPIS' overall flexibility and adaptability as researchers aimed to understand policy-maker decision-making processes across outer and inner contexts and achieve statewide implementation of a complex policy innovation (Crable et al., 2022a, 2022b).

Healthcare access and quality gap

The US opioid epidemic began in 1993, and since then more than 932,000 individuals have died from a drug overdose, most of which involved prescription opioids, heroin, and/or synthetic and illicitly manufactured fentanyl (Centers for Disease Control and Prevention, 2021). The opioid epidemic is creating an unprecedented need for substance use treatment across the United States, especially among lower-income, publicly insured populations (Donohue et al., 2020).

In the United States, health insurance is provided by a mix of privately financed market coverage that individuals and families purchase, and two publicly financed and government-administered programmes: Medicare, which serves adults aged 65 years and older, and Medicaid, which provides health benefits for individuals younger than 65 years of age whose financial situation would be characterized as low income and thus they qualify for free or low-cost health coverage. Medicaid members are disproportionally represented in both non-fatal and fatal opioid-related overdose rates, but state-run Medicaid programmes have traditionally offered few substance use treatment services in their benefit array (Grogan et al., 2016).

Innovation

In 2015, the federal agency overseeing all state-run Medicaid programmes created a policy opportunity for states to revise their benefits and adopt evidence-based care continuums for substance use treatment. Care continuums include early intervention (e.g. screening, brief intervention and referral to treatment), withdrawal management, outpatient, inpatient and recovery support services (e.g. peer supports, educational and housing supports) and are designed to support individuals throughout their unique substance use treatment and recovery processes over time via gradations in the intensity of care provided. Before the 2015 federal policy opportunity, most state Medicaid programmes had never included full substance use treatment care continuum services in their benefit arrays. States' decisions to adopt new care continuums provided an opportunity to study statewide implementation of multiple EBPs packaged as unique policy innovations across three US states.

Study approach

The EPIS framework was used to guide an observational, qualitative study examining the translation of this federal policy opportunity into state-level Medicaid benefit arrays in three US states (Crable et al., 2022a, 2022b). The study also described state-contracted substance use treatment providers' experiences delivering these services.

EPIS constructs informed questions included in the semi-structured interview guide, the deductive analysis and the resulting themes generated from interview data and policy document review.

EPIS phases

The EPIS phases provided language to organize key decision points and implementation activities of Medicaid programme policy makers and service providers over time (Crable et al., 2022a, 2022b). During the Exploration phase, state Medicaid programme leaders examined the need for substance use treatment and decided on the types of new services that would be included in benefit arrays. In the Preparation phase, state Medicaid programmes identified funding to pay for new benefits, contracted with providers to deliver services and planned strategies to mitigate implementation barriers. Providers delivered new services to Medicaid members with varying degrees of fidelity during the Implementation phase, and state Medicaid programmes planned training and funding strategies to support the Sustainment phase. Researchers documented 29 distinct implementation strategies used by state Medicaid programme staff over the four EPIS phases (Crable et al., 2022a).

EPIS constructs

This study demonstrates how EPIS can be used to describe the interactions of multi-level outer and inner contexts. The multi-level outer context included federal and state environments. Federal agency leadership created a policy opportunity to influence state-run Medicaid programmes to change their benefit arrays. State leadership, including governors and state legislature, were required to approve and fund any Medicaid programme changes. State substance use treatment services and funding environments described funds to pay for new services. Inter-organizational environments described how state agencies and provider organizations interacted during implementation. The sociopolitical environment and media attention are outer context adaptations used to capture the politicization and stigma associated with the opioid epidemic and receipt of Medicaid services. The inner context represents individual Medicaid programmes with distinct leadership and organizational characteristics that could influence their programmatic decision to implement new substance use treatment services. Researchers adapted the inner context to include a service environment construct describing each programme's existing benefit array and provider network, which had an impact on the scope of policy change required to implement new benefits and the number of providers that needed to be trained to deliver new benefits such as substance use treatment services to Medicaid members (Crable et al., 2022a).

Innovation factors described the substance use treatment care continuums implemented by each state (i.e. the innovation). Researchers described the complexity of assessing innovation fit. New services were desired by state programmes, service providers and clients to address the opioid epidemic, but providers struggled to achieve fidelity when delivering complex substance use treatment care continuum services (innovation characteristics). Several bridging factors were used to align inner context benefit design with outer context service delivery environments (Crable et al., 2022a). For example, Medicaid programmes revised provider contracts and service manuals to improve innovation fit. Medicaid programmes also increased reimbursement rates to entice providers to contract with Medicaid and deliver new services (Crable et al., 2022a). Contract and service manual revisions complemented implementation strategies that focused on training and educating providers and facilitated the initial implementation efforts. But increased reimbursement rates were insufficient bridging factors to achieve statewide adoption of new services (Crable et al., 2022a).

Case 3: Youth Functioning and Organizational Success for West African Regional Development (Youth FORWARD, Sierra Leone)

This case study highlights the use of EPIS in global implementation research conducted in a low-income, post-conflict setting. This case study also describes how EPIS can capture the multi-level influences of implementation partners across governmental organizations and non-governmental organizations (NGOs).

Healthcare access or quality gap

Within the last two decades, youths living in Sierra Leone have experienced adversity, including the trauma of living through an 11-year civil war, the Ebola virus disease epidemic, the global COVID-19 pandemic and its social and economic consequences, and several climate change-related natural disasters including deadly mudslides (Bond et al., 2022). All these factors are associated with higher rates of traumatic stress reactions, anxiety and depression, among other behavioural health needs (Hopwood et al., 2021). Mental health and substance use treatment needs are prevalent among Sierra Leoneans, but an estimated 98% of people with identified treatment needs are not receiving care (Alemu et al., 2012). Evidence-based behavioural health programmes that fit the population health needs, resources, and infrastructure constraints of Sierra Leone's conflict-affected regions are needed.

The Youth Functioning and Organizational Success for West African Regional Development (Youth FORWARD) collaboration served as an implementation science hub to create partnerships between researchers and practitioners and increase access to evidence-based mental health services for young people (Betancourt et al., 2021). Youth FORWARD supported the implementation of the Youth Readiness Intervention (YRI), an evidence-based and group-based mental health intervention proven to be effective for addressing transdiagnostic consequences of trauma and life disruption, including emotion dysregulation and inter-personal functioning. Youth FORWARD tested an innovative strategy for reaching vulnerable youth by linking YRI to livelihood initiatives in the country (e.g. employment, entrepreneurship) and was implemented in conjunction with the Government of Sierra Leone, a European development agency, and its subcontracted implementation partners. Funded by the US National Institute of Mental Health, the Youth FORWARD team and its research partners used the EPIS framework to help engage key stakeholders and implement YRI as part of a preexisting youth-focused entrepreneurship training programme (Betancourt et al., 2021; Bond et al., 2022).

Study approach

The researchers conducted a hybrid type II effectiveness-implementation study using a cluster randomized control trial design to study the implementation of YRI in three districts of Sierra Leone (Bond et al., 2022). The EPIS framework was used to inform qualitative interview guides for individual and focus group discussions with policy makers and programme staff about system- and organizational-level factors influencing implementation and the overall fit of the YRI with local populations and service delivery contexts. Semi-structured interviews with agency leaders and YRI implementers were conducted to describe implementation activities and outcomes, including the overall acceptability, appropriateness, and feasibility of YRI. A combination of inductive and deductive qualitative analysis techniques was used to generate qualitative themes linked to the phases and constructs of the EPIS framework.

EPIS phases

The EPIS phases were used to organize implementation process activities across the multi-partner team. During the Exploration phase, Sierra Leone's broad country-level context was evaluated to identify mental health needs and the potential fit for YRI. Researchers identified unmet needs for youth mental health services and government agencies and health systems focused their attention on addressing the immediate needs of the Ebola epidemic. Limited short-term behaviour-change funding was provided to NGOs via a European development agency and used primarily for livelihood activities. Although a "psychosocial" component of this programming was envisioned, an evidence-based model was not included. During the Preparation phase, partners planned how to best integrate the evidence-based YRI into the ongoing entrepreneurship training programme and service delivery system. YRI was implemented with funding from the European development agency in concert with the Government of Sierra Leone National Youth Commission (NAYCOM). Implementation activities included assessing the ideological fit between the YRI and the existing NAYCOM and the entrepreneurship training approach supported by the European development agency. A process similar to the ICT model described in the first case study, called the Collaborative Team Approach, was used to support YRI implementation. The Collaborative Team Approach relied on stakeholders from the European development agency, NAYCOM, the entrepreneurship programme service provision agency contracted to provide services, YRI experts from an NGO that had run the previous YRI research trials and academic research partners to plan and implement Youth FORWARD. Similar to the ICT model, Collaborative Team Approach seed teams of local experts were responsible for training and supervising YRI providers. The Implementation phase focused on understanding the role of YRI facilitator supervision and implementation outcomes. Sustainment phase activities focused on continued efforts to integrate YRI with other educational and entrepreneurial programmes for youth. However, sustainment depends largely on government commitment and continued funding for mental health programmes such as YRI.

EPIS constructs

Sierra Leone's broad country-level context is identified as the outer context and was adapted to consider how historical traumas, rates of unemployment, underemployment, gender issues, and a limited service environment might have an impact on YRI implementation on a greater scale. Outer context leadership included the constitutional republic's presidential and parliamentary members who were elected just before the study began. Leadership within the new government were keen to prioritize youth issues but were overwhelmed with responding to weaknesses in the health system as the country recovered from the Ebola virus disease outbreak within a health system already destroyed by 11 years of civil war. The inter-organizational environment and network (i.e. EPIS inter-connections and linkages) included pre-existing government organizations, NGOs and academic partners working together to build capacity in the public health system to enhance access to mental health services. Service environments and policies included policies related to mental health, youth health and training needs. Funding/contracting described the contracted labour force funded by short-term grants to support behaviour-change interventions, including livelihood skills and mental health and psychosocial support services. Researchers also considered how competition for service contracts funded by a European partner agency affected the service context of YRI implementation; contracting rules precluded the use of inter-agency approaches because regulations stipulated the funding of only a single agency for implementation.

An NGO responsible for Youth FORWARD implementation was selected through competitive service contract applications as the inner context platform for service delivery. The study aimed to integrate YRI into the Youth FORWARD programming, and the YRI Collaborative Team Approach had little influence on the agency that was selected. Once the agency was contracted by the European funder, seed teams based at the NGO, with experience in the YRI (as in the ICT study in case 1), were responsible for ensuring the quality and fidelity monitoring of YRI implementation by the newly contracted agency.

Outer context funding and contracting arrangements became important bridging factors to support the integration of YRI into the inner context entrepreneurship programming and the larger absorption of the YRI into other outer context service sectors related to the mission of NAYCOM. Innovation factors described the YRI programme components that were designed to address transdiagnostic issues common in youth exposed to violence. Innovation fit characterized YRI's compatibility with existing entrepreneurship programming and NAYCOM's goals for human capital and support services to youth. YRI seed team experts supported new YRI facilitators to adapt features of the YRI to ensure responsivity to the unique needs of young women compared with young men because the YRI intervention was delivered in same-gender groups. In each of the three districts in which Youth FORWARD operated, plan-do-study-act cycles were used to identify implementation barriers, propose innovative solutions for overcoming them, test these innovations, and share lessons learned across district teams to foster district cross-site learning.

Future opportunities to advance EPIS-guided research

As demonstrated by the case studies, EPIS has substantial utility for guiding implementation research on diverse health topics and innovations, in domestic, high- income, and low-and-middle-income country settings. The EPIS phases provide useful process components that are practical for bench marking the decisions and actions of cross-context stakeholders throughout the fits and starts of implementation. The non-linear nature of the EPIS phases reminds implementers to focus on and plan for sustainment from the beginning, considering which outer and/or inner context and innovation factors may support or hinder sustainment, and which bridging factors can support sustainment goals over time. The Exploration and Preparation phases are currently understudied (Moullin et al., 2019). Additional research on the specific decisions and activities that stakeholders engage in during the Exploration and Preparation phases is needed to improve our understanding of how these pre-implementation actions affect implementation and sustainment outcomes.

Much of the existing EPIS-driven research focuses on implementation. Additional research on how EPIS guides pre-implementation research and practice is needed. One current study is using EPIS to understand the determinants across the Preparation and Implementation phases that influence how legislators write and implement tax proposals that allocate funding for mental health services (Purtle and Stadnick, 2020; Purtle et al., 2022). Researchers are using data on identified determinants to craft implementation strategies to improve the tax design process and increase access to tax-funded EBPs. In addition, EPIS is being utilized in studies incorporating team effectiveness research to improve implementation and service processes (McGuier et al., 2023). In addition, recent work has integrated issues of equity and power with the EPIS framework (Stanton et al., 2022).

Future research should also investigate how EPIS can support dissemination research. Researchers are currently using EPIS to guide the investigation of how decision makers across different public and privately funded insurance agencies use evidence- and non-evidence-based sources to make decisions about which medications are included in benefit arrays, and how evidence-use behaviours influence the design of utilization management policies that limit access to specific medication types (Crable et al., 2023). Researchers are using EPIS to define the multi-level inner contexts of each agency. Survey research with decision makers will reveal the extent to which different outer and inner context factors and bridging factors act as determinants, mechanisms or intermediaries to influence their agency-level evidence-use behaviours. These findings will inform the development of dissemination strategies tailored to each agency, across EPIS phases, to increase evidence-informed decision-making processes (Crable et al., 2023). Additional research testing the utility of EPIS for D&I research across non-linear implementation phases is encouraged. Such future research is critical for enhancing our knowledge of new applications for EPIS to guide scientific study and practice across different populations, settings and topic areas.

There is increasing interest in investigating the multifaceted roles that health policy can play in D&I efforts. The emergent sub-field of policy D&I purports to resolve knowledge gaps about when, how and why policy makers use evidence to inform policy, how evidence-based policies are implemented and sustained, as well as methods to de-implement policies that are ineffective or cause harm to individuals or society. Researchers recently developed specific recommendations for conceptualizing the role(s) of policy, policy makers and political and policy-making entities within EPIS' outer and inner contexts (Crable et al., 2022c). Recommendations for optimizing EPIS (and other theories, models and frameworks) for policy D&I research provide guidance for identifying bridging factors that align multi-level outer and inner contexts, including formal arrangements or relational ties with intermediaries, such as lobbyists or researchers who share information with policy makers, and processes that dictate how evidence is communicated to policy makers. Recommendations also describe how researchers can use EPIS to examine how policy innovation factors influence the implementation and sustainment of evidence-based policies and their downstream impact on population health outcomes (Crable et al., 2022c). Future research should operationalize and test the utility of these recommendations in EPIS-guided policy D&I research.

A non-exhaustive list of example implementation questions that can be investigated across EPIS phases is provided in Table 13.2 to further aid researchers and practitioners in future applications of EPIS.

Table 13.2 Example research questions to investigate across Exploration, Preparation, Implementation, Sustainment (EPIS) phases.

Non-linear EPIS phases	Example questions to investigate in each phase
Exploration	How do stakeholders (outer or inner context) understand the needs of clients, communities and/or providers? What are those needs?
	Which level(s) are important to consider (e.g. policy, system, community, organization, teams, individual)?
	How do stakeholders generate support to do something about those unmet needs?
	Which types of innovations are considered to address the identified needs? How are those practices understood and vetted?
Preparation	What is the existing implementation climate, culture and infrastructure? How might it need to be bolstered to support implementation?
	Which stakeholders need to be involved in planning and implementing the implementation object?
	What types of resources are needed to support implementation and sustainment?
Implementation	Who are the implementers?
	How are implementation strategies being used (e.g. as planned/with fidelity, or are adaptations needed)?
	What types of outer/inner context spanning relationships, formal arrangements, processes or resources support implementation (to align multi-level contexts for implementation)?
	What are the implementation, service and client outcomes, and potential unintended consequences (e.g. the implementation efforts' impact on the workforce)?
Sustainment	What are the implementation, service and client outcomes, potential long-term benefits or unintended consequences?

References

Aarons, G.A., Fettes, D.L., Hurlburt, M.S., Palinkas, L.A., Gunderson, L., Willging, C.E. (2014) Collaboration, negotiation, and coalescence for interagency-collaborative teams to scale-up evident-based practice. *Journal of Clinical Child & Adolescent Psychology* 43, 915–928. https://doi.org/10.1080/15374416.2013.876642

Alemu, W., Funk, M., Gakurah, T., Bash-Taqi, D., Bruni, A., Sinclair, J., et al. (2012) *WHO proMIND: Profiles on Mental Health in Development, Sierra Leone*. Geneva: World Health Organization.

Betancourt, T.S., Hansen, N., Farrar, J., Borg, R.C., Callands, T., Desrosiers, A., et al. (2021) Youth Functioning and Organizational Success for West African Regional Development (Youth FORWARD): study protocol. *Psychiatric Services* 72, 563–570. https://doi.org/10.1176/appi.ps.202000009

Bond, L., Farrar, J., Borg, R.C., Keegan, K., Journeay, K., Hansen, N., et al. (2022) Alternate delivery platforms and implementation models for bringing evidence-based behavioral interventions to scale for youth facing adversity: a case study in West Africa. *Implementation Science Communications* 3, 16. https://doi.org/10.1186/s43058-022-00259-5

Centers for Disease Control and Prevention. (2021) Wide-ranging online data for epidemiologic research (WONDER). https://wonder.cdc.gov/ (accessed 22 May 2023).

Chaffin, M., Hecht, D., Bard, D., Silovsky, J. F., & Beasley, W. H. (2012) A statewide trial of the SafeCare home-based services model with parents in Child Protective Services. *Pediatrics*, 129(3), 509–515.

Chaffin, M., Hecht, D., Aarons, G.A., Fettes, D., Hurlburt, M., Ledesma, K. (2016) EBT fidelity trajectories across training cohorts using the Interagency Collaborative Team strategy. *Administration and Policy in Mental Health and Mental Health Services Research* 43, 144–156. https://doi.org/10.1007/s10488-015-0627-z

Crable, E.L., Benintendi, A., Jones, D.K., Walley, A.Y., Hicks, J.M., Drainoni, M.L. (2022a) 'Translating Medicaid policy into practice: policy implementation strategies from three US states' experiences enhancing substance use disorder treatment. *Implementation Science* 17, 3. https://doi.org/10.1186/s13012-021-01182-4

Crable, E.L., Jones, D.K., Walley, A.Y., Hicks, J.M., Benintendi, A., Drainoni, M.L. (2022b) How do Medicaid agencies improve substance use treatment benefits? Lessons from three states' 1115 waiver experiences. *Journal of Health Politics, Policy and Law* 47, 497–518. https://doi.org/10.1215/03616878-9716740

Crable, E.L., Lengnick-Hall, R., Stadnick, N.A., Moullin, J.C., Aarons, G.A. (2022c) 'Where is "policy" in dissemination and implementation science? Recommendations to advance theories, models, and frameworks: EPIS as a case example. *Implementation Science* 17, 80. https://doi.org/10.1186/s13012-022-01256-x

Crable, E.L., Grogan, C.M., Purtle, J., Roesch, S.C., Aarons, G.A. (2023) Tailoring dissemination strategies to increase evidence-informed policymaking for opioid use disorder treatment: study protocol. *Implementation Science Communications* 4, 16. https://doi.org/10.1186/s43058-023-00396-5

Donohue, J., Raslevich, A.C., Cole, E. (2020) Medicaid's role in improving substance use disorder treatment. Milbank Memorial Fund. Retrieved from www.milbank.org/wp-content/uploads/2020/09/Primer_Fund_Donohue_v8.pdf (accessed 12 September 2023).

Gershater-Molko, R. M., Lutzker, J. R., & Wesch, D. (2003) Project SafeCare: Improving health, safety, and parenting skills in families reported for, and at-risk for child maltreatment. *Journal of family violence*, 18, 377–386.

Grogan, C.M., Andrews, C., Abraham, A., Humphreys, K., Pollack, H.A., Smith, B.T., et al. (2016) Survey highlights differences in Medicaid coverage for substance use treatment and opioid use disorder medications. *Health Affairs (Millwood)* 35, 2289–2296. https://doi.org/10.1377/hlthaff.2016.0623

Hopwood, H., Sevalie, S., Herman, M.O., Harris, D., Collet, K., Bah, A.J., et al. (2021) The burden of mental disorder in Sierra Leone: a retrospective observational evaluation of programmatic data from the roll out of decentralised nurse-led mental health units. *International Journal of Mental Health Systems* 15, 31. https://doi.org/10.1186/s13033-021-00455-1

Hurlburt, M., Aarons, G.A., Fettes, D., Willging, C., Gunderson, L., Chaffin, M.J. (2014) Interagency collaborative team model for capacity building to scale-up evidence-based practice. *Child and Youth Services Review* 39, 160–168. https://doi.org/10.1016/j.childyouth.2013.10.005

Lengnick-Hall, R., Willging, C., Hurlburt, M., Fenwick, K., Aarons, G.A. (2020) Contracting as a bridging factor linking outer and inner contexts during EBP implementation and sustainment: a prospective study across multiple US public sector service systems. *Implementation Science* 15, 43. https://doi.org/10.1186/s13012-020-00999-9

McGuier, E.A., Aarons, G.A., Byrne, K.A., Campbell, K.A., Keesin, B., Rothenberger, S.D., et al. (2023) Associations between teamwork and implementation outcomes in multidisciplinary cross-sector teams implementing a mental health screening and referral protocol. *Implementation Science Communications* 4, 13. https://doi.org/10.1186/s43058-023-00393-8

Moullin, C., Dickson, K.S., Stadnick, N.A., Rabin, B., Aarons, G.A. (2019) Systematic review of the Exploration, Preparation, Implementation, Sustainment (EPIS) framework. *Implementation Science* 14, 1. https://doi.org/10.1186/s13012-018-0842-6

Purtle, J., Brinson, K., Stadnick N.A. (2022) Earmarking excise taxes on recreational cannabis for investments in mental health: an underused financing strategy. *JAMA Health Forum* 3, e220292. https://doi.org/10.1001/jamahealthforum.2022.0292

Purtle, J., Stadnick, N.A. (2020) Earmarked taxes as a policy strategy to increase funding for behavioral health services. *Psychiatric Services* 71, 100–104. https://doi.org/10.1176/appi.ps.201900332

Skolarus, T.A., Lehmann, T., Tabak, R.G., Harris, J., Lecy, J., Sales, A.E. (2017) Assessing citation networks for dissemination and implementation research frameworks. *Implementation Science* 12, 97. https://doi.org/10.1186/s13012-017-0628-2

Stanton, M.C., Ali, S.B.; The SUSTAIN Center Team (2022) A typology of power in implementation: building on the Exploration, Preparation, Implementation, Sustainment (EPIS) framework to advance mental health and HIV health equity. *Implementation Research and Practice* 3, 26334895211064250. https://doi.org/10.1177/26334895211064250

Willging, C.E., Green, A.E., Gunderson, L., Chaffin, M., Aarons, G.A. (2015) From a "perfect storm" to "smooth sailing": policymaker perspectives on implementation and sustainment of an evidence-based practice in two states. *Child Maltreatment* 20, 24–36. https://doi.org/10.1177/1077559514547384

Willging, C.E., Gunderson, L., Green, A.E., Jaramillo, E.T., Garrison, L., Ehrhart, M.G., et al. (2018) Perspectives from community-based organizational managers on implementing and sustaining evidence-based interventions in child welfare. *Human Service Organizations Management, Leadership and Governance* 42, 359–379. https://doi.org/10.1080/23303131.2018.1495673

14 Applying the Consolidated Framework for Implementation Research

Caitlin Reardon, Shari Rogal, Rachel Rosenblum, Andrea Nevedal and Matthew Chinman

Introduction

This chapter demonstrates how the Consolidated Framework for Implementation Research (CFIR) (Damschroder et al., 2009, 2022b) was applied in three different projects, highlighting different methods for achieving the same end, identifying barriers and facilitators to implementation of evidence-informed practices. Originally, using CFIR relied on traditional in-depth qualitative methods consisting of conducting and transcribing interviews, using directed content analysis to code transcripts in qualitative software, aggregating coded data by construct in detailed case memos, and rating constructs as −2 (strong barrier) to +2 (strong facilitator) to implementation (Damschroder et al., 2011, 2017a, 2017b; Cannon et al., 2019). However, this approach is time and resource intensive, therefore new approaches have evolved to better meet the needs of rapid and/or resource-constrained projects.

The cases described in this chapter applied CFIR in different settings with different innovations (Table 14.1). In addition, the cases varied in terms of their overall purpose and research design: Cases 1 and 2 used CFIR post-implementation to understand

Table 14.1 Case comparison: innovation and setting.

CFIR domains	Case 1	Case 2	Case 3
Innovation	CHOICE (school-based substance-use prevention programme)	Diverse evidence-informed practices developed by Veterans Health Administration staff	Early palliative care consultation for patients with a new cancer diagnosis
Inner setting and outer setting	Boys and girls clubs in southern California and settings outside of the boys and girls clubs	Veterans Health Administration facilities across the United States and settings outside Veterans Health Administration facilities	Outpatient palliative care clinics across the United States and settings outside the palliative care clinics
Individuals: deliverers	Boys and girls club staff	Veterans Health Administration Staff	Oncologists and palliative care clinicians

DOI: 10.4324/9781003318125-16

CFIR *domains*	*Case 1*	*Case 2*	*Case 3*
Individuals: recipients	Youth attending boys and girls clubs	Veterans Health Administration staff and veteran patients receiving care in Veterans Health Administration facilities	Patients with a new advanced solid cancer diagnosis
Implementation process	Getting To Outcomes (Chinman et al., 2004) support	Diffusion of Excellence: external implementation support	Not applicable (data collection was before active implementation)

implementation outcomes and case 3 used CFIR pre-implementation to inform implementation strategy development. Cases 1 and 2 used qualitative data collection methods, but case 1 used the traditional in-depth approach and case 2 used a rapid approach to analyse and rate the qualitative data. In contrast, case 3 used CFIR with a quantitative approach, collecting data with a recently developed CFIR survey. After the presentation of each case, the trade-offs associated with the different approaches are discussed (see Table 14.2 for a comparison of each case based on research design and trade-offs).

Case 1: Using CFIR to conduct a post-implementation evaluation: semi-structured interviews and traditional in-depth qualitative analysis

This case used CFIR in a 29-site, cluster-randomized, controlled trial comparing two groups of community-based agencies (i.e. boys and girls clubs [BCGs]) implementing an evidence-informed substance-use prevention programme (CHOICE) twice over a 2-year period (Chinman et al., 2016). The intervention group ($n = 14$ sites) received an implementation strategy called Getting To Outcomes (GTO) and the control group ($n = 15$ sites) did not receive additional implementation support. Before this study, GTO had been shown to build knowledge and skills among community practitioners to select, plan, implement and self-evaluate evidence-informed practices; improve implementation of practices (e.g. adherence to programme curricula) and improve youth outcomes (Acosta et al., 2013; Chinman et al., 2013a, 2013b, 2016). However, the trial was designed to replicate earlier GTO findings and better understand which barriers were addressed by GTO. The team hypothesized that GTO's focus on goal setting, planning, evaluation and quality improvement would improve the CFIR-defined implementation process constructs: planning and reflecting and evaluating. The study aimed to empirically determine which barriers were addressed by the implementation strategy (GTO), answering a mechanistic implementation science question.

The innovation: CHOICE

CHOICE is a substance-use prevention programme for middle-school youth involving five 30-minute sessions based on social learning (Bandura, 1977), decision making (Kahneman and Tversky, 2000) and self-efficacy theories (Bandura, 1997). Delivered using motivational interviewing (Miller and Rollnick, 2013), CHOICE uses role plays to teach resistance skills and provide education. Two randomized trials of CHOICE found the programme was associated with reductions in alcohol and marijuana use (D'Amico and Edelen, 2007; D'Amico et al., 2012).

The inner and outer settings

The inner setting was each BGC that was implementing CHOICE; BGCs provide youth programming ranging from recreation in gyms to leadership, character education, health and wellness, and academic programmes. BGCs are often free-standing and may include multiple sites (i.e. geographic locations). The outer setting included the local, state and national settings around the BGCs.

The individuals: Deliverers

Deliverers included BGC full- and part-time staff ($n = 7$–10), ranging from an executive director to programme staff that worked directly with youth.

The individuals: Recipients

Recipients were youth attending the BGC. Across two cohorts of middle-school youth, (year 1, $n = 356$; year 2, $n = 253$), about half identified as girls. About two thirds were Latine ethnicity and the remaining one third were a mix of several other races/ethnicities.

The implementation process: Getting To Outcomes

Rooted in the social cognitive theory of behavioural change (Fishbein and Ajzen, 1975; Ajzen and Fishbein, 1977; Bandura, 2004), GTO supports implementation by increasing knowledge and skills around key planning and evaluation tasks. These key tasks are organized into GTO's 10-step approach that practitioners can apply to any programme (e.g. goal setting, planning, evaluation, quality improvement and sustaining) (Livet and Wandersman, 2005). The GTO logic model states that improved performance of these steps can improve practice fidelity, and in turn, improve outcomes (Durlak and DuPre, 2008). GTO is supported by a manual, training, and proactive and ongoing technical assistance (Chinman et al., 2004). Using existing staff, BGC sites in both groups were asked to implement CHOICE once a year for 2 years with a different group of middle-school youth each year (2014–2016). BGC staff collected fidelity and youth outcome data, which were then incorporated to improve the plan for a second round of CHOICE implementation.

Data collection: Implementation determinants

Semi-structured interviews based on CFIR were conducted at each site ($n = 28$ at GTO sites, $n = 21$ at control sites) between years 2 and 3 with BGC staff to assess barriers and facilitators to CHOICE implementation. In addition, data on BGC staff demographics and background were collected at baseline. GTO dose (i.e. hours of technical assistance) was collected in years 1 and 2 while GTO was active; data on GTO performance (i.e. 12 items that assessed how well sites performed key tasks aligned with the GTO steps) were collected in years 1–3; year 3 was 1 year after GTO support ended.

Data collection: Implementation outcomes

CHOICE fidelity (curricula adherence and delivery quality) was assessed by trained outside observers in about 40% of CHOICE sessions. In addition, the continuation of CHOICE was assessed in years 3 and 4 (1 and 2 years after GTO support ended, respectively).

Data analysis

A traditional in-depth qualitative approach was used in this case (i.e. CFIR-based directed content analysis; Hsieh and Shannon, 2005) to code and rate data from interview transcripts. Transcripts were coded independently in qualitative software by two analysts, and a consensus approach was used to finalize the codes. Data were then aggregated by construct in detailed site-level memos, in which data for each construct were summarized and rated. Ratings were based on two factors: (1) valence (positive or negative influence on implementation) and (2) strength (weak or strong influence on implementation). Summaries and ratings were then copied into an MS Excel CFIR construct by site matrix, with cases ordered by implementation outcomes, for case and cross-case analysis and interpretation.

Results

By year 2, GTO sites had significantly higher fidelity (i.e. ratings of CHOICE curricula adherence and quality of delivery). Two years after the end of active GTO support, GTO sites were more likely to have continued implementing CHOICE. The CFIR constructs planning (which includes goal setting) and reflecting and evaluating were rated higher for GTO sites (versus non-GTO sites), whereas the culture construct was rated lower for GTO sites (versus non-GTO sites) because GTO sites had more challenges with staff turnover. An aggregate measure of all CFIR barriers and facilitators was significantly associated with GTO performance and CHOICE fidelity; that is, the more facilitators and the fewer barriers, the better GTO performance and CHOICE fidelity.

Reflections on the use of CFIR

CFIR's inclusion in the trial elucidated mechanisms by which GTO worked. For example, GTO improved constructs in CFIR's implementation process domain, a key GTO focus, which in turn improved the implementation of CHOICE, including helping GTO sites mitigate the impact of having more staff turnover than non-GTO sites. In addition, overcoming CFIR barriers overall was associated with both stronger performance of activities contained in the GTO steps and curricular fidelity. Implementation science continues to investigate ways to empirically match implementation strategies with barriers, and these findings contribute to that body of knowledge.

Case 2: Using CFIR to conduct a post-implementation evaluation: semi-structured interviews and rapid qualitative analysis

CFIR was used in this case to identify barriers and facilitators to the successful replication of multiple evidence-informed practices in the Veterans Health Administration Diffusion of Excellence (DoE) initiative. The DoE was designed to identify and disseminate evidence-informed practices developed by Veterans Health Administration employees

(Nevedal et al., 2020). First, evidence-informed practices are submitted by employees to the DoE's annual Shark Tank Competition; second, Veterans Health Administration facility or network leaders bid on practices that they want to implement; and third, practices are replicated in additional facilities with external implementation support (Nevedal et al., 2020). Results were shared with the DoE leadership to guide the refinement of DoE processes for future cohorts.

The innovation: diverse evidence-informed practices

The fourth cohort of Shark Tank included ten evidence-informed practices (Reardon et al., 2021), including innovations at patient, staff, and system levels. Examples of each type of practice are provided.

- Patient-level practice: Advanced Comprehensive Diabetes Care (ACDC) is a "nurse-administered telehealth intervention for veterans with poor diabetes control despite standard diabetes care" (VA Diffusion Marketplace, 2013).
- Staff-level practice: Stay-In-Veterans Affairs (SIVA) is "modeled after an industry best practice referred to as 'Stay Interviews', which involve questions designed to encourage dialogue between a supervisor and employee" to improve employee retention (VA Diffusion Marketplace, 2017b).
- System-level practice: Machine Learning Decision Support (MLDS) is a platform that identifies "anomalies in clinician benefit decisions involved in billing events with high precision" (VA Diffusion Marketplace, 2017a).

The inner and outer settings

The inner setting was each Veterans Health Administration facility that was implementing an evidence-informed practice. The Veterans Health Administration is the largest integrated healthcare system in the United States; it has over 1000 medical centres, community-based outpatient clinics, and other entities, and serves 9.6 million enrolled US military veterans. The outer setting included the broader Veterans Health Administration network as well as local, state, and national settings.

The individuals: Deliverers

Deliverers included Veterans Health Administration staff who were leading evidence-informed practices for other staff (e.g. Veterans Health Administration supervisors in SIVA) or patients (e.g. the telehealth nurses in ACDC).

The individuals: Recipients

Recipients included Veterans Health Administration staff who were receiving an evidence-informed practice from other Veterans Health Administration staff (e.g. Veterans Health Administration employees in SIVA) or patients receiving an evidence-informed practice from Veterans Health Administration staff (e.g. veterans with diabetes in ACDC).

The implementation process

The DoE provided 6 months of external implementation support for teams that were replicating an evidence-informed practice in a new facility (Nevedal et al., 2020). After each facility identified an implementation lead, they attended training and met with the practice developer and an external implementation facilitator to develop an implementation plan. During implementation, the external facilitator helped teams overcome barriers and provided project management expertise, including coordinating weekly meetings and tracking tasks and milestones.

Data collection: Implementation determinants

Semi-structured telephone interviews were conducted using an interview guide based on CFIR (Nevedal et al., 2021). An external evaluation team conducted interviews with 72 participants involved in replicating practices across 16 facilities (3–6 interviews per facility).

Data collection: Implementation outcomes

The interview inquired about implementation outcomes emerged from the interviews and the extent to which practice components were or were not implemented. A three-level ordinal scale was used for the coding: no implementation, partial implementation, and full implementation.

Data analysis

A rapid qualitative approach was used in this case (i.e. CFIR-based directed content analysis; Hsieh and Shannon, 2005) to analyse and rate data from interview notes and audio recordings. The primary analyst wrote detailed notes during the interviews and immediately coded them into an MS Excel CFIR construct by facility matrix, and then a secondary analyst listened to audio recordings and edited the matrix. Analysts used a codebook with deductive CFIR constructs as well as inductive codes not captured in CFIR that were relevant to the evaluation. The analysts met weekly to adjudicate differences and refine the codebook.

The primary analyst reviewed matrix summaries to determine a rating for each CFIR construct and wrote a high-level summary for each facility, and then the secondary analyst reviewed and edited the matrix. Similar to case 1, ratings were determined based on two factors: (1) valence (positive or negative influence on implementation) and (2) strength (weak or strong influence on implementation). The analysts met weekly to adjudicate differences in ratings. The matrix was ordered by implementation outcomes and used for case and cross-case analysis and interpretation. For additional detail on this approach compared with the traditional in-depth approach using CFIR, see Nevedal et al. (2021).

Results

Similar to previous DoE cohorts (Nevedal et al., 2020), the extensive implementation support provided by the DoE resulted in implementation success, unless the team encountered insurmountable barriers related to engaging innovation deliverers or obtaining available resources. In this cohort, there was confusion around the staffing and resources necessary to implement some of the evidence-informed practices, and feedback to DoE leadership included additional criteria for presenting an evidence-informed practice in Shark Tank and bidding on a practice.

Reflections on the use of CFIR

The traditional in-depth approach (CFIR-based directed content analysis) using interview transcripts was used to evaluate the implementation of evidence-informed practices in previous DoE cohorts (Nevedal et al., 2020) (the same approach used in case 1). When comparing the approaches across cohorts (which had similar interview audio hours), it was found that the rapid approach (CFIR-based directed content analysis using notes and audio recordings) was less time intensive and eliminated transcription costs, yet was effective in meeting evaluation objectives with rigour (Nevedal et al., 2021).

Although this rapid approach was beneficial for this team, researchers should consider the level of team expertise in CFIR. Although some previous literature suggests that traditional in-depth qualitative analysis requires more intense training than rapid analysis (Neal et al., 2015; Gale et al., 2019), this rapid approach may be more suited to researchers who already have a strong foundation in CFIR, allowing them to rapidly code qualitative data into CFIR constructs in real time. However, even for skilled researchers, rapid analysis intensified the effort and cognitive load during the initial coding phase; for example, a 3-hour calendar block was required to conduct the interview and code the data.

Researchers should also consider what level of detail is needed for data analysis and the presentation of results (Neal et al., 2015). As articulated in previous research, rapid approaches using notes and audio recordings provide a "big picture" view, yielding a lower level of detail than transcript-based approaches (Neal et al., 2015). However, although the rapid approach provided less detail, it allowed the team to see both the overall patterns and the important details in the data more rapidly and efficiently (i.e. seeing both the forest and the trees). However, for a project that requires a high level of detail and/or long quotations, the rapid approach may not be appropriate.

Case 3: Using CFIR to assess context and inform implementation strategy development: surveys and quantitative analysis

This case used CFIR to conduct a context assessment to inform the development of strategies to improve the implementation of early palliative care for patients with newly diagnosed advanced solid cancer in the United States (Rosenblum et al., 2022). Early palliative care is an evidence-informed practice intended not to cure but to improve the quality of life and patient-centredness of care for people living with a serious illness (e.g. advanced cancer). However, this practice has not been widely adopted by oncology clinicians (Hausner et al., 2021); as a result, the team developed a CFIR-based survey to understand key barriers and facilitators to future active implementation.

The innovation: early palliative care consultation for patients with a new cancer diagnosis

Since 2016, the American Society of Clinical Oncology has recommended that all patients with new diagnoses of advanced solid cancer receive dedicated specialty palliative care services concurrent with cancer-directed therapy within 8 weeks of diagnosis (Ferrell et al., 2017). Specialty palliative care is provided by a trained palliative care expert, rather than by the oncology or primary care team.

The inner and outer settings

The inner setting was each surveyed outpatient specialty palliative care clinic; these clinics are associated with National Cancer Institute-Designated Cancer Centers in the

United States. They receive referrals from oncologists and are led by palliative care clinicians. The outer setting included the broader context of academic medicine in the United States.

The individuals: Deliverers

The deliverers were oncology and palliative care clinicians.

The individuals: Recipients

The recipients were patients with a recent diagnosis of advanced solid cancer.

The implementation process

Not applicable; the recommendation for early specialty palliative care was provided in published guidelines but not actively implemented before data collection.

Data collection

Working with CFIR developers, the team developed a CFIR-based survey to administer to clinicians. The survey asked respondents to rate their agreement with statements presented as facilitators on a Likert scale, ranging from +2 (representing strong agreement) to −2 (representing strong disagreement). For three statements, the respondents were asked to elaborate on their Likert score selection with an open text response. The constructs selected and tailored for this project were those that were deemed to be relevant by palliative care and oncology clinicians, who were consulted for the development of the survey. Items were revised iteratively to assess determinants of early palliative care implementation with parenthetical examples that were anticipated to be relevant to the respondents. The survey was then sent electronically to oncology and outpatient palliative care clinician leaders at each eligible outpatient clinic. Responses were collected in Qualtrics.

Data analysis

Data were analysed descriptively, summarizing the frequency of survey item responses according to the Likert score level and identifying the most agreed upon facilitators and barriers among all respondents. A total composite score was calculated for each site by summing the Likert scores of all 31 survey items and was used to compare clinics of different sizes and maturity.

Results

Forty ($n = 60$; 67%) eligible sites responded to the survey; most informants were palliative care clinicians rather than oncologists (Rosenblum et al., 2022). The most common barriers endorsed were related to the following CFIR constructs: difficulties engaging innovation deliverers (i.e. palliative care clinicians), limited available resources (i.e. clinic space), absence of performance measure pressure, and inadequate interdisciplinary networks and communication. Although clinic size and maturity were not significantly associated with the total composite score, the most frequently reported barriers did differ when stratified by these site characteristics.

Reflections on the use of CFIR

The high response rate to the survey demonstrates the acceptability of this approach to clinicians. The survey provided rapid data from multiple respondents that could be used to quickly identify patterns and differences between types of sites and informants. Because surveys require few resources to collect and analyse data, this approach is feasible in busy academic medical settings. Future work will help clarify how respondents interpreted the questions and how that could be improved. Plans also include assessing the construct validity of survey items by comparing them with data collected using semi-structured interviews. Methods to optimize the survey constructs and to summarize the data are also needed. These data were evaluated using the total composite score, ratios of facilitators to barriers, and domain aggregates, with advantages and limitations associated with each method. Evaluating the associations of each score with implementation success will further elucidate the methods of analysis and survey items that are most important to collect.

Concluding remarks

CFIR is an important implementation science framework and, as demonstrated in this chapter, an adaptable one. CFIR can be used to empirically explain the mechanisms of action of implementation strategies through traditional in-depth qualitative methods (case 1); CFIR can be used to provide feedback to interested parties on an implementation effort more quickly through more rapid qualitative methods (case 2); and CFIR can be used to assess context and quickly diagnosis implementation barriers through quantitative survey methods, potentially informing the development of implementation strategies (case 3).

Each approach involves trade-offs in terms of the burden on respondents, resource intensity (researcher time and transcription cost), researcher expertise, data richness and rigour (Table 14.2). The traditional in-depth qualitative CFIR approach (i.e. case 1) is the most resource intensive, yet yields the richest data, and would be most appropriate for use in theory building, which was a goal of case 1 using GTO. The rapid qualitative CFIR approach (i.e. case 2) is less resource intensive, requiring fewer analyst hours and eliminating the cost of transcription, but requires experienced analysts to simultaneously conduct interviews and code notes. This rapid approach yields data on the bigger picture (i.e. less rich) compared with traditional in-depth qualitative analysis. The burden on respondents is the same for these two methods. The survey CFIR approach (i.e. case 3) is the least resource intensive and minimizes participant burden but does not yield qualitative data. In addition, the CFIR-based survey needs to be validated against semi-structured interviews to ensure construct validity.

The cases also highlight how different approaches may have different levels of utility depending on whether the evidence-informed practice is completely new to the implementing setting (cases 1 and 2) or somewhat known to the organization but not used as much as it could be (case 3). When a practice is completely new, it may be challenging to ask about perceptions of barriers in the absence of experience with the practice, and thus it may make more sense to ask after implementation has started. As in case 3, when the practice is known but underutilized, asking about barriers at the start allows respondents to draw upon actual experience with the practice, and using a survey makes data collection an efficient way to link barriers to potential implementation strategies.

Table 14.2 Case comparison: trade-offs based on research design.

	Case 1	Case 2	Case 3
Research design			
Purpose	Post-implementation evaluation	Post-implementation evaluation	Pre-implementation context assessment (to inform strategy development)[a]
Data collection approach	Semi-structured interviews	Semi-structured interviews	Survey
Data analysis approach	Traditional in-depth qualitative analysis	Rapid qualitative analysis	Quantitative analysis
	Coding: CFIR-based directed content analysis using interview transcripts	Coding: CFIR-based directed content analysis using interview notes and audio recordings	Descriptive statistics and associations with clinic characteristics
	Rating: Strength and valence assessments based on full construct data in case memos	Rating: Strength and valence assessments based on construct summaries in a matrix	
Trade-offs			
Participant burden	High (45- to 60-minute interview)	High (45- to 60-minute interview)	Low (5- to 10-minute survey)
Analyst hours	High	Medium	Low
Analyst CFIR expertise	Medium-high	High (simultaneous data collection and coding with no transcript)	Low
Transcription delay + cost	Yes	No	N/A
Data richness	High (transcript + recording; lengthy quotations)	Medium-high (recording only; short quotations)	Limited qualitative data (three Likert statements with an open-text box)
Rigour	High	High	Medium (survey not validated against interview)

[a] The recommendation for early specialty palliative care was provided in published guidelines but not actively implemented before data collection.

These conclusions are consistent with findings from a 2020 survey completed by 134 CFIR users about the framework (Damschroder et al., 2022a, 2022b). Following Flottorp et al.'s (2013) "sensibility" criteria for determinant frameworks (comprehensiveness, relevance, applicability, simplicity, logic, clarity, usability, suitability, usefulness), two of the lowest-rated criteria were simplicity and usability, suggesting that the availability of a CFIR survey would be a useful complement to the qualitative approaches. In addition, over 40% and 25% of respondents had recommendations to add or remove domains/constructs, respectively.

CFIR's adaptability makes for an expansive future research agenda for the framework. For example, it will be important to compare data from the different methods discussed in this chapter, especially the traditional in-depth qualitative approach versus the survey approach. The authors are planning to collect both survey and in-depth interview data from the same respondents, which will allow for psychometric validity comparisons between the two methods. If found to be comparable, it would then be possible to experiment with using a combination of interviews and surveys in the same project, perhaps matching different methods to different respondents. Evaluating which CFIR constructs predict implementation outcomes across different evidence-informed practices is another worthy research pursuit. Empirical methods are needed to more efficiently match CFIR barriers to implementation strategies beyond the gut instinct, convenience, and "kitchen sink" approaches often adopted by clinicians or the complex methods (e.g. concept mapping and implementation mapping) often adopted by implementation science experts.

Acknowledgements

We acknowledge Sandra Gibson for her assistance with the preparation of this chapter.

References

Acosta, J., Chinman, M., Ebener, P., Malone, P.S., Paddock, S., Phillips, A., et al. (2013) An intervention to improve program implementation: findings from a two-year cluster randomized trial of assets-getting to outcomes. *Implementation Sci* 8, 87. https://doi.org/10.1186/1748-5908-8-87

Ajzen, I., Fishbein, M. (1977) Attitude-behavior relations: a theoretical analysis and review of empirical research. *Psychological Bulletin* 84, 888–918. https://doi.org/10.1037/0033-2909.84.5.888

Bandura, A. (1977) Self-efficacy: toward a unifying theory of behavioral change. *Psychological Review* 84, 191–215. https://doi.org/10.1037/0033-295X.84.2.191

Bandura, A. (1997) *Self-Efficacy: The Exercise Of Control*. New York: WH Freeman/Times Books/ Henry Holt.

Bandura, A. (2004) Health promotion by social cognitive means. *Health Education & Behavior* 31, 143–164. https://doi.org/10.1177/1090198104263660

Cannon, J.S., Gilbert, M., Ebener, P., Malone, P.S., Reardon, C.M., Acosta, J., et al. (2019) Influence of an implementation support intervention on barriers and facilitators to delivery of a substance use prevention program. *Prevention Science* 20, 1200–1210. https://doi.org/10.1007/s11121-019-01037-x

Chinman, M., Imm, P., Wandersman, A. (2004) *Getting To Outcomes 2004: Promoting Accountability Through Methods and Tools for Planning, Implementation, and Evaluation*. Santa Monica, CA: Rand Corporation.

Chinman, M., Acosta, J., Ebener, P., Burkhart, Q., Malone, P.S., Paddock, S.M., et al. (2013a) Intervening with practitioners to improve the quality of prevention: one-year findings from a randomized trial of assets-getting to outcomes. *Journal of Primary Prevention* 34, 173–191. https://doi.org/10.1007/s10935-013-0302-7

Chinman, M., Acosta, J., Ebener, P., Driver, J., Keith, J., Peebles, D. (2013b) Enhancing Quality Interventions Promoting Healthy Sexuality (EQUIPS): a novel application of translational research methods. *Clinical and Translational Science* 6, 232–237. https://doi.org/10.1111/cts.12031

Chinman, M., Acosta, J., Ebener, P., Malone, P.S., Slaughter, M.E. (2016) Can implementation support help community-based settings better deliver evidence-based sexual health promotion programs? a randomized trial of Getting to Outcomes(R). *Implementation Science* 11, 78. https:// doi.org/10.1186/s13012-016-0446-y

D'Amico, E.J., Edelen, M.O. (2007) Pilot test of project choice: a voluntary afterschool intervention for middle school youth. *Psychology of Addictive Behaviors* 21, 592–598. https://doi.org/10.1007/s11121-011-0269-7

D'Amico, E.J., Tucker, J.S., Miles, J.N., Zhou, A.J., Shih, R.A., Green Jr., H.D. (2012) Preventing alcohol use with a voluntary after-school program for middle school students: results from a cluster randomized controlled trial of choice. *Prevention Science* 13, 415–425. https://doi.org/10.1007/s11121-011-0269-7

Damschroder, L.J., Aron, D.C., Keith, R.E., Kirsh, S.R., Alexander, J.A., Lowery, J.C. (2009) Fostering implementation of health services research findings into practice: a consolidated framework for advancing implementation science. *Implementation Science* 4, 50. https://doi.org/10.1186/1748-5908-4-50

Damschroder, L.J., Goodrich, D.E., Robinson, C.H., Fletcher, C.E., Lowery, J.C. (2011) A systematic exploration of differences in contextual factors related to implementing the move! weight management program in VA: a mixed methods study. *BMC Health Services Research* 11, 248. https://doi.org/10.1186/1472-6963-11-248

Damschroder, L.J., Reardon, C.M., Auyoung, M., Moin, T., Datta, S.K., Sparks, J.B., et al. (2017a) Implementation findings from a hybrid III implementation-effectiveness trial of the Diabetes Prevention Program (DPP) in the Veterans Health Administration (VHA). *Implementation Science* 12, 94. https://doi.org/10.1186/s13012-017-0619-3

Damschroder, L.J., Reardon, C.M., Sperber, N., Robinson, C.H., Fickel, J.J., Oddone, E.Z. (2017b) Implementation evaluation of the Telephone Lifestyle Coaching (TLC) program: organizational factors associated with successful implementation. *Translational Behavioral Medicine* 7, 233–241. https://doi.org/10.1007/s13142-016-0424-6

Damschroder, L.J., Reardon, C.M., Opra Widerquist, M.A., Lowery, J. (2022a) Conceptualizing outcomes for use with the Consolidated Framework For Implementation Research (CFIR): the CFIR outcomes addendum. *Implementation Science* 17, 7. https://doi.org/10.1186/s13012-021-01181-5

Damschroder, L.J., Reardon, C.M., Widerquist, M.A.O., Lowery, J. (2022b) The updated Consolidated Framework for Implementation Research based on user feedback. *Implementation Science* 17, 75. https://doi.org/10.1186/s13012-022-01245-0

Durlak, J.A., Dupre, E.P. (2008) Implementation matters: a review of research on the influence of implementation on program outcomes and the factors affecting implementation. *American Journal of Community Psychology* 41, 327–350. https://doi.org/10.1007/s10464-008-9165-0

Ferrell, B.R., Temel, J.S., Temin, S., Alesi, E.R., Balboni, T.A., Basch, E.M., et al. (2017) Integration of palliative care into standard oncology care: American Society of Clinical Oncology Clinical Practice Guideline Update. *Journal of Clinical Oncology* 35, 96–112. https://doi.org/10.1200/JCO.2016.70.1474

Fishbein, M., Ajzen, I. (1975) *Belief, Attitude, Intention, and Behavior: An Introduction to Theory and Research*. Reading, MA: Addison-Wesley.

Flottorp, S.A., Oxman, A.D., Krause, J., Musila, N.R., Wensing, M., Godycki-Cwirko, M., et al. (2013) A checklist for identifying determinants of practice: a systematic review and synthesis of frameworks and taxonomies of factors that prevent or enable improvements in healthcare professional practice. *Implementation Science* 8, 35. https://doi.org/10.1186/1748-5908-8-35

Gale, R.C., Wu, J., Erhardt, T., Bounthavong, M., Reardon, C.M., Damschroder, L.J.et al. (2019) Comparison of rapid vs in-depth qualitative analytic methods from a process evaluation of academic detailing in the Veterans Health Administration. *Implementation Science* 14, 11. https://doi.org/10.1186/s13012-019-0853-y

Hausner, D., Tricou, C., Mathews, J., Wadhwa, D., Pope, A., Swami, N., et al. (2021) Timing of palliative care referral before and after evidence from trials supporting early palliative care. *Oncologist* 26, 332–340. https://doi.org/10.1002/onco.13625

Hsieh, H.F., Shannon, S.E. (2005) Three approaches to qualitative content analysis. *Qualitative Health Research* 15, 1277–1288. https://doi.org/10.1177/1049732305276687

Kahneman, D., Tversky, A. (2000) *Choices, Values, and Frames*, New York: Cambridge University Press. https://doi.org/10.1017/CBO9780511803475

Livet, M., Wandersman, A. (2005) Organizational functioning: facilitating effective interventions and increasing the odds of programming success. In: Fetterman, D.M., Wandersman, A. (Eds.), *Empowerment Evaluation Principles in Practice*. New York: Guilford Press.

Miller, W.R., Rollnick, S. (2013) *Motivational Interviewing: Helping People Change*. 3rd edition. New York: Guilford Press.

Neal, J.W., Neal, Z.P., Vandyke, E., Kornbluh, M. (2015) Expediting the analysis of qualitative data in evaluation: a procedure for the Rapid Identification of Themes from Audio Recordings (RITA). *American Journal of Evaluation* 36, 118–132. https://doi.org/10.1177/1098214014536601

Nevedal, A.L., Reardon, C.M., Jackson, G.L., Cutrona, S.L., White, B., Gifford, A.L., et al. (2020) Implementation and sustainment of diverse practices in a large integrated health system: a mixed methods study. *Implementation Science Communications* 1, 61. https://doi.org/10.1186/s43058-020-00053-1

Nevedal, A.L., Reardon, C.M., Opra Widerquist, M.A., Jackson, G.L., Cutrona, S.L., White, B.S. et al. (2021) Rapid Versus traditional qualitative analysis using the Consolidated Framework for Implementation Research (CFIR). *Implementation Science* 16, 67. https://doi.org/10.1186/s13012-021-01111-5

Reardon, C., Nevedal, A., Widerquist, M.A.O., Arasim, M., Jackson, G.L., White, B., et al. (2021). Sustainment of diverse evidence-informed practices disseminated in the Veterans Health Administration (VHA): initial development and piloting of a pragmatic instrument. Preprint. https://doi.org/10.21203/rs.3.rs-951440/v2 (accessed 3 November 2022).

Rosenblum, R.E., Rogal, S.S., Park, E.R., Impagliazzo, C., Abdulhay, L.B., Grosse, P.J., et al. (2022) National survey using CFIR to assess early outpatient specialty palliative care implementation. *Journal of Pain and Symptom Management* 65, e175–e180. https://doi.org/10.1016/j.jpainsymman.2022.11.019

VA Diffusion Marketplace (2013) *Advanced Comprehensive Diabetes Care (ACDC)*. https://marketplace.va.gov/innovations/advanced-comprehensive-diabetes-care-acdc (accessed 2 November, 2022).

VA Diffusion Marketplace (2017a) *Machine Learning Decision Support (MLDS)*. https://marketplace.va.gov/innovations/utilizing-machine-learning-uml (accessed 2 November 2022).

VA Diffusion Marketplace (2017b) *Stay in VA*. https://marketplace.va.gov/innovations/rn-stay-interviews-a-nurse-retention-strategy (accessed 2 November 2022).

15 Applying the integrated Promoting Action on Research Implementation in Health Services framework

Sarah C. Hunter, Gillian Harvey and Alison L. Kitson

Introduction

The integrated Promoting Action on Research Implementation in Health Services (i-PARIHS) framework was developed as a practical tool to help clinicians or managers get evidence or research into practice. Originally developed as the PARIHS framework, it was generated inductively through case studies of attempts to implement clinical guidelines (Kitson et al., 1998, 2008; Rycroft-Malone et al., 2002, 2004a). The i-PARIHS framework is a revision of the PARIHS framework, developed through multiple iterations from being used by clinicians and researchers (Harvey and Kitson, 2015, 2016).

This chapter illustrates the flexibility of the i-PARIHS framework by showing how it can be applied at different stages of the implementation process (pre-implementation, conducting implementation and post-implementation). Research has outlined how appropriately and comprehensively applying implementation frameworks is one of many challenges faced by researchers and clinicians (Birken et al., 2017; Lynch et al., 2018). Facilitation, enacted by one or more individuals in facilitator roles, is a distinguishing feature of the i-PARIHS framework (Harvey and Kitson, 2015). However, this can be a difficult role to operationalize, particularly for new or novice users of i-PARIHS, due to the context-responsive and iterative nature of facilitation.

The three cases presented in this chapter reflect some of the different ways in which i-PARIHS can be applied. Cases 1 and 2 use i-PARIHS prospectively and case 3 uses i-PARIHS retrospectively. Case 1 uses solely qualitative measures, whereas cases 2 and 3 draw upon multiple methods. A mixed-method analysis is applied in case 3. Case 1 outlines a pre-implementation project, case 2 outlines an implementation project, and case 3 outlines a post-implementation evaluation. A facilitation process is applied only in case 2. However, despite not operationalizing the facilitation construct, the other two cases ultimately reflect and conclude the importance of facilitation. Table 15.1 provides a high-level overview of the background information for each project.

Table 15.1 Summary of each case.

	Case 1	*Case 2*	*Case 3*
Intervention and key references	Management of traumatic brain injury behaviour (Block et al., 2023)	Oral healthcare intervention (Lewis et al., 2022; Murray et al., 2023)	Specialized vestibular physiotherapy (Ip et al., 2022)
Project dates	2022	2020–2022	2018–2019

(Continued)

DOI: 10.4324/9781003318125-17

Table 15.1 (Continued)

	Case 1	Case 2	Case 3
Purpose	Prospective pre-implementation planning	Prospective implementation study	Retrospective post-implementation evaluation
Aims	Investigate staff's perceptions of barriers and enablers to implementing evidence-informed approaches in the management of traumatic brain injury behaviour in an acute hospital setting	Co-design, implement and evaluate an oral healthcare intervention for older adults in a geriatric evaluation unit	Evaluate the process of implementing specialized vestibular physiotherapy (SPV) in an emergency department from the clinician's perspective
Method	Qualitative	Multi-methods	Mixed-method
Data collection	Semi-structured focus groups	Context assessment, semi-structured interviews, and clinical audits	Surveys, semi-structured interviews, and focus groups
Data analysis	Inductive and deductive thematic analysis	Context assessments were analysed using narrative descriptions, interviews were analysed using content analysis, and audits were analysed using percentages	Quantitative data were analysed using descriptive statistics and qualitative data were analysed using thematic analysis

Case 1: Using i-PARIHS prospectively for pre-implementation planning

This case used i-PARIHS in a pre-implementation study to understand staff perspectives on managing challenging behaviours following a traumatic brain injury (TBI) in the acute care setting.

- Problem: guideline recommendations for managing challenging behaviours following acute TBI are poorly implemented in acute hospital settings.
- Innovation: implementation of clinical guideline recommendations for behaviour management of challenging behaviours following acute TBI.
- Context: acute hospital and subacute specialized inpatient brain injury rehabilitation unit in Australia.
- Recipients: multi-disciplinary staff.
- Facilitation: no facilitation roles or processes undertaken.

Application of i-PARIHS

This project formed part of a broader PhD study focused on implementing clinical guideline recommendations for the management of challenging behaviours following TBI within the context of acute inpatient hospital settings. As part of the background literature review for this PhD, it was identified that there is limited research on the factors that enhance or impede the implementation of evidence-informed improvements for TBI behaviour management within the context of acute care. Therefore, it was identified that there was a need for systematic exploration into the barriers, enablers and contextual factors that may influence the implementation of TBI behaviour management in the acute care setting.

This study used the i-PARIHS framework to conduct pre-implementation focus groups with staff to investigate barriers and enablers to implementing evidence-informed approaches in TBI behaviour management. Specifically, i-PARIHS was used to identify the innovation-related, recipient and contextual barriers and enablers to enable the development of a tailored implementation plan to improve TBI behaviour management in the acute hospital setting.

Data collection

Focus groups were conducted with multi-disciplinary staff from both an acute and subacute context to investigate staff (recipient) perspectives of barriers and enablers. The acute hospital setting was a major trauma hospital with a 16-bed neurosurgery unit for patients with TBI requiring neurosurgery intervention and care within the intensive care unit, high-dependency ward and neurosurgery ward. The subacute rehabilitation setting was a specialized state-wide brain injury rehabilitation unit with 24 beds for patients recovering from TBI with a rehabilitative focus in preparation for discharge to the community setting. Participants included staff from both settings to gain perspectives on TBI behaviour management throughout the recovery phase in acute settings with transition to inpatient rehabilitation. Semi-structured question guides were developed to facilitate discussion during the focus groups. The question guides were developed considering the constructs of the i-PARIHS framework.

Data analysis

Transcripts from the focus groups were initially coded inductively using an iterative process, focusing on descriptive content and processes reported by participants. Second-round coding was completed using a deductive approach, mapping against the i-PARIHS constructs of innovation, recipients and context. Themes were generated that best represented the barriers and enablers for the implementation of evidence-informed TBI behaviour management in the acute setting.

Reflections

This case used i-PARIHS in the pre-implementation phase to understand the system, organizational, clinician and patient contextual factors to inform a specific and tailored implementation approach to facilitate successful adoption of evidence into practice. By doing this, the authors were able to identify likely barriers and enablers before implementation. Key barriers related to the innovation and context included limited applicability of the evidence (staff felt that aspects of the behaviour management approach were difficult to apply in the unpredictable context of an acute ward) and hospital

systems and resources (staff felt the focus was on acute intervention and not prevention), and the overstimulating and unsecured hospital context did not align with the
behaviour management approach. Key enablers related to the recipients (staff felt a
commitment to person-centred care and reflected on supportive teamwork). By applying i-PARIHS to systematically understand the barriers and enablers, this case was able
to develop and recommend a robust implementation approach that highlighted the
need for facilitation to improve evidence-informed TBI behaviour management in the
hospital setting.

Case 2: Using i-PARIHS prospectively for conducting an implementation project

This case used i-PARIHS prospectively in an implementation study to implement and
evaluate an oral healthcare intervention for older adults in an acute hospital.

- Problem: hospitalized older adults are at high risk of poor oral health, which carries
  an increased risk of systemic infection and malnutrition affecting overall health, psy-
  chological health, quality of life, and well-being.
- Innovation: implementation of clinical guideline recommendations for oral healthcare
  for older adults in the acute care setting.
- Context: geriatric evaluation and management ward in an acute Australian hospital.
- Recipients: multi-disciplinary ward staff and hospitalized older adults.
- Facilitation: internal-external model of facilitation based on i-PARIHS.

Application of i-PARIHS

This project was a partnership between a university, a hospital, and a state-wide dental
service and focused on implementing clinical guideline recommendations for oral healthcare for older adults in one geriatric evaluation and management ward in an acute hospital. This project used i-PARIHS to inform the overall implementation and evaluation of
the oral healthcare intervention.

i-PARIHS was used to assess the context and recipients at multiple time points and
informed a multi-level facilitation approach. The multi-level facilitation approach navigated individuals and teams through the complex change processes involved, both at the
local ward level and the system-wide level, and the contextual challenges encountered.
Facilitation included two internal novice facilitators (one nurse and one speech patholo-
gist), four external experienced facilitators (based at the university and dental service)
and an external expert facilitator (based at the university). This facilitation team was
supported by a project reference group that included various staff at the hospital in leadership roles.

The facilitation approach allowed for an examination of baseline oral healthcare
practice, identification of gaps against clinical guideline recommendations, and the
development of multi-disciplinary team strategies to implement and sustain evidence-
based practice. The facilitation approach also allowed the project team to build
capacity in the hospital workforce to undertake future implementation projects, inclusive of undertaking context assessments and tailoring evidence and implementation
strategies.

Data collection

To evaluate the feasibility and success of the implementation project, data were collected from multiple sources using various methods:

1 The context was assessed at three time points (pre-, mid-, and post-implementation) by the internal novice facilitators, with support from one of the external experienced facilitators, using the Mi-PARIHS Facilitation Planning Tool (Hunter et al., 2023). The Mi-PARIHS Facilitation Planning Tool (Hunter et al., 2023) was developed to support the assessment of the implementation context and the development of tailored implementation and facilitation strategies. This project used the tool to evaluate how the inner context of the local ward level, the inner context organization level, and the outer context of the broader healthcare system shaped the experience of recipients (ward staff and patients) and the uptake of the innovation.

2 Semi-structured interviews were conducted at three time points (pre-, mid- and post-implementation) with the recipients, both staff and hospitalized older adults:

   (a) Staff interviews focused on perceptions of the implementation project with respect to the contextual barriers and enablers, the process of facilitation, and the acceptability and feasibility of the innovation.
   (b) Hospitalized older adult interviews focused on their oral health literacy, beliefs, and experiences while in hospital.

3 A project-specific audit tool was developed to measure oral healthcare practice against best-practice standards, and this was conducted at two time points (pre- and post-implementation).

Data analysis

A multi-method approach was taken to analyse the quantitative and qualitative data. Narrative descriptions were written summarizing the context at each time point. Both staff and hospitalized older adult interviews were analysed using descriptive content analysis. Audit data results were tabulated and compliance against best practice was analysed as percentages. Key findings and implementation success were considered in the discussion.

Reflections

This case identified the importance of pre-implementation planning at an early stage (Murray et al., 2023). In this example, the management of the health service was interested in improving oral healthcare for older patients and therefore engaged the research team to support the implementation of clinical guideline recommendations. However, local ward staff were not engaged from the beginning and subsequently felt the project was pushed on them. This created significant contextual barriers from the outset. In addition, despite the planned comprehensive model of facilitation, COVID-19-related restrictions resulted in the external facilitators not being able to go on site. This left the internal novice facilitators with limited support. Positively, the use of i-PARIHS in this case highlighted the need to facilitate changes at both the local level and the system level to make impactful and sustainable changes.

Case 3: Using i-PARIHS retrospectively for post-implementation data analysis

This case used i-PARIHS retrospectively in a mixed-methods process evaluation to understand the process of implementing specialized vestibular physiotherapy in an emergency department.

- Problem: failure to accurately diagnose and treat benign paroxysmal peripheral vertigo (BPPV) during an initial presentation can result in adverse outcomes for patients. BPPV can be diagnosed and treated using specialized vestibular physiotherapy, however, it is not routinely implemented in the emergency department context.
- Innovation: implementation of specialized vestibular physiotherapy in the emergency department context.
- Context: specialized vestibular physiotherapy was implemented in one emergency department of an acute tertiary metropolitan Australian hospital.
- Recipients: clinicians with direct experience in implementing the specialized vestibular physiotherapy service in the emergency department at the study site.
- Facilitation: no facilitation roles or processes were undertaken.

Application of i-PARIHS

This project, a process evaluation, formed part of a larger project focused on evaluating the implementation of specialized vestibular physiotherapy in the emergency department (Lloyd et al., 2020). In the pilot implementation project, no implementation framework was used, and the specialized vestibular physiotherapy was evaluated against usual care through a pre-post design (Lloyd et al., 2020). The innovation introduced in this study was having physiotherapists routinely assess and treat people presenting with BPPV, rather than the usual care of medical intervention only. The pilot project found that this innovation was safe and feasible, and had a positive impact on adherence to evidence-based practice (Lloyd et al., 2020).

In the process evaluation, i-PARIHS was used to examine a secondary aim of understanding the implementation context. To achieve this, i-PARIHS was applied retrospectively after the completion of the pilot project (Lloyd et al., 2020) to understand how specialized vestibular physiotherapy functioned in the Australian emergency department and identify any barriers or enablers to the implementation process. Specifically, a researcher with implementation expertise, who was not involved in the pilot project, joined the project team to support the application of i-PARIHS to evaluate the implementation process.

Data collection

Data were collected by purposive sampling of clinicians who had direct experience with implementing the specialized vestibular physiotherapy service in the emergency department trial (Lloyd et al., 2020) as well as study team members who were crucial to the design and implementation of the service (Lloyd et al., 2020). The following data were collected from these participants:

1 The Organisational Readiness for Change Assessment (ORCA) (Helfrich et al., 2009) is a 77-item checklist designed to operationalize the constructs of the PARIHS framework (Kitson et al., 1998, 2008; Harvey et al., 2002; Rycroft-Malone et al., 2004b). The ORCA was completed to understand the factors influencing the implementation process.

2 Implementation outcome measures, not originally developed for i-PARIHS, were used to evaluate implementation success. To support analysis against the i-PARIHS framework, the items on each of the measures were categorized against the i-PARIHS constructs of facilitation, innovation, recipients and context. The implementation outcome measures were:

- Acceptability of Intervention Measure (AIM) (Weiner et al., 2017).
- Feasibility of Intervention Measure (FIM) (Weiner et al., 2017).
- Intervention Appropriateness Measure (IAM) (Weiner et al., 2017).

3 Qualitative data were collected via semi-structured interviews and focus groups. Both were based on the i-PARIHS constructs and then general reflections on the implementation process were discussed.

Data analysis

A convergent parallel model of mixed methods was used to analyse the quantitative and qualitative data (Cresswell and Plano, 2018). This involves concurrent collection of the qualitative and quantitative data and both are given equal value when analysing and interpreting the results (Cresswell and Plano, 2018). The quantitative data were presented against the i-PARIHS constructs and the qualitative focus group and interview data were coded against an i-PARIHS codebook. Both quantitative and qualitative findings for each i-PARIHS construct were integrated for a final mixed-methods analysis outlining implementation success.

Reflections

The application of i-PARIHS in this retrospective process evaluation of an implementation study identified the clinician and research team perspectives on implementing specialized vestibular physiotherapy in an emergency department. A variety of barriers and enablers to the implementation process were identified by some of the participants and these spanned the multiple domains of i-PARIHS. For example, the roles of leadership and champions were identified as crucial for successful facilitation. This was identified even though a facilitation process or role was not used in the pilot project (Lloyd et al., 2020).

This case demonstrates successful application of i-PARIHS retrospectively. The initial pilot project did not have an implementation framework informing the design or evaluation (Lloyd et al., 2020). Usually when this happens, project teams refer to an implementation framework superficially in their discussion to make sense of their findings (Bergström et al., 2020). However, this project team designed a separate process evaluation that used i-PARIHS in the planning, data collection, analysis and interpretation to ensure a rigorous and systematic retrospective application of i-PARIHS (Ip et al., 2022) to understand the findings of the initial pilot project (Lloyd et al., 2020).

The reference to the ORCA checklist (Helfrich et al., 2009) as operationalizing the i-PARIHS framework was notable (Harvey and Kitson, 2015, 2016). However, it was actually developed to operationalize the original PARIHS framework (Kitson et al., 1998, 2008; Rycroft-Malone et al., 2002, 2004a). The confusion between the PARIHS and i-PARIHS frameworks is not uncommon and is evident in published articles (Tuepker et al., 2018).

Reflections and future research

The case studies presented in this chapter are examples of the diverse ways in which PhD students, novice facilitators and/or clinicians and novice implementation researchers can use and apply the i-PARIHS framework in their projects. We hope to encourage first-time or novice users by demonstrating how i-PARIHS, although capable of guiding large-scale, complex implementation projects, can also be used in smaller-scale or pilot projects. However, we wanted to demonstrate that this does not mean the framework cannot be applied in flexible or creative ways, and so we have showcased that i-PARIHS can be applied successfully at the pre-implementation, implementation and post-implementation stages to inform, guide and understand implementation processes. We have also highlighted how i-PARIHS can be used in qualitative, multi-method and mixed-method designs.

We have highlighted the ways in which i-PARIHS can be used in discrete projects, but it is important to reflect on the impact this has on sustainability. Discrete projects that have an input of resources, driven by academics or researchers, with a defined beginning and end, often result in the intervention or evidence not being maintained or sustained once the project ends. Facilitation is a mechanism that supports sustainability (Harvey and Kitson, 2015). As identified in case 2, facilitation allowed the project team to build capacity in the workforce to not only support sustainability but also undertake future implementation projects.

Therefore, as we have discussed elsewhere, facilitation is crucial and needs to be embedded across the pre-implementation, implementation and post-implementation phases (Harvey and Kitson, 2020). Although these phases may appear sequential, in practice, the process is much more iterative because barriers and enablers may shift or new ones arise that may necessitate a return to earlier phases (Harvey and Kitson, 2020).

This chapter has reinforced the importance of the facilitation construct within i-PARIHS. Although cases 1 and 3 did not include a facilitation role or process within their study, both identified how crucial facilitation is. Case 1, a pre-implementation study, which resulted in the development of a tailored implementation approach, recommended that facilitation was crucial to managing the complex barriers and enablers that were identified. Case 3, a post-implementation process evaluation, identified that the leadership and local champions were the crucial elements for successful implementation (Ip et al., 2022), even though no formal facilitation role or process was used in the implementation study (Lloyd et al., 2020). Case 2, an implementation study, did have a multi-level facilitation approach, which was critical for successful implementation (Lewis et al., 2022). Therefore, it remains true that the facilitation construct is required to harness the enablers and manage the barriers at the innovation, recipient and context levels. We maintain that i-PARIHS should ideally be used prospectively with deliberate attention to facilitation processes.

We recognize that first-time or novice users of i-PARIHS are likely to apply it in a discrete project to build their capacity and confidence in using the framework. Therefore, we recommend that, when using the framework for the first few times, surround yourself with a team of experienced implementation researchers to support operationalization of the facilitation construct and improve the chances of sustainability. In addition, we are committed to encouraging use of the framework and are therefore continuing to develop a suite of practical resources for using i-PARIHS in planning, conducting and evaluating implementation projects (Harvey and Kitson, 2020; Hunter et al., 2023).

References

Bergström, A., Ehrenberg, A., Eldh, A.C., Graham, I.D., Gustafsson, K., Harvey, G., et al. (2020) The use of the PARIHS framework in implementation research and practice—a citation analysis of the literature. *Implementation Science* 15, 68. https://doi.org/10.1186/s13012-020-01003-0

Birken, S.A., Powell, B.J., Shea, C.M., Haines, E.R., Alexis Kirk, M., Leeman, J., et al. (2017) Criteria for selecting implementation science theories and frameworks: results from an international survey. *Implementation Science* 12, 124. https://doi.org/10.1186/s13012-017-0656-y

Block, H., Bellon, M., Hunter, S.C., George, S. (2023) Barriers and enablers to managing challenging behaviours after traumatic brain injury in the acute hospital setting: a qualitative study. *BMC Health Services Research* 23, 1266. https://doi.org/10.1186/s12913-023-10279-z

Cresswell, J., Plano, C. (2018) *Designing and Conducting Mixed Methods Research*. New York: Sage.

Harvey, G., Kitson, A. (2015) *Implementing Evidence-Based Practice in Healthcare: A Facilitation Guide*. Abingdon, Oxon: Routledge. https://doi.org/10.4324/9780203557334

Harvey, G., Kitson, A. (2016) PARIHS revisited: from heuristic to integrated framework for the successful implementation of knowledge into practice. *Implementation Science* 11, 33. https://doi.org/10.1186/s13012-016-0398-2

Harvey, G., Kitson, A. (2020) Promoting action on research implementation in health services: the integrated-PARIHS framework. In: Nilsen, P., Birken, S.A. (Eds.), *Handbook on Implementation Science*. Cheltenham, UK: Edward Elgar. https://doi.org/10.4337/9781788975995.00012

Harvey, G., Loftus-Hills, A., Rycroft-Malone, J., Titchen, A., Kitson, A., Mccormack, B., et al. (2002) Getting evidence into practice: the role and function of facilitation. *Journal of Advanced Nursing* 37, 577–588. https://doi.org/10.1046/j.1365-2648.2002.02126.x

Helfrich, C.D., Li, Y.-F., Sharp, N.D., Sales, A.E. (2009) Organizational readiness to change assessment (ORCA): development of an instrument based on the promoting action on research in health services (PARIHS) framework. *Implementation Science* 4, 38. https://doi.org/10.1186/1748-5908-4-38

Hunter, S.C., Kim, B., Kitson, A.L. (2023) Mobilising implementation of i-PARIHS (Mi-PARIHS): development of a facilitation planning tool to accompany the integrated Promoting Action on Research Implementation in Health Services framework. *Implementation Science Communications* 4, 2. https://doi.org/10.1186/s43058-022-00379-y

Ip, K., Lloyd, M., Luscombe, A., Hitch, D. (2022) Implementing specialised vestibular physiotherapy in an emergency department: a process evaluation. *Implementation Science Communications* 3, 63. https://doi.org/10.1186/s43058-022-00313-2

Kitson, A., Harvey, G., Mccormack, B. (1998) Enabling the implementation of evidence based practice: a conceptual framework. *Quality in Health Care* 7, 149–158. https://doi.org/10.1136/qshc.7.3.149

Kitson, A.L., Rycroft-Malone, J., Harvey, G., Mccormack, B., Seers, K., Titchen, A. (2008) Evaluating the successful implementation of evidence into practice using the PARIHS framework: theoretical and practical challenges. *Implement ationScience* 3, 1. https://doi.org/10.1186/1748-5908-3-1

Lewis, A., Murray, J., Hunter, S.C., Conroy, T., Kitson, A., Splawinski, Z., et al. (2022) *REDUCE (tRanslating knowlEDge for fUndamental CarE): missed oral healthcare: it takes a team*

(Whittaker Smiles): Project Report. Adelaide: Flinders University. https://researchnow-admin. flinders.edu.au/ws/portalfiles/portal/65084162/REDUCE_missed_oral_healthcare_Project_ Report_June_2022.pdf (accessed 12 July 2023). https://doi.org/10.25957/g0y8-m635

Lloyd, M., Luscombe, A., Grant, C., Karunajeewa, H., Klim, S., Wijeratne, T., et al. (2020) Special-ised vestibular physiotherapy in the emergency department: a pilot safety and feasibility study. *Emergency Medicine Australasia* 32, 860–863. https://doi.org/10.1111/1742-6723.13569

Lynch, E.A., Mudge, A., Knowles, S., Kitson, A.L., Hunter, S.C., Harvey, G. (2018) "There is nothing so practical as a good theory": a pragmatic guide for selecting theoretical approaches for implementation projects. *BMC Health Services Research* 18, 857. https://doi.org/10.1186/ s12913-018-3671-z

Murray, J., Hunter, S.C., Splawinski, Z., Conroy, T. (2023) Lessons learned from the preimplemen-tation phase of an oral health care project. *JDR Clinical, Translational Research* 8, 299–301. https://doi.org/10.1177/23800844221083966

Rycroft-Malone, J., Kitson, A., Harvey, G., Mccormack, B., Seers, K., Titchen, A., et al. (2002) Ingredients for change: revisiting a conceptual framework. *Quality & Safety in Health Care* 11, 174–180. https://doi.org/10.1136/qhc.11.2.174

Rycroft-Malone, J., Harvey, G., Seers, K., Kitson, A., Mccormack, B., Titchen, A. (2004a) An exploration of the factors that influence the implementation of evidence into practice. *Journal of Clinical Nursing* 13, 913–924. https://doi.org/10.1111/j.1365-2702.2004.01007.x

Rycroft-Malone, J., Seers, K., Titchen, A., Harvey, G., Kitson, A., McCormack, B. (2004b) What counts as evidence in evidence-based practice? *Journal of Advanced Nursing* 47, 81–90. https:// doi.org/10.1111/j.1365-2648.2004.03068.x

Tuepker, A., Elnitsky, C., Newell, S., Zaugg, T., Henry, J.A. (2018) A qualitative study of imple-mentation and adaptations to progressive tinnitus management (PTM) delivery. *PLoS One* 13, e0196105. https://doi.org/10.1371/journal.pone.0196105

Weiner, B.J., Lewis, C.C., Stanick, C., Powell, B.J., Dorsey, C.N., Clary, A.S., et al. (2017) Psycho-metric assessment of three newly developed implementation outcome measures. *Implementation Science* 12, 108. https://doi.org/10.1186/s13012-017-0635-3

16 Applying the Tailored Implementation for Chronic Disease checklist

Anne Sales, Signe Flottorp and Michel Wensing

Introduction

The Tailored Implementation for Chronic Diseases (TICD)checklist (Flottorp et al., 2013) is the most recently published consolidated implementation determinant framework. Our goal in this chapter is to illustrate the use of the TICD checklist in three case studies. The primary use of this checklist, as with most of the determinant frameworks, is to design and tailor implementation strategies (also referred to as implementation interventions). Frameworks that catalogue strategies are different from those that catalogue determinants, making the use of determinants complex. There are no one-to-one mappings of determinants to strategies, in part because multiple determinants may be mapped onto one or more strategies, and multiple strategies may map to one or more determinants. Multiple theoretical causal mechanisms may underlie each determinant, and the same is true of implementation strategies. In addition, the effect of a determinant is often, if not always, modified or mediated by the context or environment in which the practice takes place in ways that are difficult to predict.

In this chapter, we demonstrate how the TICD checklist was applied in three different projects (Table 16.1) by showing which constructs from each domain were included in planning, designing and tailoring implementation strategies. Despite its origins in primary care, it has been used across multiple settings for different kinds of implementation efforts. We selected the three case studies to illustrate the range of uses and the benefits and challenges of using a consolidated implementation determinant framework to design and tailor implementation strategies.

Table 16.1 Overview of case studies using the Tailored Implementation for Chronic Diseases (TICD) checklist.

TICD domains and constructs	Case 1	Case 2	Case 3
Guideline or innovation (the "thing" to be implemented)	Six recommendations for treating older patients with depression in Norwegian primary care settings	Six recommendations for improving the risk for cardiovascular disease in Dutch primary care settings	Guideline recommendations for high-quality care for mechanically ventilated patients with acute respiratory distress syndrome (focus here is on lung protective ventilation)

(Continued)

DOI: 10.4324/9781003318125-18

Table 16.1 (Continued)

TICD domains and constructs	Case 1	Case 2	Case 3
Guideline factors	Accessibility of the recommendation	Little flexibility in recommendations	Observability; accessibility; clarity
Individual health professional factors	Self-efficacy; domain knowledge; intention and motivation	Clinical inertia; presence of practice nurses	Intention and motivation; agreement with the recommendation; expected outcome; skills needed to adhere; awareness and familiarity with recommendation; knowledge about own practice
Patient factors	Patient behaviour; patient preferences; patient motivation; patient beliefs and knowledge	Patient knowledge, motivation, behaviour	Patient needs
Professional interactions	None noted	Communication between primary care and hospital settings	Team processes; communication and influence; workflow and processes of care[a]
Incentives and resources	Availability of necessary resources; non-financial incentives and disincentives; financial incentives and disincentives	Time for counselling of patients; information materials for patients	Continuing education system; quality assurance and patient safety systems; information system; availability of necessary resources
Capacity for organizational change	Priority of necessary change	None noted	Assistance for organizational changes; regulations, rules and policies; capable leadership; mandate, authority, accountability
Social, political and legal factors	None noted	None noted	Legislation; contracts

[a]This was developed based on the interview data from this study. It is not a construct originally included in the TICD when it was first published, but there were repeated references to "workflow and processes of care" in the interviews.

Case 1: Implementing guideline recommendations for treatment of depression among older adults in Norwegian primary care settings

Context and gap in care

Several papers on this study have been published (Aakhus et al., 2014a, 2014b, 2015), including the results of the pragmatic cluster randomized trial used to evaluate the outcomes of the study, both in terms of implementation and patient-focused outcomes (Aakhus et al., 2016). The problem being addressed is a common one in primary care, where older adults are often not treated appropriately for depression. Depression is known to co-occur with many other chronic illnesses and can complicate the treatment of those diseases adequately if depression is left untreated. This was a multi-level implementation effort targeting individuals in Norwegian municipalities, general practitioners in municipalities, and older adults diagnosed with mild to severe depression and their families and caregivers.

Innovation

The goal was to implement six guideline recommendations for treating depression in older adults: social contact, collaborative care plan, depression care manager, counselling, prescribing psychotherapy and/or treatment with anti-depressants when appropriate (for severe or recurrent depression).

Study approach

This study was one of five projects within the overall TICD programme and initially assessed determinants of practice through the TICD checklist. The implementation strategies were selected and tailored within the research team. The study design for evaluating the effect of the tailored strategies was a pragmatic, cluster-randomized trial.

Methods of assessing determinants

Multiple methods were used, including brainstorming, structured focus groups with key stakeholders, structured individual interviews with additional stakeholders, and a mailed survey of clinicians and nurses. These processes yielded 352 determinants, which were reduced to 99 by stakeholders through prioritization processes. Of these, 21 determinants related to the six recommendations to be implemented were deemed important by the research team, and they developed probes to use with stakeholders through structured group sessions and interviews. These were ranked by the stakeholders on five-point scales assessing plausibility (the importance of the determinant in influencing practice) and feasibility (the extent to which the determinant could be modified). The determinants were mapped to each of the six recommendations to be implemented.

Methods for selecting implementation strategies

The research team drafted an implementation strategy plan based on input from stakeholders, which was assessed by stakeholders through brainstorming sessions, both individually and in groups. From this input, the research team developed an extensive logic model and ultimately derived specific strategies to support the implementation of each of the six recommendations.

Each of the six guideline recommendations had its own implementation strategies. Most implementation strategies were delivered online, most through a comprehensive website that included support for administrators to develop a collaborative care plan for older adults with depression; content for the collaborative care plan to tailor it for each community; templates, manuals and pamphlets for health professionals in each municipality; pamphlets for patients and their relatives; and a comprehensive website with educational materials for individuals in many roles and levels within general practices and in the municipalities. In addition, outreach visits to general practitioners were made to provide information about depression and the six recommendations as well as discuss possible adaptations to local conditions.

Methods of evaluating the effect of implementation strategies

Eighty of 428 municipalities, which are the governing units for primary care in Norway, were randomized to either intervention or control arms in a pragmatic, cluster-randomized controlled trial. All general practitioners in the intervention municipalities were offered the implementation strategy, and all general practitioners in both arms were invited to participate in data collection. Patients ≥65 years old who had been diagnosed with depression and who had consulted their practitioner within the last 6 months were identified through electronic medical records, and lists of these patients were provided through software systems to the general practitioners caring for them.

Case 2: Delivery of tailored approaches to implementing six recommendations to improve cardiovascular risk management in primary care in the Netherlands

Context and gap in care

This study was also part of the TICD programme of multiple implementation trials in five European countries. Several papers have been published describing the protocol (Huntink et al., 2013), methods and process evaluation (Huntink et al., 2014, 2015, 2016), and the results of the cluster randomized trial (van Lieshout et al., 2016). The focus was on implementing six guideline recommendations to improve cardiovascular risk. The primary target group for implementation was practice nurses in primary care practices in the Netherlands.

Innovation

The goal was to implement six guideline recommendations to improve cardiovascular care, including improving blood pressure management for patients at high risk for cardiovascular disease and those with established disease (two recommendations); decreasing low-density lipoprotein cholesterol to recommended levels for patients at high risk for cardiovascular disease and those with established disease (two recommendations); promoting lifestyle change for patients with cardiovascular disease as well as those at high risk; and creating a risk profile for patients with chronic kidney disease.

Study approach

Determinants were assessed much as in case 1 and worked through assessment of importance and modifiability to select determinants to focus on. The implementation strategies were selected and tailored based on these determinants and on suggestions for strategies from primary care providers. The evaluation design was a cluster randomized trial targeting behaviour change by practice nurses within primary care practices.

Methods of assessing determinants

The methods were similar to those described in case 1. In this case, the key selection attributes were perceived importance of the determinants and the degree to which they were perceived to be modifiable or changeable.

Methods for selecting implementation strategies

Group interviews with healthcare providers and patients were used to select implementation strategies to address the assessed determinants. These interviews started with a brief oral presentation of the main determinants of practice.

The interviews produced a total of 181 implementation strategies suggested for addressing the identified and prioritized determinants. These were narrowed down by the research team to a set deemed feasible to deploy, which included mandatory training in motivational interviewing for practice nurses to improve patient motivation; an enhanced online educational module for nurses on cardiovascular risk management and support for patient self-management; grouping patients by the presence of depressive symptoms that can affect their ability to take in new knowledge and change behaviour; goal-setting and self-monitoring for patients without depressive symptoms; and patients with depressive symptoms, referral to physical exercise groups to support overcoming depression through physical activity. Logic models, as in case 1, were used to map determinants to strategies. The implementation strategies were introduced in person to each practice through a study visit using a standardized script to ensure that the same information was provided to each practice nurse.

Methods of evaluating the effect of implementation strategies

A full-scale process evaluation was conducted as part of the evaluation of the effectiveness of the implementation strategies. This included an evaluation of audiotapes of sessions between the practice nurses and patients in which motivational interviewing was used to increase patient motivation to engage in behaviour change. These recordings were scored by professional motivational interviewing trainers to assess the nurses' fidelity to motivational interviewing principles and core skills. A knowledge-based questionnaire was administered to the practice nurses to assess their knowledge both of cardiovascular risk management and other aspects of the strategies, including motivational interviewing. Questionnaires were also administered to patients identified as high cardiovascular risk or with existing cardiovascular disease, covering the referral part of the implementation strategy and whether they used this advice. Furthermore, interviews were conducted with all the practice nurses to assess their experiences of the strategies. Interviews were also conducted with a sample of patients who had visited one of the intervention practices during the intervention period. Practices were randomly allocated to either the intervention or control arm, and patients were selected within each practice who were identified as being at high risk of cardiovascular disease or had been diagnosed with it. Medical records of selected patients were audited to assess patient-level outcomes.

Case 3: Implementing guideline-based recommendations for improving care for mechanically ventilated patients in acute respiratory failure and acute respiratory distress syndrome in critical care units in the United States

Context and gap in care

Mechanical ventilation, delivered in the context of critical care using machines to regulate and support breathing, is an essential life-saving therapy for patients with acute respiratory failure. However, it can result in serious adverse outcomes if used for too long and without appropriate safeguards to prevent lung damage from excessive ventilation pressure. Optimizing the duration of mechanical ventilation through evidence-based practices is critical to ensuring optimal outcomes for mechanically ventilated patients. The goal of this project was to define a set of evidence-based practices that span the continuum of mechanical ventilation from initiation to weaning or liberation from mechanical ventilation and develop implementation strategies to support their implementation in routine critical care practice. This case study remains a work in progress, and we describe our work as currently completed.

Innovation

The first step was to review recently published critical care guidelines to assess recommendations for care across the continuum of mechanical ventilation (Ervin et al., 2020). The team conducted multiple rounds of surveys to assess those that were considered most important and most feasible to implement, ultimately prioritizing 11 of the 30 identified initially (Ervin et al., 2022). The focus in this case is on lung protective ventilation, a recommendation to tailor the volume and pressure of ventilation to the body size of the individual receiving care, thus reducing the likelihood of lung injury. This recommendation was uniformly regarded as important and feasible to implement (Ervin et al., 2022).

Study approach

After completing survey rounds to determine priorities among the initial 30 recommendations, the team conducted site visits and interviews with administrators and clinicians in five critical care settings across four health systems. The team interviewed clinical leaders, physicians, nurses, and respiratory therapists in all settings, using an interview guide developed based on the TICD, covering all seven domains, to elicit determinants of current practice that indicated both opportunities (facilitators) and challenges (barriers) to implementing the 11 prioritized recommendations. The interview data were coded using template analysis (Skolarus et al., 2019), initially using the TICD as the codebook and adding constructs and definitions as needed. Future steps will include developing implementation strategies using the electronic health record as both a data source and vehicle for delivering strategies.

Methods of assessing determinants

As previously described, interviews were used to assess determinants. One of the constructs in Table 16.1 for case 3 was developed based on the interview data from this study. It is not a construct originally included in the TICD when it was first published, but there were repeated references to "workflow and processes of care" in the interviews. This makes sense in the context of critical care, compared with primary care; processes of care and complex workflows that may require ongoing interactions and negotiations among healthcare professionals providing team-based care are common in critical care settings and may dominate providers' consciousness more than in primary care. This is an example of the need to be flexible when analysing data related to determinants of practice, because different settings and contexts may require additional codes and constructs to ensure full coverage of relevant determinants.

Methods for selecting implementation strategies

The development and design of implementation strategies are not yet complete. The focus is on digitally enabled strategies that will address key determinants identified in the interviews. One important point that came up frequently was the lack of knowledge of current practice, noted under the Individual Health Professional Factors domain. Interview participants could not reliably describe the average duration of mechanical ventilation in their units, for example, and they could not state the proportion receiving lung-protective ventilation beyond general estimates ("most", "usually"). A clear candidate strategy for addressing this lack of knowledge of own current practice is audit with feedback, with the audit conducted through data extraction from electronic health records and feedback delivered digitally through email or some form of dashboard or both.

Methods of evaluating the effect of implementation strategies

The plan is to evaluate effectiveness using a sequential, multiple assignment, randomized trial (SMART) design (Necamp et al., 2017), evaluating both implementation and clinical intervention outcomes in a hybrid type 3 trial (Curran et al., 2012).

Benefits and challenges in using consolidated implementation determinant frameworks in tailoring implementation strategies

We have identified three case studies that illustrate methods of using the TICD, the most recent consolidated determinant framework in the published implementation literature. These three case studies illustrate how to use the framework, but it is important to consider the benefits and challenges of using determinant frameworks to design and then tailor or adapt implementation strategies.

We believe that the most important benefit to using these frameworks, among which we include not only the TICD but also the Consolidated Framework for Implementation Research (Damschroder et al., 2009) and the Theoretical Domains Framework (Michie et al., 2005), is that they provide a systematic checklist to ensure that important domains and factors that have been shown through empirical research to be important in determining whether implementation is likely to be successful are included. Related to this, they provide structure for reporting on the wide range of determinants, that is, the barriers and facilitators that are critical to understanding whether implementation will succeed. The current consolidated frameworks should be used as checklists in making assessments of the context within which a problem or gap exists.

A major issue with all the current frameworks is that the meaning of the constructs or factors that are included in the checklist is not always easy to find in the existing literature. None of the available frameworks should be considered the "final list" of factors because they are all intermediate products of developing research. Many of the constructs are identified within the context of a specific study and require going to the reports of that study to understand the meaning of the terms. Others derive from the many underlying disciplines from which implementation science draws its content, such as psychology, organizational and management studies, engineering, sociology, anthropology, economics, and other social sciences. Understanding the meanings of the terms in the frameworks is not trivial, and many of them are multi-faceted, leading to their being used in different ways in different studies. The terms may not be mutually exclusive, and the lack of common definitions makes it difficult to read across studies and assess commonalities and differences. Even when studies use a common framework, one cannot generally assume that the same definitions are used for all terms.

Related to this is a problem of semantic structure. Although determinant frameworks are all organized into domains with related constructs within each domain, the domains are generally created idiosyncratically within each framework, embodying a structure that does not rest on common definitions but on the specific knowledge and understanding of the groups that created them. Even though there are relationships among the determinant frameworks, particularly for the TICD, which is consolidated across existing frameworks, these relationships cannot be readily discerned or assessed and reconciling across studies using different frameworks is difficult.

One of the great strengths of the TICD programme of research, described by Wensing et al. (2011), is the systematic nature of the entire programme of research, with careful standardization of approaches. This has rarely been done in implementation research; reviewing the papers produced through this large-scale programme of research may be a useful introduction to the field.

Other potential uses of the TICD checklist

Although the most important use of determinant frameworks is to design and tailor or adapt implementation strategies, there are other uses. Change in determinants may be a relevant outcome for an implementation study, particularly those determinants that play broad roles in influencing implementation success, such as organizational capacity for change, also called readiness to change, or health professionals' attitudes towards guidelines. Considering use of the TICD to monitor change over time in specific constructs as implementation progresses may be beneficial.

An ongoing challenge is how to take the information from the determinants assessed and map these effectively and appropriately to strategies designed either to overcome negative determinants or barriers, or to enhance the effect of positive determinants, or facilitators. As yet, there are no straightforward approaches to accomplishing this important step, although the ongoing interactions with key stakeholders who can provide critical information about the feasibility of specific strategies in the organizational context of the places where implementation is being conducted, and the use of some form of logic model to create visual and logical linkages between determinants and strategies seem promising approaches. Implementation research logic models have recently been described that build on the approaches used in the TICD projects and focus on the mechanisms of action of strategies (Smith et al., 2020), possibly enhanced through an additional focus on mechanisms of action of determinants (Sales et al., 2021). However, without additional development in the field of implementation science, this issue is likely to continue to pose problems in designing implementation strategies.

References

Aakhus, E., Granlund, I., Odgaard-Jensen, J., Wensing, M., Oxman, A.D., Flottorp, S.A. (2014a) Tailored interventions to implement recommendations for elderly patients with depression in primary care: a study protocol for a pragmatic cluster randomised controlled trial. *Trials* 15, 16. https://doi.org/10.1186/1745-6215-15-16

Aakhus, E., Oxman, A.D., Flottorp, S.A. (2014b) Determinants of adherence to recommendations for depressed elderly patients in primary care: a multi-methods study. *Scandinavian Journal of Primary Health Care* 32, 170–179. https://doi.org/10.3109/02813432.2014.984961

Aakhus, E., Granlund, I., Oxman, A.D., Flottorp, S.A. (2015) Tailoring interventions to implement recommendations for the treatment of elderly patients with depression: a qualitative study. *International Journal of Mental Health Systems* 9, 36. https://doi.org/10.1186/s13033-015-0027-5

Aakhus, E., Granlund, I., Odgaard-Jensen, J., Oxman, A.D., Flottorp, S.A. (2016) A tailored intervention to implement guideline recommendations for elderly patients with depression in primary care: a pragmatic cluster randomised trial. *Implementation Science* 11, 32. https://doi.org/10.1186/s13012-016-0397-3

Curran, G.M., Bauer, M., Mittman, B., Pyne, J.M., Stetler, C. (2012) Effectiveness-implementation hybrid designs: combining elements of clinical effectiveness and implementation research to enhance public health impact. *Medical Care* 50, 217–226. https://doi.org/10.1097/MLR.0b013e3182408812

Damschroder, L.J., Aron, D.C., Keith, R.E., Kirsh, S.R., Alexander, J.A., Lowery, J.C. (2009) Fostering implementation of health services research findings into practice: a consolidated framework for advancing implementation science. *Implementation Science* 4, 50. https://doi.org/10.1186/1748-5908-4-50

Ervin, J.N., Rentes, V.C., Dibble, E.R., Sjoding, M.W., Iwashyna, T.J., Hough, C.L., et al. (2020) Evidence-based practices for acute respiratory failure and acute respiratory distress syndrome: a systematic review of reviews. *Chest* 158, 2381–2393. https://doi.org/10.1016/j.chest.2020.06.080

Ervin, J.N., Dibble, M.R., Rentes, V.C., Sjoding, M.W., Gong, M.N., Hough, C.L., et al. (2022) Prioritizing evidence-based practices for acute respiratory distress syndrome using digital data: an iterative multi-stakeholder process. *Implementation science* 17, 82. https://doi.org/10.1186/s13012-022-01255-y

Flottorp, S.A., Oxman, A.D., Krause, J., Musila, N.R., Wensing, M., Godycki-Cwirko, M., et al. (2013) A checklist for identifying determinants of practice: a systematic review and synthesis of frameworks and taxonomies of factors that prevent or enable improvements in healthcare professional practice. *Implementation science* 8, 35. https://doi.org/10.1186/1748-5908-8-35

Huntink, E., Heijmans, N., Wensing, M., van Lieshout, J. (2013) Effectiveness of a tailored intervention to improve cardiovascular risk management in primary care: study protocol for a randomised controlled trial. *Trials* 14, 433. https://doi.org/10.1186/1745-6215-14-433

Huntink, E., van Lieshout, J., Aakhus, E., Baker, R., Flottorp, S., Godycki-Cwirko, M., et al. (2014) Stakeholders' contributions to tailored implementation programs: an observational study of group interview methods. *Implementation Science* 9, 185. https://doi.org/10.1186/s13012-014-0185-x

Huntink, E., Wensing, M., Klomp, M.A., van Lieshout, J. (2015) Perceived determinants of cardiovascular risk management in primary care: disconnections between patient behaviours, practice organisation and healthcare system. *BMC Family Practice* 16, 179. https://doi.org/10.1186/s12875-015-0390-y

Huntink, E., Wensing, M., Timmers, I. M., & van Lieshout, J. (2016). Process evaluation of a tailored intervention programme of cardiovascular risk management in general practices. *Implementation Science* 11, 164. https://doi.org/10.1186/s13012-016-0526-z

Michie, S., Johnston, M., Abraham, C., Lawton, R., Parker, D., Walker, A., et al. (2005) Making psychological theory useful for implementing evidence based practice: a consensus approach. *Quality & Safety in Health Care* 14, 26–33. https://doi.org/10.1136/qshc.2004.011155

Necamp, T., Kilbourne, A., Almirall, D. (2017) Comparing cluster-level dynamic treatment regimens using sequential, multiple assignment, randomized trials: regression estimation and sample size considerations. *Statistical Methods in Medical Research* 26, 1572–1589. https://doi.org/10.1177/0962280217708654

Sales, A.E., Barnaby, D.P., Rentes, V.C. (2021) Letter to the editor on "The Implementation Research Logic Model: a method for planning, executing, reporting, and synthesizing implementation projects" (Smith JD, Li DH, Rafferty MR. The Implementation Research Logic Model: a method for planning, executing, reporting, and synthesizing implementation projects. Implementation Science 2020;15:84. https://doi.org/10.1186/s13012-020-01041-8). *Implementation Science* 16, 97. https://doi.org/10.1186/s13012-021-01169-1

Skolarus, L.E., Neshewat, G.M., Evans, L., Green, M., Rehman, N., Landis-Lewis, Z., et al. (2019) Understanding determinants of acute stroke thrombolysis using the tailored implementation for chronic diseases framework: a qualitative study. *BMC Health Services Research* 19, 182. https://doi.org/10.1186/s12913-019-4012-6

Smith, J.D., Li, D.H., Rafferty, M.R. (2020) The Implementation Research Logic Model: a method for planning, executing, reporting, and synthesizing implementation projects. *Implementation Science* 15, 84. https://doi.org/10.1186/s13012-020-01041-8

van Lieshout, J., Huntink, E., Koetsenruijter, J., Wensing, M. (2016) Tailored implementation of cardiovascular risk management in general practice: a cluster randomized trial. *Implementation Science* 11, 115. https://doi.org/10.1186/s13012-016-0460-0

Wensing, M., Oxman, A., Baker, R., Godycki-Cwirko, M., Flottorp, S., Szecsenyi, J., et al. (2011) Tailored Implementation For Chronic Diseases (TICD): a project protocol. *Implementation Science* 6, 103. https://doi.org/10.1186/1748-5908-6-103

17 Applying the Practical, Robust Implementation and Sustainability Model

Katy E. Trinkley, Rebecca J. Guerin, James Pittman, Amy G. Huebschmann, Russell E. Glasgow and Borsika A. Rabin

Introduction

The Practical, Robust Implementation and Sustainability Model (PRISM) is an implementation science framework that consists of contextual domains, as well as the broadly utilized Reach, Effectiveness, Adoption, Implementation and Maintenance (RE-AIM) outcomes (Feldstein and Glasgow, 2008; Glasgow et al., 1999, 2019; Rabin et al., 2022). The PRISM domains consider the multi-level recipient characteristics and their perspectives on the intervention, the external environment, and the implementation and sustainability infrastructure. PRISM can be used across each phase of a project's lifecycle (i.e. pre-implementation planning, implementation, evaluation and sustainment) to support activities associated with all these phases. A conceptual overview and description of the components of PRISM are provided in Chapter 6.

Here, we describe different ways in which PRISM has been and can be applied across diverse populations, situations and settings. Some of the unique features of PRISM are illustrated using case study examples: (1) it promotes health equity (Shelton et al., 2020; Fort et al., 2023); (2) it can be used once or iteratively across the different phases of a project to guide and document adaptations (Rabin et al., 2018; Glasgow et al., 2020, 2022; Maw et al., 2022); (3) it supports designing for Dissemination and Sustainability.(Kwan et al., 2022). In these examples, we also highlight how PRISM can be used pragmatically to fit different types of projects; used with other theories, models or frameworks; and as a process, determinant, and/or evaluation framework (Holtrop et al., 2021; Rabin et al., 2022).

We summarize three applications of PRISM as case study examples and highlight some of the unique features of PRISM (Table 17.1) and the different ways it is or has been applied in each of the case studies. Then, Table 17.2 illustrates the different ways in which PRISM was or is proposed to be applied during the planning, implementation and sustainment phases of each case example.

Case 1: A randomized trial comparing two different clinical decision support tools to improve prescribing for heart failure

PRISM was used in the planning, implementation and evaluation/sustainment phases of the project. Specifically, PRISM was used to guide and assess a randomized controlled trial across 28 primary care clinics that compared two clinical decision support (CDS) alerts for 6 months: a CDS customized to the local context and a commercial CDS developed to meet the general needs of health systems (Trinkley et al., 2021). Both CDSs were

DOI: 10.4324/9781003318125-19

Table 17.1 Description of how key features of the Practical, Robust Implementation and Sustainability Model (PRISM) were applied to each case study.

PRISM feature	Heart failure clinical decision support (CDS) example	Occupational Safety and Health Administration (OSHA) 10-hour course example	eScreening example
For equity	Engaged diverse clinicians and patients to promote representation of different perspectives	Engaged diverse partners (school administrators, teachers, students) to ensure multiple participant characteristics and varied perspectives represented	Specific questions on the PRISM survey that addressed alignment between the intervention and perspectives of patients who have historically experienced disparities
For different settings, issues, populations	For primary care clinicians in a large integrated healthcare system using an electronic health record to address gaps in evidence-based prescribing for heart failure	Providing workplace safety and health training to young people who are at increased risk of experiencing life-altering, occupational injuries delivered in their usual health sciences school context (career and technical education programmes)	Veterans Health Affairs (VHA) transition clinics, screening for mental health and suicide risk of veterans enrolling in VHA for healthcare
To guide and document adaptations (e.g. used iteratively, with the Framework for Reporting Adaptations and Modifications to Evidence-based interventions [FRAME])	A proactive plan to monitor adaptations and document contextual drivers	Proactive plan to iteratively assess, implement and document adaptations along with contextual drivers based on FRAME	Proactive plan to iteratively assess, implement and document adaptations along with contextual drivers

Used pragmatically (e.g. portions of it, adapting measures, combining with other theories, models and frameworks)	Given the limitations of electronic health record data availability, used an imprecise denominator for the reach outcome to determine the proportion of patients reached. Modified the adoption outcome to measure whether clinicians dismissed the alert, given they did not have the choice to see the alert. Used PRISM as the overarching framework – also integrated a framework for the established best practices in clinical decision support design	Although all PRISM domains will be assessed, some domains will receive less attention/focus (e.g. implementation and sustainability infrastructure)	Developed a code book for qualitative analysis with pragmatic definitions and examples for each PRISM context domain and RE-AIM measure. Use of iterative PRISM as an implementation strategy for action planning. Developed a brief PRISM survey to assess PRISM domains
To design for dissemination and sustainability	Designed the alerts to be automated and integrated within routine workflows. Built the alerts using technical approaches that minimized the need for future build maintenance (e.g. Health Level 7 standards, RxNorm nomenclature)	Designed the training materials to be readily adapted for use in other school contexts. Building a suite of knowledge and tools for replicating the programme in other school districts	The external facilitator worked with the team to develop a plan that would meet their unique needs and fit current resources to ensure it was sustainable
As a process, determinant, or evaluation framework	Process, determinant, and evaluation	Process, determinant, and evaluation	Process, determinant, and evaluation
For different phases of implementation	Used at all three phases	Used at all three phases	Used at all three phases

Table 17.2 Comparison of how the Practical, Robust Implementation and Sustainability Model (PRISM) was or is planned to be applied across the different phases.

	Planning phase: study design	*Implementation phase: study conduct*	*Sustainment phase: evaluation and scaling*
Heart failure clinical decision support (CDS) example	PRISM used to: guide systematic consideration of context and alignment with the CDS, including multi-level partner engagement; develop relevant and pragmatic outcome measures. PRISM's Implementation and Sustainability Infrastructure domain was leveraged to "design for Dissemination and Sustainability"	Adaptations were proactively evaluated with a plan to document	Planned a mixed methods evaluation guided by PRISM and PRISM's RE-AIM outcomes; disseminated the findings; scaled the customized CDS to all primary care clinics previously receiving the commercial CDS
Occupational Safety and Health Administration (OSHA) 10-hour course example	PRISM used to: develop study aims; develop pragmatic outcome measures; guide systematic and ongoing assessment of context and alignment: assess initial and ongoing potential for reaching key RE-AIM outcomes. An extensive database was developed to ensure systematic and longitudinal use of PRISM	PRISM used to: categorize and proactively monitor and document adaptations and periodic reflections; guide engagement with key partners to identify areas for better alignment with context and develop adaptation strategies; guide fidelity checks and reflections to enhance RE-AIM outcomes	Multi-method evaluation guided by PRISM outcomes; prioritizing identification of barriers and opportunities for long-term programme sustainment and scale up from the programme
eScreening example	PRISM used to: develop study aims; select components of the implementation strategy; develop pragmatic outcome measures	PRISM interviews were used to inform external facilitation. PRISM was used to categorize and proactively monitor adaptations and periodic reflections	Mixed methods evaluation guided by PRISM outcomes; disseminated findings; results to inform enterprise-wide implementation of eScreening nationally

implemented in the electronic health records (EHRs) to alert primary care clinicians during an office visit and recommend prescription of an evidence-based β-blocker medication for patients with a diagnosis of heart failure with reduced ejection fraction (HFrEF) who were not already prescribed a β-blocker. β-Blockers are evidence-based treatments indicated for patients with HFrEF and are strongly recommended by guidelines in the United States and globally (Heidenreich et al., 2022). Unfortunately, prescription of β-blockers for these patients remains suboptimal (Greene et al., 2018; Allen et al., 2021). Thus evidence-based interventions such as CDS alerts can be used to address this gap in care. The best approach to designing CDS alerts was unclear before this study. Many health systems relied on commercially available alerts supplied by the EHR vendor that were not tailored to the local context of the health system. In this study, we experimentally evaluated the effect of customizing a CDS based on PRISM to the local context compared with a commercially available CDS; the use case was prescription of β-blockers for patients with HFrEF.

Methods and strategies to apply PRISM

During the planning phase, PRISM was used to inform the design and develop the customized CDS to maximize its alignment with the local health system's context while also considering external factors such as national guidelines and planning for sustainability. Before implementation, we engaged patients, clinicians and several levels of operational leadership to systematically assess the local context. Specifically, we engaged (Trinkley et al., 2020):

- Patients who would be affected by the recommendations of the CDS to ensure the recommendations were patient-centred. We conducted focus groups with diverse patients with HFrEF to understand patient preferences and priorities (PRISM domains: patient perspectives and characteristics).
- Clinicians who were potential end-users of the CDS to understand their informational needs and preferences for how the CDS was designed and integrated within their EHR workflows. Clinicians were recruited from diverse types of primary care settings (academic, rural, community), specialties (geriatrics, family medicine, internal medicine) and disciplines (advanced practice providers, physicians). We engaged clinicians in three ways. First, we conducted a series of focus groups to get high-level understanding of how the CDS should be designed. We then developed prototypes of the CDS, iteratively shared them with individual clinicians and made revisions based on their input. Finally, we built the CDS in EHR test environments and iteratively conducted usability testing interviews with the clinicians to develop a version of the CDS that was deemed acceptable (PRISM domains: staff perspectives and characteristics).
- Operational leaders, including clinic-level medical directors and managers and system-level informatics leaders to garner support and approval to implement the CDS within the EHR, as well as ensure alignment with their priorities and resource allocation (PRISM domains: leadership perspectives and characteristics).

During these partner engagement activities, we also worked with the partners to define pragmatic RE-AIM outcome measures that were both relevant to the different perspectives and feasible to measure. Some of the original RE-AIM outcomes were not practical to collect, given resource constraints or limitations in data availability. More details of how we adapted the RE-AIM outcomes are described in the Findings section and Table 17.2.

When considering PRISM's external environment domain, key factors included established best practices in CDS design and the HFrEF guidelines. The framework for best practices in CDS design was embedded within the PRISM domains and offered more granular direction on contextual factors to consider as the customized CDS was designed to align with the local context.

We also used implementation strategies to optimize alignment of the CDS with PRISM's implementation and sustainability infrastructure domain. The CDS was designed to be automated and to fit within routine clinical workflows. Automation mitigated the need for manual labour, and workflow integration minimized the effort that busy clinicians needed to make in their already limited time. The CDS was also built using technical approaches (no custom code) and standards (e.g. RxNorm nomenclature, HL7) that minimize the need for ongoing maintenance over time.

During the implementation or study conduct phase of this project, we developed a plan to monitor for and document adaptations that occurred and the contextual reasons for them. This plan included proactively monitoring clinician free-text comments to the CDS and the CDS performance via standard reporting logs.

During the evaluation or sustainment phase, we conducted a sequential mixed methods evaluation to evaluate and compare the two CDSs. This evaluation included RE-AIM outcome data collected from the EHR and qualitative data obtained via interviews with clinicians exposed to one of the CDSs. The interviews were guided by PRISM to understand the contextual drivers for the RE-AIM outcomes. During this evaluation, we also explored ways to optimize the sustainability of the CDS and identify ways to scale it to other guideline-recommended medications and settings.

Findings

Over the 6-month period, the customized CDS alert was triggered or reached 61 unique patients and the commercial CDS reached only 26 patients. Because of data limitations, we were unable to define a precise denominator for reach. Instead of reporting the proportion of patients with HFrEF who were indicated for a β-blocker, we reported the proportion of patients with HFrEF for whom the CDS alerted.

Clinician adoption (62% versus 29%; $p < 0.001$) and effectiveness of changing prescribing (14% versus 0%, $p < 0.006$) were significantly higher with the customized CDS than the commercial CDS. Clinician adoption was defined as whether the clinician did something other than dismiss the CDS outright. For the RE-AIM outcome of adoption, we modified it from the usual definition of adoption for two reasons: (1) it better aligns with the terminology used in the informatics literature, and (2) clinics and clinicians did not have a choice about adopting it. The CDS interrupted their workflow whether they wanted it or not.

For the RE-AIM outcome of implementation, we did not identify any adaptations to either CDS. With respect to maintenance, these findings prompted the health system to switch all clinics from the commercial CDS to the customized CDS, which has now been sustained for more than 2 years.

Of the 21 clinicians interviewed to understand the PRISM domain of clinician perspectives, 19 (90%) indicated one of the two CDSs should be continued and most (74% of 19) wanted the customized CDS to be continued. The reasons the five clinicians wanted the commercial CDS to be continued were also the reasons why the other

14 clinicians felt it should not be continued. Most of the clinicians felt the CDS should not allow a quick dismissal given the importance of prescribing these medications and felt the commercial CDS was too brief and did not provide enough information to inform decision making.

Case 2: Implementing the Occupational Safety and Health Administration (OSHA) 10-hour training for young workers

Case 2 uses PRISM across the planning, implementation and evaluation/sustainment phases of a multi-method, hybrid type 2 effectiveness-implementation trial. In this example, PRISM guides the simultaneous evaluation of the effectiveness and implementation of an industry-standard, workplace safety and health training: the Occupational Safety and Health Administration (OSHA) 10-hour training for general industry (US Department of Labor, n.d.). In this study, the OSHA 10-hour training was adapted for US high school career and technical education (CTE) students in the health sciences pathway in one of the largest US public school districts. School-based, workplace safety and health training is needed because adolescents and young adults in the United States are injured at twice the rate of adults (>25 years of age) on the job (Guerin et al., 2020). Research (Boini et al., 2017) indicates that occupational safety and health education provided to young people while in secondary school may be protective against future work-related injury and should be part of a comprehensive, public health strategy for protecting young workers. The OSHA 10-hour training has been delivered in US high schools (Shendell et al., 2017), especially in the context of CTE programmes, but the courses are not tailored to the needs and learning styles of younger workers. Nor has the effectiveness and implementation of an OSHA 10-hour course been systematically studied in a large US public school district.

Case 2 uses a waitlist randomized control design with roughly 30 CTE teachers in the health sciences, who are delivering the tailored OSHA 10-hour course to approximately 2000 CTE students over 2 study years. A multi-level, longitudinal, multi-method, multi-perspective approach is being used for data collection for study teachers trained to deliver the intervention, CTE students, school administrators and training partners. The core components of the programme include:

- Teacher training to become an OSHA-authorized instructor (e.g. paperwork before and after to be completed by teachers, and attending 2 weeks of training).
- Content of the OSHA-10 training curriculum as designed and provided (e.g. lessons, activities).
- Preparation and delivery of the OSHA 10-hour training curriculum (e.g. reviewing and tailoring slides, preparing for class, delivering class content).
- Administrative tasks associated with teaching the OSHA 10-hour training and being an OSHA-authorized instructor (e.g. logging student hours, maintaining records, distributing OSHA 10 cards to students).
- Ongoing support from external facilitators (partners from a national teachers' union).

Methods and strategies to apply PRISM

In the planning phase, we developed a multi-level and multi-component implementation strategy bundle to optimize the alignment of the OSHA 10-hour training with the school setting. The bundle was informed by PRISM's context domains to maximize the RE-AIM outcomes. These context domains include perception of the intervention by teachers and administrators; administrator, teacher and student characteristics; implementation and sustainability infrastructure within the schools and school district; and the external environment consisting of national educational policy and practices.

To ensure systematic, multi-level use of PRISM throughout the lifecycle of the study, we also developed a database to map all qualitative (interviews, focus groups) and quantitative (surveys) items/instruments with one or more PRISM construct (i.e. PRISM context domains and RE-AIM outcomes). The database includes a total of 628 unique items with multiple constructs addressed across more than one phase (pre-implementation, implementation, evaluation/sustainment) allowing for longitudinal assessment. Furthermore, constructs are often measured at several levels (i.e. administrator, teacher, student), allowing for a multi-level perspective. For PRISM context domains, most items were associated with Recipient characteristics ($n = 300$). For RE-AIM outcomes, most items were tagged as Effectiveness ($n = 407$) followed by Implementation ($n = 70$).

Beginning in planning and continuing through the implementation phase, we are conducting iterative PRISM assessments (Rabin et al., 2018; Glasgow et al., 2020, 2022; Maw et al., 2022) with follow-up debrief meetings with study teachers, school administrators and members of the research team after each iteration. The iterative PRISM assessment is a survey that asks participants to rate various aspects of the OSHA 10-hour training programme, including anticipated adoption, implementation, reach, effectiveness and maintenance on a 4-point scale. The survey also asks how well the programme fits with the contextual characteristics of key groups (i.e. students, teachers, administrators, and programme partners) and settings (i.e. the district CTE health science programme) as well as the implementation and sustainability infrastructure and external environment. Results from the surveys are summarized and used in a discussion format with various partners. The key goals of this activity are to (1) provide a baseline and ongoing assessment of context and potential for achieving key implementation and effectiveness outcomes; (2) identify challenge areas for achieving the desired implementation and effectiveness goals and develop strategies to improve these areas; and (3) identify areas with opportunities for better alignment of the OSHA 10-hour training programme with the context and develop strategies to achieve this alignment.

We are also using the PRISM RE-AIM outcomes to iteratively track adaptations in a web-based tool (i.e. RedCap) using methodology developed by Rabin and colleagues based on the RE-AIM enriched, expanded Framework for Reporting Adaptations and Modifications to Evidence-based interventions (FRAME) (Rabin et al., 2018; McCreight et al., 2019; Stirman et al., 2019; McCarthy et al., 2021). Adaptations are documented (on a bimonthly basis by the research team via periodic reflections and/or field notes) if changes made to the programme might have an impact on implementation outcomes (e.g. reach of students, adoption by teachers, sustained use); programme outcomes; or how the programme is being delivered in the current or a different setting. Modifications to the study design, data collection, instruments and analysis are also being monitored and documented.

Group interviews with teachers, administrators and OSHA training partners are being conducted after each implementation cycle. These semi-structured interviews are guided by PRISM and focused on exploring key lessons learned and opportunities to improve the contextual alignment of the OSHA 10-hour training programme with the local setting.

These interviews aim to understand contextual drivers of the RE-AIM outcomes and plan for Sustainability and Dissemination.

After completion of programme delivery (evaluation/sustainment phase), we will again administer the iterative PRISM assessment. Information from the iterative PRISM assessment, emphasizing PRISM's implementation and sustainability infrastructure domain, will inform the ongoing delivery of the OSHA 10-hour training programme within the current school district and identify strategies needed to successfully scale the programme out to other school districts with optimal alignment and outcomes. We will also conduct semi-structured group and individual interviews with teachers, administrators and training partners. These interviews will be guided by PRISM and will facilitate our understanding of the multi-level barriers and opportunities to long-term programme sustainment and scale out.

We will also conduct a longitudinal analysis of the data collected throughout the lifecycle of the programme. PRISM will be used to guide the analytic plan, presentation of findings and development of action items to support sustained use and scale out of the programme. An implementation guide structured by PRISM is being developed to support these activities so that the programme can be implemented on an ongoing basis or scaled up or out to other school settings.

Findings

For the iterative PRISM assessment in the planning phase, three study teachers, two school administrators and four members of the research team ($n = 9$) completed the survey and participated in a 90-minute debrief session. Areas with lower average scores and several "don't know" responses were highlighted for discussion. Open-text comments from participants were also summarized. Preliminary results from the pre-implementation iterative PRISM surveys indicate lower average scores on the RE-AIM domains of adoption at the setting and implementer levels and also maintenance. For the PRISM context domains, the scores were relatively high overall, with slightly lower scores on programme characteristics from the perspective of the students and programme characteristics from the perspective of teachers (e.g. "How well does the OSHA 10-hour Training Program as currently planned align with the expectations and perspectives of students [and teachers] from the CTE Health Science Program?") The debrief session provided additional context for the survey results. These data are being used to operationalize strategies to improve programme implementation and to describe and characterize context longitudinally throughout the research lifecycle. The research is in progress and data are not yet available for the RE-AIM outcomes.

Case 3: Evaluating the implementation and effectiveness of screening software to aid suicide prevention in veterans

Case 3 used PRISM across the planning, implementation, and evaluation/sustainment phases. Specifically, PRISM was used to guide an eight-site, mixed-method, hybrid type-II implementation trial evaluating the effectiveness and RE-AIM implementation outcomes of an electronic screening programme (eScreening) for suicide prevention. eScreening was developed for use in the Veterans Health Administration (VHA). The programme was implemented in clinics where veterans initially enrol for VHA care using a multi-component implementation strategy that was informed by PRISM during the planning phase (Pittman et al., 2021a) The multi-component implementation strategy consisted of external and internal facilitation and training components. Eight diverse VHA sites were paired into four two-site cohorts and randomized to determine implementation order using a stepped-wedge design. Veterans account for a disproportionate number of all known suicides in the United States, with 20%–22% ending their lives (Nelson et al., 2015; Veterans Administration/Department of Defense, 2019). Screening for suicide risk at the first contact with a health system is a best practice in the national Zero Suicide framework (Labouliere et al., 2018) and vital to enhancing access to appropriate care. Transition programmes in the VHA are positioned to screen newly enrolled veterans at the critical moment of enrolment in health care. Unfortunately, many veterans who present for the first time in the VHA with recent suicidal thoughts do not receive same-day comprehensive suicide risk evaluation (Pittman et al., 2017). In this study, we assessed eScreening as a tool to evaluate the rate and speed of initial mental health and suicide risk screening in transition programmes and examined the feasibility, acceptability and impact of our multi-component implementation strategy consisting of software provision, training/support, external/internal facilitation and a modified rapid process improvement workshop (Pittman et al., 2021b).

Methods and strategies to apply PRISM

PRISM was used in multiple ways during the planning phase. We used PRISM to develop a pre-implementation interview guide that we used with the staff involved in the implementation of eScreening to gather contextual information about each implementation site's organizational context. We then used the data to inform the focus of the external facilitation activities. The study interviewer used field notes and reviewed insights with the lead investigator and the external facilitator supporting implementation on a weekly basis.

We also developed a 29-item quantitative PRISM survey that we used with the staff to assess PRISM's contextual domains at each site to identify factors that may predict greater or lesser implementation success defined by PRISM's RE-AIM outcomes.

Beginning in the planning phase and throughout the study, we used PRISM to assess implementation. Similar to case 2, we developed a study-specific web-based (i.e. Qualtrics) adaptation tracker to capture information about adaptations made to the study, the eScreening programme and the implementation strategies. We also created a web-based tool for staff to use weekly to capture periodic reflections based on observations from training, facilitation or other factors. Both tools were modified from those used previously (Glasgow et al., 2020, 2022; Maw et al., 2022). Each of these included a question to identify which element(s) of PRISM the adaptation or reflection were relevant to the entry.

During the implementation phase, we used PRISM in two primary ways. We selected and used the modified rapid process improvement workshop as a key component of the implementation strategy. The modified rapid process improvement workshop was a multiple-day process that engaged multi-level organizational partners (i.e. managers and staff) to tailor the implementation of eScreening into the site-specific workflow and context. Partners addressed PRISM's contextual domains of patient and organizational characteristics and perspectives, as well as external factors (e.g. policies, COVID-19 process changes) that could facilitate or impede implementation. The external facilitator worked with the team to develop a plan that would meet their unique needs and resources (Implementation and Sustainability infrastructure) so that by the end, they had a plan with specific roles, responsibilities and deadlines for implementation.

During the second half of the implementation phase, we used a study-specific version of the iterative PRISM assessment (Glasgow et al., 2020; Estabrooks et al., 2021) (for details, see case 2) to make adjustments to the implementation process. The external facilitator conducted a 2-hour meeting with the site partners to review the scores, identify areas of potential improvement and develop an action plan. The adaptations that were needed were documented using the process developed during the pre-implementation phase.

During the evaluation/sustainment phase, we conducted post-implementation interviews with the staff participants using an interview guide based on PRISM. We also developed a PRISM codebook to assist with qualitative data analysis. Data from the interviews along with data from the adaptations and reflections will be used to improve our understanding of the contextual factors that affected the implementation of eScreening, what impact these factors had, and how implementation can be improved as eScreening is deployed to all VHA sites nationally.

Findings

The mean overall score from the initial administration of the 29-item survey across participants and sites was 3.95 (0.42 standard deviation) and the mean PRISM domain scores across participants and sites ranged from 3.5 (0.40 standard deviation) for patient characteristics to 4.1 (0.22 standard deviation) for organizational characteristics. Fifty-three adaptations have been documented using the adaptation tracker with 44 (83%) related to a PRISM contextual domain. Of 88 periodic reflections documented, 71 (81%) were related to a PRISM contextual domain. Seven sites completed the iterative PRISM assessment during the implementation phase and attended group meetings with an average of 5.6 (range, 4–8) participants. PRISM domains were broadly dispersed across clinics.

Lessons learned and future directions

These case examples highlight how PRISM can be applied in different ways and pragmatically to meet the needs of different implementation teams and types of projects at each stage of a project's life cycle. PRISM can be used to systematically align or adapt a project to fit with the context, enhance equitable outcomes and plan for sustainability and dissemination. Diverse partner perspectives are represented in these examples, demonstrating how PRISM can be used to consider and promote equity in research studies (Fort et al., 2023).

The meaningful assessment of PRISM domains requires partner engagement. These case examples emphasize the value of iterative, ongoing partner engagement to implement course corrections and adaptations in a systematic way and to consider how modifications may positively or negatively affect outcomes. PRISM also emphasizes equity in other ways by considering the representativeness of outcomes across different settings and populations, including for those who have historically been disadvantaged or who are from low-resource backgrounds (Fort et al., 2023).

To facilitate widespread use of the iterative PRISM assessment and PRISM more generally, the recently developed and publicly available iPRISM webtool (www.prismtool.

org) can be accessed. This webtool guides users through the process of operationalizing PRISM at each phase of a project. It is currently being used by English- and Spanish-speaking individuals and teams with and without implementation science experience for diverse types of projects within the United States and Latin America. Key features of the iPRISM webtool include embedded education, examples and an interactive design that prompts users to complete a series of PRISM assessment questions that are then summarized in visual feedback displays to identify and prioritize strategies or adaptations and develop action plans. In addition to the webtool, there are a number of resources available, including a guidebook (https://medschool.cuanschutz.edu/accords/cores-and-programs/dissemination-implementation-science-program/resources-services#Resources-Services-InteractiveTools) and website (https://re-aim.org) to assist users through the process of using PRISM (Guerin et al., 2022).

PRISM is a pragmatic and comprehensive framework that can be used in different projects, settings and phases of a project, including planning and ongoing evaluation. Over time, new ways of using PRISM have continued to emerge, including its use to promote health equity (Fort et al., 2023) and to iteratively identify and address areas in which contextual alignment or anticipated outcomes are suboptimal. PRISM is used to both assess and inform adaptations, although it is not yet known whether it enhances sustainment. An ongoing area of emphasis is to make PRISM more accessible and intuitive for diverse audiences, including non-English speakers. These initial efforts to increase the accessibility of PRISM appear to be effective, but more work is needed to continue to simplify and adapt PRISM to and for different audiences. In future work, we will evaluate the use of PRISM with an equity lens and the iPRISM webtool for diverse situations and settings, and under different conditions, such as with different amounts of facilitation.

References

Allen, L.A., Venechuk, G., McIlvennan, C.K., Page II, R.L., Knoepke, C.E., et al. (2021) An electronically delivered, patient-activation tool for intensification of medications for chronic heart failure with reduced ejection fraction: the EPIC-HF trial. *Circulation* 143, 427–437. https://doi.org/10.1161/circulationaha.120.051863

Boini, S., Colin, R., Grzebyk, M. (2017) Effect of occupational safety and health education received during schooling on the incidence of workplace injuries in the first 2 years of occupational life: a prospective study. *BMJ Open* 7, e015100. https://doi.org/10.1136/bmjopen-2016-015100

Estabrooks, P.A., Gaglio, B., Glasgow, R.E., Harden, S.M., Ory, M.G., Rabin, B.A., et al. (2021) Editorial: Use of the RE-AIM framework: translating research to practice with novel applications and emerging directions. *Frontiers in Public Health* 9, 691526. https://doi.org/10.3389/fpubh.2021.691526

Feldstein, A.C., Glasgow, R.E. (2008) A practical, robust implementation and sustainability model (PRISM) for integrating research findings into practice. *Joint Commission Journal on Quality and Patient Safety* 34, 228–243. https://doi.org/10.1016/s1553-7250(08)34030-6

Fort, M.P., Manson, S.M., Glasgow, R.E. (2023) Applying an equity lens to assess context and implementation in public health and health services research and practice using the PRISM framework. *Frontiers in Health Services* 3, 1139788. https://doi.org/10.3389/frhs.2023.1139788.

Glasgow, R.E., Vogt, T.M., Boles, S.M. (1999) Evaluating the public health impact of health promotion interventions: the RE-AIM framework. *American Journal of Public Health*.89, 1322–1327. https://doi.org/10.2105/AJPH.89.9.1322

Glasgow, R.E., Harden, S.M., Gaglio, B., Rabin, B., Smith, M.L., Porter, G.C., et al. (2019) RE-AIM planning and evaluation framework: adapting to new science and practice with a 20-year review. *Frontiers in Public Health* 7, 64. https://doi.org/10.3389/fpubh.2019.00064.

Glasgow, R.E., Battaglia, C., McCreight, M., Ayele, R.A., Rabin, B.A. (2020) Making implementation science more rapid: use of the RE-AIM framework for mid-course adaptations across five health services research projects in the Veterans Health Administration. *Frontiers in Public Health* 8, 194. https://doi.org/10.3389/fpubh.2020.00194

Glasgow, R.E., Fort, M.P., Paniagua, A., Maw, A.M., Huebschmann, A.G., Trinkley, K.E., et al. (2022) Applying the PRISM framework to guide iterative and responsive adaptations. Presented at Academy Health and National Institute of Health 15th Annual Conference on the Science of Dissemination and Implementation, Washington, DC.

Greene, S.J., Butler, J., Albert, N.M., DeVore, A.D., Sharma, P.P., Duffy, C.I., et al. (2018) Medical therapy for heart failure with reduced ejection fraction: the CHAMP-HF registry. *Journal of the American College of Cardiology* 72, 351–366. https://doi.org/10.1016/j.jacc.2018.04.070

Guerin, R.J., Reichard, A.A., Derk, S., Hendricks, K.J., Menger-Ogle, L.M., Okun, A.H. (2020) Nonfatal occupational injuries to younger workers - United States, 2012–2018. *MMWR. Morbidity and Mortality Weekly Report* 69, 1204–1209. https://doi.org/10.15585/mmwr. mm6935a3

Guerin, R.J., Glasgow, R.E., Tyler, A., Rabin, B.A., Huebschmann, A.G. (2022) Methods to improve the translation of evidence-based interventions: a primer on dissemination and implementation science for occupational safety and health researchers and practitioners. *Safety Science* 152, 105763. https://doi.org/10.1016/j.ssci.2022.105763

Heidenreich, P.A., Bozkurt, B., Aguilar, D., Allen, L.A., Byun, J.J., Colvin, M.M., et al. (2022) 2022 AHA/ACC/HFSA Guideline for the Management of Heart Failure: a report of the American College of Cardiology/American Heart Association Joint Committee on Clinical Practice Guidelines. *Circulation* 145, E895–E1032. https://doi.org/10.1161/CIR.0000000000001063

Holtrop, J.S., Estabrooks, P.A., Gaglio, B., Harden, S.M., Kessler, R.S., King, D.K., et al. (2021) Understanding and applying the RE-AIM framework: clarifications and resources. *Journal of Clinical and Translational Science* 5, e126. https://doi.org/10.1017/CTS.2021.789

Kwan, B.M., Brownson, R.C., Glasgow, R.E., Morrato, E.H., Luke, D.A. (2022) Designing for dissemination and sustainability to promote equitable impacts on health. *Annual Review of Public Health* 43, 331–335. https://doi.org/10.1146/annurev-publhealth-052220-112457

Labouliere, C.D., Vasan, P., Kramer, A., Brown, G., Green, K., Rahman, M., et al. (2018) "Zero Suicide" – a model for reducing suicide in United States behavioral healthcare. *Suicidologi* 23, 22. https://doi.org/10.5617/suicidologi.6198.

Maw, A.M., Morris, M.A., Glasgow, R.E., Barnard, J., Ho, P.M., Ortiz-Lopez, C., et al. (2022) Using iterative RE-AIM to enhance hospitalist adoption of lung ultrasound in the management of patients with COVID-19: an implementation pilot study. *Implementation Science Communications* 3, 89. https://doi.org/10.1186/S43058-022-00334-X.

McCarthy, M.S., Ujano-De Motta, L.L., Nunnery, M.A., Gilmartin, H., Kelley, L., Wills, A., et al. (2021) Understanding adaptations in the Veteran Health Administration's Transitions Nurse Program: refining methodology and pragmatic implications for scale-up. *Implementation Science* 16, 71. https://doi.org/10.1186/S13012-021-01126-Y

McCreight, M.S., Rabin, B.A., Glasgow, R.E., Ayele, R.A., Leonard, C.A., Gilmartin, H.M., et al. (2019) Using the Practical, Robust Implementation and Sustainability Model (PRISM) to qualitatively assess multilevel contextual factors to help plan, implement, evaluate, and disseminate health services programs. *Translational Behavioral Medicine* 9, 1002–1011. https://doi.org/10.1093/TBM/IBZ085

Nelson, H.D., Denneson, L., Low, A., Bauer, B.W., O'Neil, M., Kansagara, D., et al. (2015) *Systematic Review of Suicide Prevention in Veterans. VA Evidence-Based Synthesis Program Reports.* Washington, DC: Department of Veterans Affairs.

Pittman, J.O.E., Floto, E., Lindamer, L., Baker, D.G., Lohr, J.B., Afari, N. (2017) VA eScreening program: technology to improve care for post-9/11 veterans. *Psychological Services* 14, 23–33. https://doi.org/10.1037/ser0000125.

Pittman, J.O.E., Lindamer, L., Afari, N., Depp, C., Villodas, M., Hamilton, A., et al. (2021a) Implementing eScreening for suicide prevention in VA post-9/11 transition programs using a stepped-wedge, mixed-method, hybrid type-II implementation trial: a study protocol. *Implementation Science Communications* 2, 46. https://doi.org/10.1186/s43058-021-00142-9.

Pittman, J.O.E., Rabin, B., Almklov, E., Afari, N., Floto, E., Rodriguez, E., et al. (2021b) Adaptation of a quality improvement approach to implement eScreening in VHA healthcare settings: innovative use of the Lean Six Sigma Rapid Process Improvement Workshop. *Implementation Science Communications* 2, 37. https://doi.org/10.1186/s43058-021-00132-x.

Rabin, B.A., McCreight, M., Battaglia, C., Ayele, R., Burke, R.E., Hess, P.L., et al. (2018) Systematic, multimethod assessment of adaptations across four diverse health systems interventions. *Frontiers in Public Health* 6, 102. https://doi.org/10.3389/fpubh.2018.00102.

Rabin, B.A., Cakici, J., Golden, C.A., Estabrooks, P.A., Glasgow, R.E., Gaglio, B. (2022) A citation analysis and scoping systematic review of the operationalization of the Practical, Robust Implementation and Sustainability Model (PRISM). *Implementation Science* 17, 62. https://doi.org/10.1186/S13012-022-01234-3

Shelton, R.C., Chambers, D.A., Glasgow, R.E. (2020) An extension of RE-AIM to enhance sustainability: addressing dynamic context and promoting health equity over time. *Frontiers in Public Health* 8, 134. https://doi.org/10.3389/fpubh.2020.00134

Shendell, D.G., Milich, L.J., Apostolico, A.A., Patti, A.A., Kelly, S. (2017) Comparing online and in-person delivery formats of the OSHA 10-hour general industry health and safety training for young workers. *New Solutions* 27, 92–106. https://doi.org/10.1177/1048291117697109

Stirman, S.W., Baumann, A.A., Miller, C.J. (2019) The FRAME: an expanded framework for reporting adaptations and modifications to evidence-based interventions. *Implementation Science* 14, 58. https://doi.org/10.1186/s13012-019-0898-y

Trinkley, K.E., Kahn, M.G., Bennett, T.D., Glasgow, R.E., Haugen, H., Kao, D.P., et al. (2020) Integrating the Practical Robust Implementation and Sustainability Model with best practices in clinical decision support design: implementation science approach. *Journal of Medical Internet Research* 22, e19676. https://doi.org/10.2196/19676.

Trinkley, K.E., Kroehl, M.E., Kahn, M.G., Allen, L.A., Bennett, T.D., Hale, G., et al. (2021) Applying clinical decision support design best practices with the Practical Robust Implementation and Sustainability Model versus reliance on commercially available clinical decision support tools: randomized controlled trial. *JMIR Medical Informatics* 9, e24359. https://doi.org/10.2196/24359.

US Department of Labor (n.d.) Program overview. Retrieved from www.osha.gov/training/outreach/overview (accessed 14 March 2023).

Veterans Administration/Department of Defense (2019) Assessment and management of patients at risk for suicide (2019) – VA/DoD clinical practice guidelines. Retrieved from www.healthquality.va.gov/guidelines/mh/srb (accessed 14 March 2023).

18 Applying Capability Opportunity Motivation – Behaviour and the Theoretical Domains Framework

Danielle D'Lima and Fabiana Lorencatto

Introduction

Implementation of anything different or new always requires someone to do something differently. This can involve adopting entirely new practices (e.g. uptake of new diagnostic tests), doing more of existing practices (e.g. increasing referral rates), doing less of existing practices (e.g. reducing inappropriate prescribing of antibiotics) or discontinuing a practice altogether (e.g. de-implementation of low-value care) (Patey et al., 2018). Such actions are all forms of human behaviour. Implementation therefore requires behaviour change, often in individual and collective behaviours as well as at organization, service and system levels (Ferlie and Shortell, 2001; Francis et al., 2012; Lorencatto, 2022).

Designing interventions to change behaviour and improve implementation processes and outcomes first requires understanding the influences (i.e. barriers and facilitators) on current and desired behaviours in the context in which they occur (Michie et al., 2014). This can be facilitated through the application of evidence-based theories, models and frameworks from behavioural science, which enable drawing from and contributing to the wider literature and evidence-base on what influences behaviour and practice change. The purpose of this chapter is to demonstrate how two such theories, models and frameworks can be used to identify influences on implementation behaviours as a step towards improving implementation.

Both Capability Opportunity Motivation – Behaviour (COM-B) and the Theoretical Domains Framework (TDF) have been applied to explore influences for a range of behaviours in the context of implementation research (Francis et al., 2012). Commonly used methods for these purposes are semi-structured interviews, focus groups and surveys. Both COM-B and the TDF can be used to inform data collection (e.g. interview or survey questions designed to elicit information on individual components/domains) and analysis (e.g. deductive qualitative coding or statistical analysis guided by the theoretical frameworks). They can also be applied in systematic reviews as a framework for synthesizing published evidence on behavioural influences.

In this chapter, three case studies are summarized using each of these three methodologies, qualitative interviews, quantitative surveys, systematic reviews, using either COM-B or the TDF as a guiding framework. The three cases are based on three published articles: case 1, Mill et al. (2023); case 2, Owens et al. (2023); case 3, Graham-Rowe et al. (2018). Further illustrative examples are given alongside each case. The chapter ends with broader reflections on the applicability of COM-B and the TDF in this context, strengths and weaknesses, and areas in which future development may benefit the field. We also offer our perspectives on the choice between COM-B and the TDF, opportunities

DOI: 10.4324/9781003318125-20

to combine the two and the selection of the most appropriate research methods in different scenarios.

Case 1: Application of COM-B to qualitatively explore an implementation challenge

This case applied COM-B to qualitatively explore influences on the use of professional practice guidelines by pharmacists in Australia. Pharmacy practice in Australia is guided by professional practice guidelines, which communicate expected pharmacist behaviours to facilitate a consistently high standard of patient care. However, such guidelines are used infrequently by pharmacists and students. A comprehensive understanding of what influences the use of pharmacists' professional practice guidelines is critical for regulators, professional organizations, guideline writers and the profession itself to ensure these guidelines are fit for purpose and support the provision of quality pharmacist care as intended. Conceptualizing the use of practice guidelines as an implementation behaviour, subject to its own influences, may aid in providing further insights into the use of these guidelines to achieve this. It will also shed light on how best to support positive behaviour change towards improved utilization of these guidelines. The aim of the study was to explore perceived influences on the use of professional practice guidelines by Australian pharmacists and to map these influences to COM-B.

Data collection

Online focus group discussions were undertaken with pharmacists (including intern pharmacists) from various practice settings and locations in Australia and with varying years of experience. The topic guide was developed by members of the research team with input from the Pharmaceutical Society of Australia project team and members of an expert advisory group. The guide covered a general discussion of the use of professional practice guidelines, followed by more specific questions about influences on their use. Question probes were guided by COM-B to ensure all potential influences were explored. The final topic guide included at least one probe linked to each of the COM-B components. Example probes included "What do you know about how to use these documents? Describe an example" for Capability, "What do you think about access to these documents? Describe an example" for Opportunity and "Do you believe that using these guidelines is/would be a good thing to do? Why/why not?" for Motivation. A presentation featuring the professional practice guidelines and discussion questions was also shared to aid participants in answering questions.

Data analysis

Data fragments, usually sentences or full participant responses were deductively coded to one or more components of COM-B using the framework method by two members of the research team independently. At least two researchers then reviewed the data coded to each COM-B component and independently coded the data fragments using an inductive approach to identify sub-themes for each component. All coding disagreements at each stage were resolved through discussion by the analysis team and a record was kept of code descriptors as they evolved. The final sub-themes identified and corresponding data fragments (charted in a matrix) were then discussed with an experienced behavioural scientist who sought clarification from the coding team on the theme descriptors to ensure internal consistency in coding and that sub-themes had been recognized under the appropriate component of COM-B. These final themes were presented back to the coding team for review and were agreed upon.

Results

Nine focus groups were conducted with a total of 45 participants. Participants ranged from intern pharmacists to pharmacists with 43 years of experience and were from community, hospital and specialty practice settings, and locations ranging from metropolitan to remote.

The study found that the use of practice guidelines by practising pharmacists was sporadic and usually prompted by situations arising in practice involving learners or patients (Opportunity) where the pharmacist was unsure how to proceed and potentially feared what would happen if they did not proceed in a guideline-concordant manner (Motivation). The use of practice guidelines was dependent on the belief that guidelines will successfully support knowing how to proceed in different situations (Motivation). Furthermore, this use of practice guidelines was also dependent on the individual pharmacist's awareness of the guidelines (Capability) and their understanding of where to find them (Capability), and facilitated by how easily they could be accessed and navigated when needed (Opportunity). Participants also expressed that they believed practice guidelines were more useful to less experienced pharmacists and for those who identified as experienced pharmacists, routine use was unnecessary (Motivation).

The use of COM-B in this qualitative study enabled a thorough, theory-informed investigation of influences on the use of professional practice guidelines by pharmacists in Australia, framed as an implementation behaviour that precedes enactment of the professional behaviours that are communicated through the guidelines themselves. The detailed understanding of what influences the use of professional practice guidelines in this context can inform implementation interventions to target and improve pharmacists' use of the guidelines going forward. This nuanced understanding of the influences, and the relationships between them, identified as a result of the use of COM-B in this qualitative study, could also be considered in the review or development of new practice guidelines both in Australia and internationally for pharmacists and other related disciplines.

Other qualitative examples using the TDF and/or COM-B

Numerous additional examples of the use of COM-B to qualitatively explore an implementation challenge have been published. These include the use of COM-B to understand influences on the implementation of weight management services in Malaysia (Blebil et al., 2022), a smoke-free policy within a mental health trust (Smith et al., 2019) and the registration of adverse drug reactions in electronic health records (Geeven et al., 2022). Qualitative examples of the use of the TDF to explore an implementation challenge are discussed in the remainder of this section. A detailed guide to using the TDF to investigate implementation problems, with an emphasis on qualitative methods, has been published (Atkins et al., 2017). This guide includes support on selecting and specifying target behaviours that are key to implementation, selecting the study design, deciding the sampling strategy, developing study materials, collecting and analysing data, and reporting findings of TDF-based studies. Examples from the implementation research literature are presented in the guide to illustrate relevant methods and practical considerations.

The TDF is commonly used in semi-structured qualitative interview studies, whereby the interview topic guide questions are structured around the 14 domains to explore the role that each domain plays in facilitating or hindering implementation in the context of interest. Example TDF-based interview questions for each domain have been published (Michie et al., 2005), and many papers reporting the findings of TDF-based interviews also publish interview topic guides as supplementary files (Patey et al., 2012). The TDF is subsequently applied during analysis as a coding framework following a combined deductive framework and inductive thematic analysis approach (Atkins et al., 2017).

Examples of this application of the TDF are listed in a thematic series on the TDF published in *Implementation Science* (Francis et al., 2012). Applications to date have focused primarily on improving the quality of healthcare, given the TDF was initially developed to explore influences on healthcare professional behaviours (Atkins et al., 2017). Examples of implementation challenges investigated qualitatively using the TDF include antibiotic prescribing in long-term care facilities (Fleming et al., 2014), delivery of early rehabilitation in critical care (Goddard et al., 2018) and delivery of community-based occupational therapy for patients with functional neurological disorders (Nicholson et al., 2022). It has also been applied to investigate potential influences on the implementation of a new clinical care bundle for the detection and management of post-partum haemorrhage, a priori, so that implementation strategies can be put in place ahead of rollout to support uptake in practice (Forbes et al., 2023).

Case 2: Application of the TDF to quantitatively explore an implementation challenge

Although the TDF has been widely used to qualitatively explore influences on implementation, there has been a recent increase in studies quantitatively applying the TDF to inform data collection and analysis using methods such as questionnaires. This is in part due to the development and publication of a TDF-based questionnaire for implementation research, which has been validated in English and Dutch (Huijg et al., 2014a, 2014b). This instrument provides a series of generic statements corresponding to each of the 14 TDF domains; the phrasing can be adapted to the specific implementation issue of interest following the TACT principle (i.e. target, action, context, timeframe) (Fishbein, 1967; Presseau et al., 2019). For example, the following item assesses the TDF domain Social/professional role and identity: "It is my responsibility as a [profession] to [A] in [C, T] with [Ta]". Applying the TACT principle to tailor this statement to the case described below would result in the statement: "It is my responsibility as a doctor to prescribe HIV PrEP [pre-exposure prophylaxis] in primary care to adolescents aged 13–18 years". Respondents rate their agreement to each item on a Likert-type scale. In turn, it is possible to use correlation and regression analyses to investigate the association between agreement scores on TDF domains and outcomes such as intention to perform the implementation behaviour of interest and/or if data are available, the actual behaviour itself (e.g. prescribing rates).

This section describes a case applying the validated TDF questionnaire to explore primary care physicians' intention to prescribe HIV PrEP to adolescents in the United States. Adolescents (aged 13–18 years) accounted for up to 21% of new HIV infections in 2019 in the United States. HIV PrEP involves a once-daily pill with demonstrated effectiveness in preventing HIV and is approved for use in adolescents. Guidelines have been produced to support clinicians with screening and assessing patient risk for HIV and subsequently offering PrEP as a preventative treatment. However, uptake remains low, with adolescents accounting for just 1.5% of PrEP usage in the United States. There has been limited research into healthcare providers' perspectives towards prescribing PrEP for this population group. Furthermore, only a handful of existing studies have drawn on theory to inform their investigation of influencing factors on PrEP prescribing practices, and many have been smaller-scale qualitative studies focusing on a limited geographic area (i.e. a single city).

This study therefore aimed to investigate this issue in a more generalizable and representative sample by conducting a TDF-based questionnaire study to explore primary care physicians' attitudes towards prescribing PrEP to sexually active adolescents in the United States and the factors that influence their intention to do so.

Data collection

An online, cross-sectional questionnaire study was conducted in July–August, 2022. Participants were licensed primary care physicians practising family medicine, internal medicine or paediatrics in the United States. They were recruited from a national panel of medical providers managed by Qualtrics, a survey management platform company. A random selection of panel members meeting the eligibility criteria were invited to participate via email. Participants were offered an incentive to take part (i.e. gift cards, cash, redeemable points). The study received ethical approval from a university institutional review board.

Participants completed a questionnaire with the following sections: (1) demographic characteristics (e.g. age, ethnicity, gender identity); (2) provider characteristics (e.g. practice speciality, geographic region); (3) sexual healthcare practices (e.g. sexual history taking, ordering tests for HIV and sexually transmitted infections for adolescents); (4) PrEP healthcare practices (e.g. if they have ever heard of PrEP and prescribed PrEP to an adolescent); and (5) factors influencing prescribing of PrEP for this population group. The latter questions were adapted from the validated TDF implementation questionnaire (Huijg et al., 2014a, 2014b), and included one belief statement for ten of the TDF domains, to which respondents rated their agreement on a 5-point Likert-type scale (1, strongly disagree; 5, strongly agree). This section also included a free-text response question to further explore the TDF domain Environmental context and resources, asking about what clinical resources they had or wish they could have to help prescribe PrEP to eligible adolescents. The outcome of interest was intention to prescribe PrEP rated on a 5-point Likert-type scale.

Data analysis

Data were checked for assumption violations, skewness, kurtosis and normality, all of which were within acceptable limits. Data were first analysed using descriptive statistics. Subsequently, Pearson and Spearman correlations were conducted to explore associations between the dependent variable (intention) and demographic characteristics, provider characteristics, PrEP and sexual healthcare practices, and the ten TDF domains. Hierarchical regressions were then conducted with significant correlations included in the model to predict intention to prescribe PrEP to sexually active adolescents. The first block included only demographic variables. The second block included demographic and sexual healthcare practice variables. The third block included the demographic variables, sexual healthcare practice variables, and all ten TDF domains. The free-text response question was analysed using inductive content analysis.

Results

In total, 770 responses were received from primary care physicians. Less than a third of respondents (30.6%) had ever prescribed PrEP to an adolescent. Nearly all respondents had heard about PrEP (90.3%) and over half (57.1%) were aware of guidelines to prescribe PrEP to adolescents (TDF domain: Knowledge). Most agreed they had the self-efficacy (69.4%) and skills (73.2%) to prescribe PrEP (TDF domains: Beliefs about capabilities and Beliefs about skills, respectively). Most (71.4%) agreed that prescribing PrEP was part of their role (TDF domain: Social/professional role and identity), that they had the necessary resources in their clinics to do so (56.5%, TDF domain: Environmental context and resources), and that they would be able to focus their attention when prescribing PrEP (74.9%, TDF domain: Memory, attention and decision processes). About half (52.6%) reported that they would be optimistic when prescribing PrEP (TDF domain: Optimism) and 41% would enjoy prescribing PrEP (TDF domain: Emotion). There was strong agreement (87%) that prescribing PrEP to sexually active adolescents would benefit public health. Only about a third of respondents (38.6%) felt supported by their colleagues to prescribe PrEP (TDF domain: Social influences). Approximately two thirds (66%) had strong intentions to prescribe PrEP to this population group in the future. All ten domains were significantly correlated with intention to prescribe PrEP to sexually active adolescents in the future. However, only eight domains were significant in subsequent hierarchical regressions: (i) knowledge, (ii) skills, (iii) social/professional role and identity, (iv) beliefs about capabilities, (v) beliefs about consequences, (vi) environmental context and resources, (vii) social influences, and (viii) emotion.

Such analyses help pinpoint the precise individual, socio-cultural and environmental factors that are influencing primary care physicians' intention to prescribe PrEP. Limitations include the cross-sectional methodology, which limits causal inferences, and the use of intention as an outcome measure. There are well-established intention-behaviour gaps (Sniehotta et al., 2005). Where possible, it would be preferable and methodologically stronger to use data on actual practice (i.e. behaviour) as the outcome of interest. Routinely collected data via electronic health records have the potential to facilitate this. Nonetheless, one benefit of quantitative TDF questionnaires is that they enable estimation of the strength of association between factors influencing the implementation challenge of interest. These findings can inform the design of more targeted, and likely effective, interventions to facilitate practice change and aid the rollout and implementation of PrEP for eligible adolescents.

Other quantitative examples using TDF and/or COM-B

The TDF has also been used to design questionnaires to explore a number of other implementation challenges, such as hand hygiene in hospitals (Gaube et al., 2021) and healthcare provider conversation skills training (Hollis et al., 2021). COM-B has also been similarly applied in questionnaire studies to identify influences on implementation challenges. A brief validated COM-B questionnaire measure has also been developed, which presents generic items that can be adapted to the specific behaviour and context of interest (Keyworth et al., 2020). A number of topic-specific questionnaires have also been developed and validated, such as a COM-B-based questionnaire for understanding dentists' management of dental caries (Abreu-Placeres et al., 2018). Examples of implementation challenges that have been investigated using COM-B-based questionnaires include orthopaedic physicians' compliance with surgical site infection prevention (Tomsic et al., 2021) and delivering smoking cessation support for patients with tuberculosis in Nepal (Warsi et al., 2019). There are also examples of COM-B and the TDF being applied concurrently in questionnaire studies, such as exploring bleeding management practices among Australian cardiac surgeons, anaesthesiologists and perfusionists (Pearse et al., 2020). Considerations for selecting between the two, or using them concurrently, are discussed later in this chapter.

Case 3: Application of the TDF to synthesize influences on an implementation challenge

Although the TDF and COM-B have predominantly been applied to primary qualitative and quantitative data collection, some recent systematic reviews have applied these behavioural and implementation science frameworks to synthesize available evidence on factors influencing practice change and implementation challenges. One example of this approach is a systematic review of influences on diabetic retinopathy screening.

Diabetic retinopathy is a leading cause of severe sight loss in people of working age globally. Effective treatments are available, but these depend on early detection. A significant proportion of diabetes-related vision loss can be prevented through a systems-level approach, which includes targeted education, well-implemented diabetic retinopathy screening programmes and timely referral pathways for further investigation, monitoring or treatment (Prothero et al., 2021). Population-wide screening programmes have been established in countries such as Ireland, Iceland and the United Kingdom, and regional and local screening programmes have been implemented in many other parts of Europe. However, screening attendance is consistently below recommended levels. Several international studies have explored the reasons why screening uptake is limited from the perspective of people with diabetes and those responsible for delivering and implementing screening (i.e. healthcare providers, service managers). This case describes a systematic review that applied the TDF to help synthesize reported influences on diabetic retinopathy screening delivery and attendance.

Data collection

A detailed protocol for this review has been published (Graham-Rowe et al., 2016) and registered in PROSPERO (CRD42016032990). In summary, six electronic databases were searched to identify the published literature with search terms related to diabetic retinopathy AND screening AND barriers or facilitators. In addition, two grey literature databases and a Google search engine were also searched. Studies were eligible for inclusion if they were published in English between 1990 and 2017 and reported primary data related to modifiable factors that might hinder or facilitate diabetic retinopathy screening attendance. Both qualitative and quantitative studies were included. Studies were excluded if they only reported non-modifiable influences (i.e. age, duration of diabetes diagnosis). Studies were double screened for inclusion.

Data analysis

Data were extracted on study characteristics (e.g. author, country, year, design, sample size). For the TDF analysis of influences, one review author identified and extracted data reporting participants' perceptions of modifiable influences on diabetic retinopathy screening. This could be either from the perspective of people with diabetes and/or healthcare professionals. A second reviewer checked the accuracy of data extraction for a random sample of 20% of the studies included. Extracted data included participant quotes from qualitative studies, quantitative findings from questionnaire studies (i.e. descriptive statistics, predictors of and associations with attendance/non-attendance) and authors' interpretive descriptions and summaries of results. In line with guidance for analysing qualitative data using the TDF (Atkins et al., 2017), extracted data on perceived influences were first coded deductively to the TDF domain they were judged to best represent (e.g. fear of pain during the procedure was coded to the TDF domain Emotion). All deductive coding was double checked by a second researcher. Next, an inductive thematic synthesis was conducted by grouping similar data points coded to each domain and generating a summary theme label representing the shared meaning among each grouping of data points. Theme labels represented a barrier and enabler of mixed influence within each domain. Important domains were identified by applying three published importance criteria: frequency (number of studies that identified each domain); elaboration (number of themes and subthemes within each domain); and expressed importance (statements from author interpretations or direct quotes emphasizing the importance of that domain) (Atkins et al., 2017).

Results

In total, 69 studies were included in the systematic review. Of these, 78% explored influences from the perspective of people with diabetes and 22% from the perspective of both healthcare professionals and people with diabetes. Reported barriers were identified within all but one TDF domain (Skills). Reported enablers were identified within all but two domains (Beliefs about capabilities and Skills). The six most important TDF domains were as follows:

- Environmental context and resources (75% of included studies): for example, accessibility of screening clinics; time constraints linked to competing demands (work, child care); cost; lack of flexibility and limited availability for scheduling appointments; long waiting times and appointments; inaccurate registers; referral issues and lack of integration among diabetes services and teams.
- Knowledge (51%): understanding of the link between diabetes and vision loss; confusion between screening and routine eye tests; lack of education and training.
- Social influences (51%): for example, doctor-patient communication (including the presence/absence of a healthcare provider recommendation to attend screening); family support; stigma.
- Memory, attention and decision processes (50%): absence of symptoms; competing health problems; forgetting.
- Beliefs about consequences (38%): the perceived necessity of screening; perceived benefit (i.e. provides valuable information on the health status of the eyes); short-term effects of screening and concern about harmful effects of the screening procedure.
- Emotions (33%): fear or anxiety; defensive responses and avoidance; emotional burden of diabetes.

This synthesis was beneficial in this topic area even though a number of primary data collection studies on influences on the behaviour of interest had already been conducted. The TDF-based synthesis resulted in the identification of a wide range of individual patient-, healthcare provider- and system-level influences on diabetic retinopathy screening delivery and uptake. This enabled the generation of a number of focused recommendations for practice to improve uptake, such as offering integrated diabetes one-stop shops in which diabetic retinopathy screening is offered at the same location and time as other diabetes appointments, healthcare provider encouragement and education around screening attendance, and improving communication materials (i.e. invitation letters) to provide reassurance around fears and concerns associated with screening (e.g. what can be done if retinopathy is detected). The synthesis of data across a large number of mixed-methods studies was facilitated through the use of the TDF. It provided a comprehensive, unifying framework to facilitate categorization and comparison of reported influences across studies. However, the ability to do so was hampered at times by the limited reporting of study findings in the studies, and the potential bias in that authors may have selectively reported findings on influences that they perceived to be more relevant, interesting, or a better fit with the original study's research question.

Other systematic review examples using TDF and/or COM-B

Numerous additional examples of TDF-based systematic reviews have recently been published: implementation of pregnancy weight management and obesity guidelines (Heslehurst et al., 2014); triage, treatment, transfer and management of acute stroke patients in emergency departments (Craig et al., 2016); and pulmonary rehabilitation referral and participation (Cox et al., 2017). COM-B has also been applied in a similar manner to synthesize evidence on behaviour change and implementation problems as part of systematic reviews. Examples include primary care practitioners' and young peoples' perceived influences on chlamydia testing in general practice (McDonagh et al., 2018) and implementing practices for the prevention of childhood obesity in primary care (Ray et al., 2022). Examples of the TDF and COM-B being used concurrently in a systematic review are also available; for example, a review to examine influences on the implementation of screening and brief interventions for alcohol use in primary care (Rosário et al., 2021); another review examining influences on mental health professionals' perceived influences on shared decision making in risk assessment and management (Ahmed et al., 2021).

Reflections on the applicability of COM-B and TDF, strengths and weaknesses from a usability perspective and areas for future research/development

Choice of methods

The three cases have provided examples of the use of COM-B and the TDF in the context of qualitative, quantitative and systematic review methods. Considerations for selecting method(s) when applying COM-B and TDF in the context of implementation are now discussed.

As with all research, the appropriate study design depends on the research question (i.e. purpose) and the state of current knowledge (i.e. scientific context) in the given field. Qualitative methods may be selected when the aim is to collect richer data on influences from a smaller sample and when little is known about the implementation behaviour(s) in the particular context. A qualitative design allows researchers to explore in greater detail providing richer data, which can be helpful when developing theory-informed interventions (i.e. they may provide better insight into the necessary content).

Quantitative methods, on the other hand, may be selected when the aim is to investigate influences in larger samples and statistically examine associations between COM-B components/TDF domains and implementation outcomes. Survey/questionnaire studies, for example, may be more appropriate when a greater amount is known about the implementation behaviour(s) and potentially relevant influencing factors, but the aim is to identify those factors in a more representative sample.

Mixed methods designs may be helpful in some instances and provide the opportunity for triangulation of data (Munafò and Davey Smith, 2018). Triangulation can be defined as the considered use of multiple methodological approaches to address one research question. The validity of findings is likely to be improved through the integration or triangulation of data. If a consistent picture of an implementation behaviour and the factors influencing it is obtained from more than one source and using more than one method, it increases confidence in the analysis. For example, Surr et al. (2020) adopted a mixed methods design combining qualitative and quantitative data from a range of sources of data to investigate influences on the implementation of dementia training. This permitted multiple perspectives to be explored across a broad range of participants and service settings using quantitative methods as well as more in-depth understanding of these factors and their implications using qualitative methods. Findings from one method may also help inform the development of data collection using an alternative method. For example, the outcomes of qualitative analysis (i.e. key themes) can be used to inform the design of the survey items (i.e. those themes become belief statements that participants rate their agreement with) (Prothero et al., 2022a, 2022b).

Systematic review methods may be selected when there is sufficient existing primary data (which may be qualitative or quantitative) about the influences on the implementation behaviour(s) of interest that may benefit from synthesis in line with a behaviour-change theory, model or framework. Synthesis of this type may enable a more holistic and theory-driven understanding of what is driving the implementation behaviour(s) and provide opportunities for the development of an intervention based on a broader dataset.

COM-B and the TDF are also potentially applicable to other research designs that have not been included in this chapter but for which methods can be further developed; for example, ethnographic observations, documentary analysis, case study designs. Ethnographic observations may be particularly well suited to exploring Opportunity in COM-B and the theoretical domains of Environmental context and resources and Social influences. We acknowledge that the selection of methods for any given project may also be influenced by pragmatic considerations, such as the available resources and expertise of the team. One option for data collection requiring fewer resources, for example, would be to conduct a structured discussion with key stakeholders, or even just the relevant staff team, based on the COM-B components and/or domains of the TDF.

Regardless of the methods chosen, the first step should always be to precisely specify whose and which behaviour is of interest. Implementation challenges are typically complex, involving multiple behaviours across different time points and requiring interprofessional effort across different roles. There will often be very different influences on these different actors and behaviours and therefore a precisely specified behaviour is essential at the outset to enable a more focused, and in turn more informative, understanding of the barriers and facilitators. Frameworks, such as the Actor, Action, Context, Target, Time framework (Presseau et al., 2019), are available to support the specification of implementation behaviours in terms of who needs to do what, differently, to/with whom, where and when.

Choice of COM-B versus TDF

We have provided examples of the use of COM-B and the TDF in the context of qualitative, quantitative and systematic review methods. However, it is worthwhile considering how to decide when and why to use each tool and in the instances when it could be appropriate to use both concurrently.

Often the end goal when exploring influences on implementation behaviours is to design interventions to change those behaviours and improve implementation outcomes. In this instance, it is beneficial to work with a theory, model or framework that links influences to behaviour-change strategies so that interventions can be developed to address the barriers and facilitators to implementation. COM-B is nested within the Behaviour Change Wheel (Michie et al., 2014), which specifies nine broad intervention types (e.g. Education, Incentivization, Modelling, Environmental restructuring) and maps these to the components of COM-B. Once selected based on the behavioural diagnosis, these intervention types can be mapped to the Behaviour Change Technique Taxonomy (Michie et al., 2013), which specifies 93 more granular techniques for changing behaviour (e.g. goal setting, self-monitoring, feedback on behaviour). These tools can guide decision making during intervention design and support more systematic, transparent and theory-based development of behaviour change and implementation interventions (Michie et al., 2014).

There are also published matrices directly pairing domains of the TDF with the intervention types and techniques in the aforementioned frameworks to suggest types of behaviour-change strategies that are likely to be effective in targeting influences within each domain (Cane et al., 2015; Johnston et al., 2021). The granularity provided by the TDF may make it an attractive choice for some when the focus is on understanding an implementation problem in depth. However, both COM-B and the TDF support the exploration of a broad range of influences on behaviour and some users may prefer the simpler nature of COM-B.

In terms of using COM-B and the TDF in parallel, researchers need to think carefully about the purpose of each and what specifically is being gained by using both tools together. If the same outcomes can be achieved with the use of just one, then we would recommend that that is sufficient. Scenarios in which it may be beneficial to use both could include the use of the TDF for granular data collection followed by the use of both TDF and COM-B for analysis to support intervention design. For example, Alexander et al. (2014) used the TDF to conduct focus groups to identify influences on the delivery of the Healthy Kids Check in Australia. Their thematic analysis involved mapping codes to the domains of the TDF and then mapping relevant TDF domains to the COM-B components. The decision to map to COM-B, as an additional stage to the analysis, was informed by their plans to map the findings to proposed interventions. The authors state that "distillation of the findings into COM-B has set the stage for developing the components of a complex intervention" (Alexander et al., 2014). Similarly, Chater et al. (2022) conducted a cross-sectional multi-country survey to investigate the determinants of nurse antimicrobial stewardship behaviours. The survey was based on the 14 domains of the TDF but their analysis also included the mapping of TDF data to COM-B to support intervention design. A further advantage of mapping to COM-B in these instances is the opportunity to explore relationships in the dataset with reference to the theoretical relationships that it proposes.

General strengths and weaknesses

COM-B and the TDF have been applied to numerous implementation problems and contexts to date, reflecting progress made towards achieving their original aims of making theory more accessible and useful to interdisciplinary researchers in implementation science and beyond and improving our understanding of behaviour-change processes in implementation (Lorencatto, 2022). As discussed, both COM-B and the TDF enable progression to intervention design, which has the potential to improve implementation outcomes using systematically developed interventions that can be clearly reported (i.e. through a logic model) and thoroughly evaluated (with a focus on both the process and outcomes).

Regarding limitations, some argue that using COM-B or the TDF to structure interview questions and analysis restricts findings to those that fit within the components/domains, thereby limiting opportunities for identifying additional influences (McGowan et al., 2020). However, a study comparing the results of interviews using the TDF versus atheoretical approaches identified that although the findings from both approaches overlapped, the TDF-based studies elicited a greater number of influences that were not mentioned in the atheoretical studies, particularly around emotional factors influencing behaviour (Dyson et al., 2011).

A further critique is that COM-B and the TDF are overly focused on individual behaviour and thus not applicable to investigating implementation problems at organizational levels (Francis et al., 2012). This argument is based on the idea of a clear dichotomy between individual and organizational/system change, which may not recognize the role of actors across the system and therefore needs to be reconsidered (Sniehotta et al., 2017). Organizational theories were among the 33 theories contributing to the development of the TDF. Organizational influences on behaviour are represented in the domains of environmental context and resources, Social influences, and Social/professional role and identity; however, some may feel these are not sufficiently elaborated. For this reason, many studies have applied the TDF concurrently alongside other determinant frameworks such as the Consolidated Framework for Implementation Research, which contains domains relating to outer contextual influences on implementation (Damschroder et al., 2009; Birken et al., 2017).

Future developments

Each COM-B component and TDF domain does not exist in a vacuum, and influences identified within each will likely interact with those in other areas (e.g. fear within the TDF domain Emotion may result from negative Beliefs about consequences). However, most COM-B and/or TDF-based studies do not discuss relationships between components/domains. Future work should move beyond generating descriptive lists of influences towards investigating and theorizing how components/domains interact for the implementation behaviour(s) of interest. A recent example of such an approach includes a TDF qualitative study of influences on opioid prescribing among family physicians (Desveaux et al., 2019). Paying greater attention to the relationships between components/domains (e.g. the relationship between Social influences and Beliefs about capabilities in the TDF) can also have positive implications for applying an intersectionality lens alongside theories, models and frameworks in implementation science. Etherington et al. (2020), for example, have developed a tool to be used alongside applications of the TDF to incorporate an intersectionality lens when identifying influences on implementation behaviours. Future work that considers interactions between COM-B components and TDF domains will support more thorough explorations of implementation behaviours as well as future refinement of theories, models and frameworks in implementation science. COM-B and the TDF should continue to be refined over time based on developments in research and practice.

References

Abreu-Placeres, N., Newton, J.T., Pitts, N., Garrido, L.E., Ekstrand, K.R., Avila, V., et al. (2018) Understanding dentists' caries management: the Com-B ICCMS questionnaire. *Community Dentistry and Oral Epidemiology* 46, 545–554. https://doi.org/10.1111/cdoe.12388

Ahmed, N., Barlow, S., Reynolds, L., Drey, N., Begum, F., Tuudah, E., et al. (2021) Mental health professionals' perceived barriers and enablers to shared decision-making in risk assessment and risk management: a qualitative systematic review. *BMC Psychiatry* 21, 594. https://doi.org/10.1186/s12888-021-03304-0

Alexander, K.E., Brijnath, B., Mazza, D. (2014) Barriers and enablers to delivery of the Healthy Kids Check: an analysis informed by the Theoretical Domains Framework and COM-B model. *Implementation Science* 9, 60. https://doi.org/10.1186/1748-5908-9-60

Atkins, L., Francis, J., Islam, R., O'Connor, D., Patey, A., Ivers, N., et al. (2017) A guide to using the Theoretical Domains Framework of behaviour change to investigate implementation problems. *Implementation Science* 12, 77. https://doi.org/10.1186/s13012-017-0605-9

Birken, S.A., Powell, B.J., Presseau, J., Kirk, M.A., Lorencatto, F., Gould, N.J., et al. (2017) Combined use of the Consolidated Framework For Implementation Research (CFIR) and the Theoretical Domains Framework (TDF): a systematic review. *Implementation Science* 12, 2. https://doi.org/10.1186/s13012-016-0534-z

Blebil, A.Q., Saw, P.S., Dujaili, J.A., Bhuvan, K., Mohammed, A.H., Ahmed, A., et al. (2022) Using COM-B model in identifying facilitators, barriers and needs of community pharmacists in implementing weight management services in Malaysia: a qualitative study. *BMC Health Services Research* 22, 929. https://doi.org/10.1186/s12913-022-08297-4

Cane, J., Richardson, M., Johnston, M., Ladha, R., Michie, S. (2015) From lists of Behaviour Change Techniques (BCTs) to structured hierarchies: comparison of two methods of developing a hierarchy of BCTs. *British Journal of Health Psychology* 20, 130–150. https://doi.org/10.1111/bjhp.12102

Chater, A.M., Family, H., Abraao, L.M., Burnett, E., Castro-Sanchez, E., Du Toit, B., et al. (2022) Influences on nurses' engagement in antimicrobial stewardship behaviours: a multi-country survey using the Theoretical Domains Framework. *Journal of Hospital Infection* 129, 171–180. https://doi.org/10.1016/j.jhin.2022.07.010

Cox, N.S., Oliveira, C.C., Lahham, A., Holland, A.E. (2017) Pulmonary rehabilitation referral and participation are commonly influenced by environment, knowledge, and beliefs about consequences: a systematic review using the Theoretical Domains Framework. *Journal of Physiotherapy* 63, 84–93. https://doi.org/10.1016/j.jphys.2017.02.002

Craig, L.E., McInnes, E., Taylor, N., Grimley, R., Cadilhac, D.A., Considine, J., et al. (2016) Identifying the barriers and enablers for a triage, treatment, and transfer clinical intervention to manage acute stroke patients in the emergency department: a systematic review using the Theoretical Domains Framework (TDF). *Implementation Science* 11, 157. https://doi.org/10.1186/s13012-016-0524-1

Damschroder, L.J., Aron, D.C., Keith, R.E., Kirsh, S.R., Alexander, J.A., Lowery, J.C. (2009) Fostering implementation of health services research findings into practice: a consolidated framework for advancing implementation science. *Implementation Science* 4, 50. https://doi.org/10.1186/1748-5908-4-50

Desveaux, L., Saragosa, M., Kithulegoda, N., Ivers, N. (2019) Understanding the behavioural determinants of opioid prescribing among family physicians: a qualitative study. *BMC Family Practice* 20, 59. https://doi.org/10.1186/s12875-019-0947-2

Dyson, J., Lawton, R., Jackson, C., Cheater, F. (2011) Does the use of a theoretical approach tell us more about hand hygiene behaviour? The barriers and levers to hand hygiene. *Journal of Infection* Prevention 12, 17–24. https://doi.org/10.1177/1757177410384300

Etherington, N., Rodrigues, I.B., Giangregorio, L., Graham, I.D., Hoens, A.M., Kasperavicius, D., et al. (2020) Applying an intersectionality lens to the theoretical domains framework: a tool for thinking about how intersecting social identities and structures of power influence behaviour. *BMC Medical Research Methodology* 20, 169. https://doi.org/10.1186/s12874-020-01056-1

Ferlie, E.B., Shortell, S.M. (2001) Improving the quality of health care in the United Kingdom and the United States: a framework for change. *The Milbank Quarterly* 79, 281–315. https://doi.org/10.1111/1468-0009.00206

Fishbein, M. (1967) Attitude and the prediction of behavior. *Readings in Attitude Theory and Measurement.* New York: Wiley, pp. 477–492.

Fleming, A., Bradley, C., Cullinan, S., Byrne, S. (2014) Antibiotic prescribing in long-term care facilities: a qualitative, multidisciplinary investigation. *BMJ Open* 4, e006442. https://doi.org/10.1136/bmjopen-2014-006442

Forbes, G., Akter, S., Miller, S., Galadanci, H., Qureshi, Z., Fawcus, S., et al. (2023) Factors influencing postpartum haemorrhage detection and management and the implementation of a new postpartum haemorrhage care bundle (E-MOTIVE) in Kenya, Nigeria, and South Africa. *Implementation Science* 18, 1. https://doi.org/10.1186/s13012-022-01253-0

Francis, J.J., O'Connor, D., Curran, J. (2012) Theories of behaviour change synthesised into a set of theoretical groupings: introducing a thematic series on the Theoretical Domains Framework. *Implementation Science* 7, 35. https://doi.org/10.1186/1748-5908-7-35

Gaube, S., Fischer, P., Lermer, E. (2021) Hand(y) hygiene insights: applying three theoretical models to investigate hospital patients' and visitors' hand hygiene behavior. *PLoS One* 16, e0245543. https://doi.org/10.1371/journal.pone.0245543

Geeven, I.P., Jessurun, N.T., Wasylewicz, A.T., Drent, M., Spuls, P.I., Hoentjen, F., et al. (2022) Barriers and facilitators for systematically registering adverse drug reactions in electronic health records: a qualitative study with Dutch healthcare professionals. *Expert Opinion on Drug Safety* 21, 699–706. https://doi.org/10.1080/14740338.2022.2020756

Goddard, S.L., Lorencatto, F., Koo, E., Rose, L., Fan, E., Kho, M.E., et al. (2018) Barriers and facilitators to early rehabilitation in mechanically ventilated patients—a theory-driven interview study. *Journal of Intensive Care* 6, 4. https://doi.org/10.1186/s40560-018-0273-0

Graham-Rowe, E., Lorencatto, F., Lawrenson, J.G., Burr, J., Grimshaw, J.M., Ivers, N.M., et al. (2016) Barriers and enablers to diabetic retinopathy screening attendance: protocol for a systematic review. *Systematic Reviews* 5, 134. https://doi.org/10.1186/s13643-016-0309-2

Graham-Rowe, E., Lorencatto, F., Lawrenson, J., Burr, J., Grimshaw, J., Ivers, N., et al. (2018) Barriers to and enablers of diabetic retinopathy screening attendance: a systematic review of published and grey literature. *Diabetic Medicine* 35, 1308–1319. https://doi.org/10.1111/dme.13686

Heslehurst, N., Newham, J., Maniatopoulos, G., Fleetwood, C., Robalino, S., Rankin, J. (2014) Implementation of pregnancy weight management and obesity guidelines: a meta-synthesis of healthcare professionals' barriers and facilitators using the Theoretical Domains Framework. *Obesity Reviews* 15, 462–486. https://doi.org/10.1111/obr.12160

Hollis, J.L., Kocanda, L., Seward, K., Collins, C., Tully, B., Hunter, M., et al. (2021) The impact of healthy conversation skills training on health professionals' barriers to having behaviour change conversations: a pre-post survey using the Theoretical Domains Framework. *BMC Health Services Research* 21, 880. https://doi.org/10.1186/s12913-021-06893-4

Huijg, J.M., Gebhardt, W.A., Crone, M.R., Dusseldorp, E., Presseau, J. (2014a) Discriminant content validity of a theoretical domains framework questionnaire for use in implementation research. *Implementation Science* 9, 11. https://doi.org/10.1186/1748-5908-9-11

Huijg, J.M., Gebhardt, W.A., Dusseldorp, E., Verheijden, M.W., Van Der Zouwe, N., Middelkoop, B.J., et al. (2014b) Measuring determinants of implementation behavior: psychometric properties of a questionnaire based on the theoretical domains framework. *Implementation Science* 9, 33. https://doi.org/10.1186/1748-5908-9-33

Johnston, M., Carey, R.N., Connell Bohlen, L.E., Johnston, D.W., Rothman, A.J., De Bruin, M., et al. (2021) Development of an online tool for linking behavior change techniques and mechanisms of action based on triangulation of findings from literature synthesis and expert consensus. *Translational Behavioral Medicine* 11, 1049–1065. https://doi.org/10.1093/tbm/ibaa050

Keyworth, C., Epton, T., Goldthorpe, J., Calam, R., Armitage, C.J. (2020) Acceptability, reliability, and validity of a brief measure of capabilities, opportunities, and motivations ("COM-B"). *British Journal of Health Psychology* 25, 474–501. https://doi.org/10.1111/bjhp.12417

Lorencatto, F. (2022) Applying the Theoretical Domains Framework: its uses and limitations. In: Rapport, F., Clay-Williams, R., Braithwaite, J. (Eds.), *Implementation Science: The Key Concepts*. Abingdon: Routledge, pp. 103–105. https://doi.org/10.4324/9781003109945-29

McDonagh, L.K., Saunders, J.M., Cassell, J., Curtis, T., Bastaki, H., Hartney, T., et al. (2018) Application of the COM-B model to barriers and facilitators to chlamydia testing in general practice for young people and primary care practitioners: a systematic review. *Implementation Science*, 13, 130. https://doi.org/10.1186/s13012-018-0821-y

McGowan, L.J., Powell, R., French, D.P. (2020) How can use of the Theoretical Domains Framework be optimized in qualitative research? A rapid systematic review. *British Journal of Health Psychology* 25, 677–694. https://doi.org/10.1111/bjhp.12437

Michie, S., Atkins, L., West, R. (2014) *The Behaviour Change Wheel. A Guide To Designing Interventions.* 1st edition. Sutton: Silverback Publishing.

Michie, S., Johnston, M., Abraham, C., Lawton, R., Parker, D., Walker, A. (2005) Making psychological theory useful for implementing evidence based practice: a consensus approach. *BMJ Quality & Safety* 14, 26–33. https://doi.org/10.1136/qshc.2004.011155

Michie, S., Richardson, M., Johnston, M., Abraham, C., Francis, J., Hardeman, W., et al. (2013) The behavior change technique taxonomy (v1) of 93 hierarchically clustered techniques: building an international consensus for the reporting of behavior change interventions. *Annals of Behavioral Medicine* 46, 81–95. https://doi.org/10.1007/s12160-013-9486-6

Mill, D., Seubert, L., Lee, K., Page, A., Johnson, J., Salter, S., et al. (2023) Understanding influences on the use of professional practice guidelines by pharmacists: a qualitative application of the COM-B model of behaviour. *Research in Social and Administrative Pharmacy* 19, 272–285. https://doi.org/10.1016/j.sapharm.2022.10.006

Munafò, M.R., Davey Smith, G. (2018) Robust research needs many lines of evidence. *Nature* 553, 399–401. https://doi.org/10.1038/d41586-018-01023-3

Nicholson, C., Francis, J., Nielsen, G., Lorencatto, F. (2022) Barriers and enablers to providing community-based occupational therapy to people with functional neurological disorder: an interview study with occupational therapists in the United Kingdom. *British Journal of Occupational Therapy* 85, 262–273. https://doi.org/10.1177/03080226211020658

Owens, C., Currin, J.M., Hoffman, M., Grant, M.J., Hubach, R.D. (2023) Implementation factors associated with primary care providers' intention to prescribe HIV PrEP to adolescents in the United States. *Journal of Adolescent Health* 73, 181–189. https://doi.org/10.1016/j.jadohealth.2023.02.007

Patey, A.M., Islam, R., Francis, J.J., Bryson, G.L., Grimshaw, J.M. (2012) Anesthesiologists' and surgeons' perceptions about routine pre-operative testing in low-risk patients: application of the Theoretical Domains Framework (TDF) to identify factors that influence physicians' decisions to order pre-operative tests. *Implementation Science* 7, 52. https://doi.org/10.1186/1748-5908-7-52

Patey, A.M., Hurt, C.S., Grimshaw, J.M., Francis, J.J. (2018) Changing behaviour "more or less" – do theories of behaviour inform strategies for implementation and de-implementation? A critical interpretive synthesis. *Implementation Science* 13, 134. https://doi.org/10.1186/s13012-018-0826-6

Pearse, B.L., Keogh, S., Rickard, C.M., Faulke, D.J., Smith, I., et al. (2020) Bleeding management practices of Australian cardiac surgeons, anesthesiologists and perfusionists: a cross-sectional national survey incorporating the Theoretical Domains Framework (TDF) and COM-B model. *Journal of Multidisciplinary Healthcare* 13, 27–41. https://doi.org/10.2147/JMDH.S232888

Presseau, J., McCleary, N., Lorencatto, F., Patey, A.M., Grimshaw, J.M., Francis, J.J. (2019) Action, actor, context, target, time (AACTT): a framework for specifying behaviour. *Implementation Science*, 14, 102. https://doi.org/10.1186/s13012-019-0951-x

Prothero, L., Cartwright, M., Lorencatto, F., Burr, J.M., Anderson, J., Gardner, P., et al. (2022a) Barriers and enablers to diabetic retinopathy screening: a cross-sectional survey of young adults with type 1 and type 2 diabetes in the UK. *BMJ Open Diabetes Research and Care* 10, e002971. https://doi.org/10.1136/bmjdrc-2022-002971

Prothero, L., Lawrenson, J.G., Cartwright, M., Crosby-Nwaobi, R., Burr, J.M., Gardner, P., et al. (2022b) Barriers and enablers to diabetic eye screening attendance: an interview study with young adults with type 1 diabetes. *Diabetic Medicine* 39, e14751. https://doi.org/10.1111/dme.14751

Prothero, L., Lorencatto, F., Cartwright, M., Burr, J.M., Gardner, P., Anderson, J., et al. (2021) Perceived barriers and enablers to the provision of diabetic retinopathy screening for young adults: a cross-sectional survey of healthcare professionals working in the UK National Diabetic Eye Screening Programme. *BMJ Open Diabetes Research and Care* 9, e002436. https://doi.org/10.1136/bmjdrc-2021-002436

Ray, D., Sniehotta, F., McColl, E., Ells, L. (2022) Barriers and facilitators to implementing practices for prevention of childhood obesity in primary care: a mixed methods systematic review. *Obesity Reviews* 23, e13417. https://doi.org/10.1111/obr.13417

Rosário, F., Santos, M.I., Angus, K., Pas, L., Ribeiro, C., Fitzgerald, N. (2021) Factors Influencing the implementation of screening and brief interventions for alcohol use in primary care practices: a systematic review using the COM-B system and Theoretical Domains Framework. *Implementation Science*, 16, 6. https://doi.org/10.1186/s13012-020-01073-0

Smith, C.A., McNeill, A., Kock, L., Shahab, L. (2019) Exploring mental health professionals' practice in relation to smoke-free policy within a mental health trust: a qualitative study using the COM-B model of behaviour. *BMC Psychiatry* 19, 54. https://doi.org/10.1186/s12888-019-2029-3

Sniehotta F., Scholz U., Schwarzer R. (2005) Bridging the intention–behaviour gap: Planning, self-efficacy, and action control in the adoption and maintenance of physical exercise. *Psychology & Health*, 20, 143–160. https://doi.org/10.1080/08870440512331317670

Sniehotta, F.F., Araújo-Soares, V., Brown, J., Kelly, M.P., Michie, S., West, R. (2017) Complex systems and individual-level approaches to population health: a false dichotomy? *Lancet Public Health* 2, e396–e397. https://doi.org/10.1016/S2468-2667(17)30167-6

Surr, C.A., Parveen, S., Smith, S.J., Drury, M., Sass, C., Burden, S., et al. (2020) The barriers and facilitators to implementing dementia education and training in health and social care services: a mixed-methods study. *BMC Health Services Research* 20, 512. https://doi.org/10.1186/s12913-020-05382-4

Tomsic, I., Ebadi, E., Gossé, F., Hartlep, I., Schipper, P., Krauth, C., et al. (2021) Determinants of orthopedic physicians' self-reported compliance with surgical site infection prevention: results of the WACH-trial's pilot survey on COM-B factors in a German university hospital. *Antimicrobial Resistance, Infection Control* 10, 67. https://doi.org/10.1186/s13756-021-00932-9

Warsi, S., Elsey, H., Boeckmann, M., Noor, M., Khan, A., Barua, D., et al. (2019) Using behaviour change theory to train health workers on tobacco cessation support for tuberculosis patients: a mixed-methods study in Bangladesh, Nepal and Pakistan. *BMC Health Services Research* 19, 71. https://doi.org/10.1186/s12913-019-3909-4

19 Applying Normalization Process Theory

Alyson Hillis

Introduction

Normalization Process Theory (NPT) provides a set of tools to support the adoption, implementation and sustainment of complex interventions. Taking a socio-technical approach, it seeks to understand how those involved in the implementation process (actors) translate their strategic intentions into behaviours and practices that change the everyday practices of others over time and in different contexts. Those who apply NPT in the implementation process aim to establish what work is done to create change; how the work gets done; and the effects of the work (May, 2006, 2013; May et al., 2007a, 2007b, 2009, 2022; May and Finch, 2009).

NPT can be applied in three ways. First, it can be used to design, conduct and analyse qualitative studies using interviews, focus groups and ethnographic techniques. More so than the quantitative application of the theory, qualitative theoretical developments of NPT address the problems of context in implementation research by analysing the properties of interventions and the adaptive normative and relational responses that emerge across time and settings within the contextual implementation process (May et al., 2016, 2022). Second, NPT can be used to design, conduct and analyse quantitative studies using the Normalization MeAsure Development (NoMAD) tool. The NoMAD instrument is the main implementation tool that applies the NPT mechanisms in quantitative research and is used to understand and predict the normalization of interventions into healthcare practice (May et al., 2011; Finch et al., 2013; Finch et al., 2018; Rapley et al., 2018). Third, NPT can be used to conduct theory-informed evidence synthesis of qualitative, quantitative or mixed-methods empirical studies. In healthcare research, NPT has been used in most therapy areas throughout the world, retrospectively in process evaluations and intervention studies as well as prospectively to enhance successful implementation (Finch et al., 2013) observed through feasibility and design studies. Due to the varying uses of NPT, it is a compatible theory for realist models and work in collaboration with other implementation theories, frameworks and strategies.

Three cases that highlight different applications of NPT in health services research are presented in this chapter (Table 19.1). The cases describe the work done by actors to determine whether change was successful in the implementation process as well as to examine the findings in each of the cases against the NPT constructs, demonstrate how NPT was applied and suggest ways in which it could have been further utilized in the design or evaluation of the interventions (Table 19.2).

DOI: 10.4324/9781003318125-21

Case 1: Implementing a video-based intervention to empower staff members in an autism care organization: a qualitative study

Video interactive guidance (VIG) uses positive video feedback to establish an organizational culture where staff feel valued and empowered. VIG has proven successful in social care and educational settings by improving verbal, non-verbal and paralinguistic interactional skills, particularly among young children and young people with autism. In theory, the multi-phase training embedded new technical skills and allowed trainees to recognize their own capabilities from the beginning of the intervention. Trainee feedback was externally accredited before moving on to the subsequent phases of the training. In addition, VIG trainers were required to film and critique themselves as a component of the intervention, encouraging collaboration between all actors based on their shared, engaging delivery of the programme. A small cohort of staff was to be trained to use VIG and then provide training to the remainder of the staff, with the intention of giving cognitive authority to participants, integrating the programme into existing roles and avoiding continual external input. This case seeks to understand how to implement VIG within specific organizational contexts, in this case, autism care in the United Kingdom, as part of a more holistic peer-support strategy (Hall et al., 2016).

Methods

Case 1 was a qualitative exploratory study. The sample included three members of staff involved in guider training (a speech and language therapist, a college tutor, and an adult home deputy manager); two were previous trainees and two were senior managers. Each participant took part in a face-to-face semi-structured interview that lasted around 30 minutes.

NPT was used to inform the interview schedule and in the analysis. Inductive thematic analysis was conducted, and the codes generated were then compared with NPT constructs in the Mechanism domain. The research team iteratively analysed the data to find the best fit between the codes generated and the NPT constructs, continually discussing the relationships within the team. The codes and constructs were then applied to the intervention's context based on the notions of "ideal conditions" and "real conditions" for the implementation of VIG. In doing so, the sustainability of VIG becomes tangible and easier to upscale. Additional methodological details are presented in Table 19.1.

The work required to embed and integrate change

Unfortunately, senior management did not provide sufficient and clear explanations as to the reasons for the implementation of VIG, and so staff members did not appreciate the purpose of the intervention or what was required of them until after they chose to join the training. Because VIG was not mandatory, those who joined had a prior interest in incorporating the intervention into their own practice and took on an advocacy role to train other members of staff. However, because the intervention was not prioritized by senior management, human resourcing barriers prevented trainers from carrying out or becoming involved in VIG alongside their daily tasks, reducing the work done to effectively pilot the intervention. The VIG intervention was successful among lower-level trainees in the staff hierarchy, who worked closely with its components, allowing staff to step out of their daily work as a form of respite to reflect on their skills, which in turn led them to feel empowered. Although they anticipated difficulty integrating VIG into their existing practice, in contrast to senior managers, they experienced increased self-esteem in technical skills as well as the confidence to suggest positive changes to daily practice, giving them agency in their role. The analysis by NPT construct is presented in Table 19.2.

Methodological and theoretical critique

NPT was used extensively in case 1, particularly in the comparison of the reciprocal relationships between the NPT constructs. The theoretical considerations in the design of the VIG training would have led to Cognitive participation being achieved through the establishment of advocates for the intervention. Yet, as the Strategic intentions were not secured before implementation, Relational restructuring and Normative restructuring, and consequently Sustainment, were unable to be realized in practice. The most notable barriers lay in the Coherence differences observed between senior management and lower-level trainees.

The authors stated that Coherence and Cognitive participation do not encompass "emotional processes through which individuals might arrive at their own understanding and involvement". Reflexive monitoring is "more representative of the collective appraisals of the worth of the intervention for an organization and appeared less helpful in capturing the personal mechanisms through which individuals make those appraisals". In addition, the authors felt that some of the more powerful quotes could not be captured in the Mechanisms domain due to the focus on collective rather than individual accounts. Other empirical research has also offered similar critique and bridged this gap by utilizing additional frameworks in tandem with NPT (Ling et al., 2012; Connell et al., 2014).

Case 2: Implementing community participation via interdisciplinary teams in primary care: an Irish case study in practice

Case 2 focused on collective participation in primary care. The authors explored service user (patients and communities) involvement in the service delivery and planning of primary care teams, with particular interest in how stakeholders within primary care teams collaborated within interdisciplinary teams and external community representatives to achieve effective community participation (Tierney et al., 2018).

Methods

Case 2 was a qualitative study in Ireland. Gatekeepers at four sites identified and invited 39 participants. Participants included 27 community representatives, five health service executive healthcare professionals working in the primary care teams, four health service executive service planners and policy makers managing the development of primary care teams and three general practitioners (GPs) working alongside primary care teams.

NPT was used during the data collection and analysis stages of the research. Around 30 face-to-face semi-structured interviews and three Participatory Learning Action focus groups were conducted with interview schedules informed by NPT. Participatory Learning Action data collection methods were used with community representatives when possible and included specific Participatory Learning Action techniques, such as flexible brainstorming. Deductive analysis using the NPT framework was undertaken, followed by asking and rating "'how strong is the implementation of community participation in primary care teams?"' and considerations of the levers and barriers of the implementation process. Findings were presented under the NPT constructs with supporting analytical questions. Additional methodological details are presented in Table 19.1.

The work required to embed and integrate change

Community representatives, managers and policy makers unanimously demonstrated a clear understanding of the new ways of working, the valuable impact that community participation would have on primary care teams, and the need to task shift for the intervention to act as a "catalyst for change". However, other members of the primary care team community, such as GPs, did not share these beliefs and demonstrated resistance to change. The participants who were invited to lead the initial implementation of community participation proved pivotal in driving the intervention and encouraging colleagues and other stakeholders to accept the changes. Others bought into community participation because it aligned with their own interests, such as ongoing community projects, professional development and strategic development of primary care. Cognitive participation was strong among the participants because community participation proved to be complementary to individual and community interests.

Additional resources were provided to coordinate the work for community participation in primary care teams. However, healthcare professionals were unable to meet the additional demands that community participation placed on top of their original role, and they lacked higher-level support to meet the intervention's requirements. Crucially, local managers described difficulty in organizing, planning and consulting on the implementation, largely based on the ineffective functioning of the existing primary care team systems, such as "tokenistic" sentiments held within the staff-level hierarchy that were shared by community representatives.

In assessing the intervention, the authors assessed individual and collective feedback, as suggested by NPT. Appraisal occurred through informal channels, with the intervention praised for raising awareness of local initiatives, empowering community representatives and supporting career development. Communal appraisal highlighted improved service delivery, networking, and resource allocation. However, the key performance indicators to measure community participation in primary care teams were considered limited and lacking in depth by participants. Overall, participants conveyed a lack of change in practice and "a sense of lost opportunity", leading participants to question the extent of the normalization of community participation in primary care teams. The analysis by NPT construct is presented in Table 19.2.

Methodological and theoretical critique

NPT was used extensively as a methodological framework for analysis and to frame the findings. Furthermore, the intervention was analysed by the strength of the four NPT Mechanism constructs, rating them from strong to weak, with working definitions developed by the authors. In classifying community participation by strength and presenting the evidence under the respective levers and barriers of the intervention, the authors were able to "[offer] the opportunity for comparable analyses of similar initiatives in other health-care jurisdictions" (Eccles et al., 2009; May and Finch, 2009; Tierney et al., 2018; McEvoy et al., 2014).

There is overlap in the use of the NPT domains, constructs, and sub-constructs. For example, if the Context constructs were considered prospectively in the design of community participation before implementation, the findings in case 2 demonstrated that they would have had a direct effect on the success of the intervention due to the impact on the Mechanisms. Where managers and GPs demonstrated their indifference to the intervention, other Individual specification and Communal specification incentives could have been provided through the Negotiating capacity and Reframing organizational logics in the Context domain. From a retrospective angle, there was also significant overlap between the Reflexive monitoring and Outcomes constructs. Clearer differentiation between these constructs would be beneficial to the overall longevity and sustainment of the intervention.

Case 3: Ready for prime time? Using Normalization Process Theory to evaluate implementation success of personal health records designed for decision making

Case 3 sought to describe the individual and collective work that service users and providers must do to integrate a personal health record (e-PHR) system into clinical practice to encourage shared decision making (SDM). This case used NPT in the pre-implementation stages of the e-PHR system for diabetes care in Canada (May et al., 2018; Davis, 2020; Davis and MacKay, 2020).

Methods

Case 3 was a mixed-methods descriptive study. Purposive, convenience and snowball sampling methods were used, and participants were recruited through posters, social media and emails. There were three study groups: 8 patients (type 1 diabetes, 18–24 years old), 11 healthcare providers and 8 organizational providers.

NPT was used in the triangulation convergence study design, with data collected concurrently and weighted equally. First, the NoMAD instrument was used "to describe the level of agreement of patients, care providers and organizational leaders". A basic psychometric evaluation was also conducted on the NoMAD instrument, using Cronbach's alpha test to determine the extent to which the NPT Mechanism constructs measured the internal consistency and reliability. Variances were found across all Mechanism constructs (20 items, $\alpha = 0.60$) as well as individual ones (ranging from $\alpha = 0.33$ to 0.80). Therefore, only Cognitive participation and Collective action underwent further analysis to determine agreement with the concepts (range from 1 [strongly disagree] to 5 [strongly agree]). Second, a practice-related outcomes survey was used to understand outcomes such as levels of potential engagement and participation in SDM and normalization of the e-PHR system. Both the instrument and the survey were delivered online. Third, following quantitative data collection, semi-structured interviews were held with individuals. NPT informed the interview schedule.

Simple descriptive statistical analysis was applied to the demographic characteristics. Both quantitative datasets were analysed using R statistical software. A deductive qualitative approach using a heuristic discovery process (concept coding, axial coding and category comparison) was undertaken for qualitative analysis. Emergent inductive themes were identified throughout the iterative process. The quantitative and qualitative datasets were integrated, and summaries were presented by the NPT Mechanism construct. Additional methodological details are presented in Table 19.1.

The work required to embed and integrate change

Before implementation, it was determined when the intervention would need to be used so that it would be beneficial to all stakeholders; planning focused on accountability, patient-orientated approaches and prioritizations to improve patient-provider relationships.

For the patients, the e-PHR system was distinguished from current ways of working because it was described as a "game-changing technology" and would provide a "sensibility of change" and "supportive approach to healthcare", through streamlining processes, improving access and communication to aid collaboration with service providers, and enabling clinicians to have a holistic understanding of the patient's condition through the intervention. Organizational providers endorsed the transfer of ownership of care onto patients, thus establishing patient-centred care. Care providers emphasized that SDM should be used to encourage compliance to care for patients because they would also be receiving more efficient care based on shared access of patient data and integrated treatment strategies.

All stakeholders demonstrated an "investment of commitment", which reflected the sharing of ownership of the work and enabling involvement for all stakeholders, while also revealing that care providers and patients would be aligned to the relational work needed to maintain the e-PHR system. Patients highlighted that SDM would enable a collaborative relationship through reciprocal understanding and communication; however, they emphasized the need for "systemic ownership" for the sustainability of the e-PHR system.

Quantitative findings demonstrated weak agreement between participant groups regarding the operational work required to normalize the intervention (patients 3.9 ± 0.33; care providers 3.4 ± 0.58; organizational providers 3.2 ± 0.44; overall 3.6 ± 0.53). The organizational providers needed to understand that the change required them to embody a "culture of care" through the e-PHR system, and the care providers questioned the ability to upskill staff, anticipating that the intervention would "expose [service delivery] gaps". All participant groups reiterated the need for planning and onboarding of all stakeholders before implementation, particularly regarding adequate resources and continual funding. Clearly designated ownership and accountability were raised by care providers and patients, but the organizational providers emphasized the need to retain "centralized control" without "stifl[ing] creativity".

Overall, the aim of the pre-implementation study was to align the e-PHR system with "current, intuitive, and acceptable ways of working", allowing access to information for the empowerment of patients, and therefore, as a means for the intervention to become normalized into daily practice. However, participants cited that normalization would only be likely with the presence of a patient-centred, team-based care culture. This was reflected in the statistical analysis (patients 4.0 ± 0.53; care providers 4.1 ± 0.54; organizational providers 3.2 ± 0.50; overall 3.9 ± 0.60).

Better health outcomes would derive from increased communication between stakeholders and a holistic understanding of patients' health through effective use of the technology across participant groups. This was due to the potential positive impact on engagement in SDM with patients (patients 4.4 ± 0.74; care providers 4.5 ± 0.52; organizational providers 4.6 ± 0.52; overall 4.5 ± 0.58) and that it would be easier for providers to support patients (patients 4.4 ± 0.52; care providers 4.3 ± 0.65; organizational providers 4.8 ± 0.46; overall 4.4 ± 0.58). Participants agreed that this shift and removal of barriers could inspire patients, allowing them to be more accountable for their own health and compliant with the intervention. The analysis by NPT constructs is presented in Table 19.2.

Methodological and theoretical critique

Case 3 is a strong theoretical paper and is one of few empirical studies that closely applied NPT to the pre-implementation stage of an intervention. It demonstrates how additional themes may sit outside the NPT framework or significantly overlap across NPT domains and constructs – a frequent critique of NPT. From a quantitative perspective, the statistical validation of the reliability and internal consistency of the Mechanism constructs strengthened the study's findings and provided additional insights into the varying perceptions of the participant groups. In addition, the authors interpreted the Reflexive

Table 19.1 Characteristics of the Normalization Process Theory (NPT) cases.

Case characteristics	Case 1	Case 2	Case 3
Context	Social care, residential, education settings and community	Primary care	Social care
Intervention	Video Interactive Guidance (VIG)	Community participation	Personal health record system for shared decision making
Study type (NPT use)	Intervention study (retrospective)	Implementation study (retrospective)	Feasibility study (pre-implementation) study (prospective)
Theory framework	NPT	NPT and Participatory Learning Action	NPT
Data collection	Qualitative (semi-structured interviews)	Qualitative (semi-structured interviews) and Participatory Learning Action focus groups	Mixed-methods (NoMAD instrument, practice-related outcomes survey and semi-structured interviews)
Data analysis	Inductive thematic analysis, with generated codes mapped onto NPT constructs	Deductive analysis using the NPT framework	Quantitative: descriptive statistics and psychometric tests. Qualitative: deductive analysis using the NPT framework
NPT codes used	Coherence, cognitive participation, collective action, reflexive monitoring	Coherence, cognitive participation, collective action, reflexive monitoring	Quantitative: cognitive participation and collective action (due to low Cronbach's alpha for other constructs). Qualitative: coherence, cognitive participation, collective action, reflexive monitoring

Table 19.2 Analysis by Normalization Process Theory (NPT) construct for each case.

Domain	Construct	Subconstruct	Case 1	Case 2	Case 3
Context	Strategic intentions		Multi-phase training embedded the skills gained by participants		It was determined when the intervention would need to be used so that it would be beneficial to all stakeholders. Planning focused on accountability, patient-orientated approaches, and prioritizations to improve patient-provider relationships
	Adaptive execution		To move to the next phase of training, feedback needed to be externally accredited		
	Negotiating capacity		Training a small cohort of staff to become trainers (or guiders) shaped organizational and relational structures		
	Reframing organizational logics				
Mechanism	Coherence	Differentiation	Intervention deemed contradictory to the existing culture	Strong evidence of effective task-shifting	The e-PHR system was distinguished from current ways of working because it was described as a "game-changing technology" and provided a "sensibility of change" and "supportive approach to healthcare"
		Communal specification	The purpose and requirements of the intervention were not communicated effectively by senior management	Community representatives, managers and policy makers demonstrated a clear understanding of the new ways of working and what the work would entail	
		Individual specification			
		Internalization	Potential value was not constructed or communicated effectively by senior management	Community participation was valued as a "catalyst for change"	
	Cognitive participation	Initiation	Multi-phase structure and advocacy pathway encouraged onboarding of staff members	Participants who led the initial community participation proved pivotal in driving the intervention	General inference of support from the managerial team
		Enrolment	Some onboarding of participants but many staff remained sceptical about embedding Video Interactive Guidance into daily tasks	Participants encouraged other stakeholders to accept changes to routine	Care providers and patients were aligned to the relational work needed to maintain the personal health record system

	Legitimation	Some staff were interested in incorporating Video Interactive Guidance	Buy-in was strong because community participation proved complementary to individual and community interests	Patients highlighted that decision making would enable a collaborative relationship through reciprocal understanding and communication
	Activation			Need identified for "systemic ownership" for the sustainability of the personal health record system
Collective action	Interactional workability	Those who took part closely followed the intervention components	Managers were unable to organize, plan and consult on implementation due to ineffective functioning of the existing primary care team system	Organizational providers needed to understand the change required to embody a "culture of care" through the personal health record system
	Relational integration	Discord reported between senior management and staff members		Care providers questioned the ability to upskill staff, anticipating that the intervention would "expose [service delivery] gaps"
	Skill-set workability	Lack of capacity to incorporate Video Interactive Guidance into daily tasks and practice	Healthcare professionals were unable to meet the demands that community participation placed on top of original roles	Care providers and patients raised the need for clearly designated ownership and accountability
	Contextual integration	Staff believed that the organization was not open to grass root strategic or operational ideas for practice	Additional resources were provided to coordinate the work for community participation in primary care teams but there was a lack of higher-level support to meet the requirements of intervention	Organizational providers endorsed the transfer of ownership of care onto patients but emphasized the need for clearer planning regarding resourcing

(*Continued*)

Table 19.2 (Continued)

Domain	Construct	Subconstruct	Case 1	Case 2	Case 3
	Reflexive monitoring	Systematization			
		Communal appraisal			
		Individual appraisal	Staff reflected on their acquired skills that contributed to their empowerment	Intervention used informal channels to measure against key performance indicators that were considered limited and lacking in depth	
		Reconfiguration	Participants experienced and anticipated difficulty integrating Video Interactive Guidance into their existing practice		
Outcome	Intervention performance		The Video Interactive Guidance intervention was successful among lower-level trainees in the staff hierarchy. Those who took part felt empowered in contrast to senior managers	Participants conveyed a lack of change in practice and "a sense of lost opportunity"	Better health outcomes would derive from increased communication between stakeholders and holistic understanding of patients' health with shared decision making due to effective use of the technology across participant groups
	Relational restructuring		Increased self-esteem of trainees in technical skills as well as confidence to suggest positive changes to daily practice, giving them agency in their role		The potential positive impact of engagement from shared decision making and the personal health record system would facilitate easier pathways to provide patient support, which would in turn encourage compliance and accountability by patients

Normative restructuring sustainment (normalization)	Until senior management are onboard, embedding and integration is limited	Normalization of community participation in primary care teams was questioned	Similar to Intervention Performance The aim of the pre-implementation study was to align the personal health record system with "current, intuitive, and acceptable ways of working". Yet normalization would only occur with the presence of a patient-centred, team-based care culture
Suggested extension in the use of NPT	The contextual considerations were theoretical and not effectively translated into practice. The core barrier was that legitimation was not achieved at management levels, leading to a lack of collective understanding and willingness to implement the Video Interactive Guidance training	Although the authors reported contextual aspects of the intervention, these were limited and would be more appropriately placed under the Mechanism constructs. Context constructs required greater attention so that the Mechanisms could be effectively operationalized by actors. Overlapping coding between the Coherence and Cognitive Participation constructs could be made clearer to ensure positive reinforcement of the intervention and provide better outcomes	Strong paper that closely applied NPT to the pre-implementation stage of the intervention. Reflexive Monitoring was interpreted as the appraisal of the intervention's performance as opposed to outlining potential available appraisal tools within the service delivery of the intervention and contextual considerations were raised in the Mechanism section rather than within the Context domain

Monitoring constructs as a performance appraisal of the e-PHR system as opposed to outlining potential available appraisal tools within the service delivery of the intervention. For example, in the themes Reflecting on value and Monitoring and adapting, the authors described how the e-PHR system would nurture engagement and collaboration by removing barriers to care and increasing care efficiency and effectiveness; yet these would arguably be more appropriately considered under the NPT Outcomes constructs of Communal appraisal and Individual appraisal.

As with the other two cases, contextual considerations were raised in the Mechanism domain. For example, multi-level implementation such as education, training (individual), auditing, resourcing (clinical), structural alignment and funding (structural) would allow the Enrolment and Legitimation of the e-PHR system so that Activation is achieved in the process. These aspects should be considered in the Context domain of NPT, notably the Strategic intentions and Reframing organizational logics constructs. If these aspects of the intervention are in place, then key individuals would be able to drive the implementation process.

Comparisons of use, considerations and future directions

The three cases provide distinct approaches to using NPT in empirical studies. There is a tendency in implementation science for studies to use every aspect of human life. However, NPT is a middle-range theory and is intended to be used as presented in the paper on theory development (May, 2006, 2013; May et al., 2007a, 2007b, 2009, 2011, 2016, 2018, 2020, 2022; May and Finch, 2009; Finch et al., 2013, 2018; Rapley et al., 2018), most notably through the NoMAD instrument for quantitative work and the Coding Manual for qualitative work (Finch et al., 2018; Rapley et al., 2018; May et al., 2022).

The breadth and applicability of NPT in healthcare research and service delivery is showcased in the differing settings, interventions and therapy areas under investigation in the three cases. They demonstrate that NPT can be used as a single framework or in collaboration with other implementation science frameworks and methodological approaches, such as Participatory Action Learning as in case 2, and that it can be used retrospectively in intervention and implementation studies or prospectively in pre-implementation designs. However, there is hesitancy around using NPT in prospective designs. It has been argued that it could potentially raise the alarm that an intervention will not be sustainable or cost-effective, and so researchers may be less inclined to test theories using such frameworks. This dilemma raises epistemological issues as to whether implementation science frameworks are able to "describe or capture, in any detail, the 'actual problem'" with the intervention (Rapley et al., 2018, p. 13). However, case 2 ascertained that "[NPTs] applicability to the different stages of system design life cycle and its valuable set of conceptual tools for the understanding of implementation as a dynamic process make it appealing" (Davis, 2020).

In general, semi-structured interviews and focus groups are used in most qualitative NPT studies, and the NoMAD instrument with descriptive and statistical analysis is the main approach for quantitative work. For qualitative data analysis, deductive techniques are used rigidly but more flexible approaches are taken when inductive thematic analysis is chosen, and the taxonomies generated are then mapped onto the NPT Mechanism constructs: "This use of NPT . . . allow[ed] us to better understand the processes and interactions, rather than the discrete things that participants say which emerge from an entirely inductive initial analysis" (Hall et al., 2016).

Furthermore, it is important to uphold theoretically informative research and encourage theory building based on the translation of theoretical to empirical work (Kislov, 2018). Across the three cases, themes were considered across multiple domains, constructs and sub-constructs. Some authors critique NPT for generating such overlapping concepts; yet they could be considered in different stages of implementation depending on the context and the intervention itself, which will inevitably be changing and adapting, and will therefore need revisiting throughout the implementation process.

By applying NPT to a protocol, design or evaluation study, researchers can clearly establish the work that is required by individual and communal actors to ensure the sustainment and high-quality performance of a successfully embedded and integrated complex intervention. The three cases only used the Mechanism constructs of NPT. As the respective theoretical papers were published after the three cases (May et al., 2022), none of the sub-constructs were utilized, and they are only incorporated here for the purposes of this chapter (see Table 19.2). Future empirical research should consider using the Context and Outcome domains, which are outlined in the Coding Manual (May et al., 2022). For example, the constructs within the Context domain of NPT should be used to "help us to understand how participants' agentic contributions to implement processes . . . interact with and are shaped by the contexts in which action takes place" (May et al., 2016). Applying NPT throughout the implementation process enables and equips researchers to holistically understand the intervention and contextual components to carry out the strategic intentions required to ignite sense-making, relational, operational and appraisal work, and therefore work towards greater performance, integrated restructuring, and normalization of any given intervention.

Acknowledgements

I would like to thank Carl May for reviewing and editing this chapter. Acknowledgements must also be given to the authors of the cases (Hall et al., 2016; Tierney et al., 2018; Davis, 2020). This report is based on independent research supported by the National Institute for Health and Care Research ARC North Thames. The views expressed in this publication are those of the author(s) and not necessarily those of the National Institute for Health and Care Research or the Department of Health and Social Care.

References

Connell, L.A., McMahon, N.E., Harris, J.E., Watkins, C.L., Eng, J.J. (2014) A formative evaluation of the implementation of an upper limb stroke rehabilitation intervention in clinical practice: a qualitative interview study. *Implementation Science* 9, 90. https://doi.org/10.1186/s13012-014-0090-3

Davis, S. (2020) Ready for prime time? Using Normalization Process Theory to evaluate implementation success of personal health records designed for decision making. *Frontiers in Digital Health* 2, 575951. https://doi.org/10.3389/fdgth.2020.575951

Davis, S., MacKay, L. (2020) Moving beyond the rhetoric of shared decision making: designing personal health record technology with young adults with type 1 diabetes. *Canadian Journal of Diabetes* 44, 434–441. https://doi.org/10.1016/j.jcjd.2020.03.009

Eccles, M.P., Armstrong, D., Baker, R., Cleary, K., Davies, H., Davies, S., et al. (2009) An implementation research agenda. *Implementation Science* 4, 18. https://doi.org/10.1186/1748-5908-4-18

Finch, T., Rapley, T., Girling, M., Mair, F., Murray, E., Treweek, S., et al. (2013) Improving the normalization of complex interventions: measure development based on normalization process theory (NoMAD): study protocol. *Implementation Science* 8, 43. https://doi.org/10.1186/1748-5908-8-43

Finch, T.L., Girling, M., May, C.R., Mair, F.S., Murray, E., Treweek, S., et al. (2018) Improving the normalization of complex interventions: part 2-validation of the NoMAD instrument for assessing implementation work based on normalization process theory (NPT). *BMC Medical Research Methodology* 18, 135. https://doi.org/10.1186/s12874-018-0591-x

Hall, A., Finch, T., Kolehmainen, N., James, D. (2016) Implementing a video-based intervention to empower staff members in an autism care organization: a qualitative study. *BMC Health Services Research* 16, 608. https://doi.org/10.1186/s12913-016-1820-9

Kislov, R. (2018) Engaging with theory: from theoretically informed to theoretically informative improvement research. *BMJ Quality & Safety* 28, 177–179. https://doi.org/10.1136/bmjqs-2018-009036

Ling, T., Brereton, L., Conklin, A., Newbould, J., Roland, M. (2012) Barriers and facilitators to integrating care: experiences from the English Integrated Care Pilots. *International Journal of Integrated Care* 12, e129. https://doi.org/10.5334/ijic.982

May, C. (2006) A rational model for assessing and evaluating complex interventions in healthcare. *BMC Health Services Research* 6, 86. https://doi.org/10.1186/1472-6963-6-86

May, C. (2013) Towards a general theory of implementation. *Implementation Science* 8, 18. https://doi.org/10.1186/1748-5908-8-18

May, C., Finch, T. (2009) Implementing, embedding, and integrating practices: an outline of Normalization Process Theory. *Sociology* 43, 535–554. https://doi.org/10.1177/0038038509103208

May, C., Finch, T., Mair, F., Ballini, L., Dowrick, C., Eccles, M., et al. (2007a) Understanding the implementation of complex interventions in health care: the normalization process model. *BMC Health Services Research* 7, 148. https://doi.org/10.1186/1472-6963-7-148

May, C.R., Mair, F.S., Dowrick, C.F., Finch, T.L. (2007b) Process evaluation for complex interventions in primary care: understanding trials using the normalization process model. *BMC Family Practice* 8, 42. https://doi.org/10.1186/1471-2296-8-42

May, C., Mair, F., Finch, T., MacFarlane, A., Dowrick, C., Treweek, S., et al. (2009) Development of a theory of implementation and integration: Normalization Process Theory. *Implementation Science* 4, 29. https://doi.org/10.1186/1748-5908-4-29

May, C.R., Finch, T., Ballini, L., MacFarlane, A., Mair, F., Murray, E., et al. (2011) Evaluating complex interventions and health technologies using normalization process theory: development of a simplified approach and web-enabled toolkit. *BMC Health Services Research* 245. https://doi.org/10.1186/1472-6963-11-245

May, C., Johnson, M., Finch, T. (2016) Implementation, context and complexity. *Implementation Science* 11, 141. https://doi.org/10.1186/s13012-016-0506-3

May, C.R., Cummings, A., Girling, M., Bracher, M., Mair, F.S., May, C.M., et al. (2018) Using Normalization Process Theory in feasibility studies and process evaluations of complex healthcare interventions: a systematic review. *Implementation Science* 13, 80. https://doi.org/10.1186/s13012-018-0758-1

May, C., Rapley, T., Finch, T. (2020) Normalization Process Theory. In: Nilsen, P., Birken, S. (Eds.), *International Handbook on Implementation Science*. Cheltenham, UK: Edward Elgar. https://doi.org/10.4337/9781788975995.00013

May, C.R., Albers, B., Bracher, M., Finch, T.L., Gilbert, A., Girling, M., et al. (2022) Translational framework for implementation evaluation and research: a normalisation process theory coding manual for qualitative research and instrument development. *Implementation Science* 17, 19. https://doi.org/10.1186/s13012-022-01191-x

McEvoy, R., Ballini, L., Maltoni, S., O'Donnell, C.A., Mair, F., MacFarlane, A. (2014) A qualitative systematic review of studies using the normalization process theory to research implementation processes. *Implementation Science* 9, 2. https://doi.org/10.1186/1748-5908-9-2

Rapley, T., Girling, M., Mair, F.S., Murray, E., Treweek, S., McColl, E., et al. (2018) Improving the normalization of complex interventions: part 1 - development of the NoMAD instrument for assessing implementation work based on normalization process theory (NPT). *BMC Medical Research Methodology* 18, 133. https://doi.org/10.1186/s12874-018-0590-y

Tierney, E., McEvoy, R., Hannigan, A., MacFarlane, A.E. (2018) Implementing community participation via interdisciplinary teams in primary care: an Irish case study in practice. *Health Expectations* 21, 990–991. https://doi.org/10.1111/hex.12692

20 Applying Reach, Effectiveness, Adoption, Implementation and Maintenance

Bethany M. Kwan, Mónica Pérez Jolles, Christina R. Studts, Jodi Summers Holtrop and Russell E. Glasgow

Introduction

Originally conceptualized as an evaluation outcomes model, Reach, Effectiveness, Adoption, Implementation and Maintenance (RE-AIM) has been used to inform research planning, quality improvement and iterative programme design and implementation in research and clinical and community settings (Kessler et al., 2013; Glasgow and Estabrooks, 2018; Kwan et al., 2019; Estabrooks et al., 2021; Glasgow et al., 2022). It can be used to evaluate the impact of interventions and implementation strategies, guide policy implementation and build partnerships (Jilcott et al., 2007; Sweet et al., 2014).

RE-AIM considers outcomes at multiple levels, in terms of both setting-level outcomes (what is the effect on the systems and personnel delivering services) and recipient-level outcomes (what is the effect on those receiving services). Both quantitative and qualitative methods can be used to assess RE-AIM domains. Quantitative data sources may include electronic health records (EHRs) or administrative data, surveys, study records and observer ratings. Numerical data are often used to describe the "what" or "to what extent" an intervention or approach worked for each domain. Conversely, qualitative methods (interviews, focus groups, observations, photo or video images) are often used to assess the "how" and "why" (Holtrop et al., 2018; Hamilton and Finley, 2019). In addition, the qualitative and quantitative data can be mixed to provide insights into the contextual circumstances under which an intervention or an implementation strategy is effective.

RE-AIM can be combined with other implementation science theories, models and frameworks. The examples in this chapter are intended to provide guidance on and help clarify these issues. The three case examples describe the application of RE-AIM in different contexts, varying in terms of settings, populations, interventions studied, implementation strategies used, study designs, use of mixed methods and the emphasis on equity.

Case 1: The Invested in Diabetes pragmatic comparative effectiveness trial of patient-driven versus standardized diabetes shared medical appointments in primary care

The Invested in Diabetes study was a 5-year cluster randomized, pragmatic comparative effectiveness study of two models of diabetes shared medical appointments (SMAs) in 22 primary care practices. The concept for the study was based on input from people living with diabetes, their care partners and representatives from clinical and community service organizations providing care for people with diabetes (Kwan et al., 2017).

DOI: 10.4324/9781003318125-22

As a pragmatic trial, participating primary care practices were non-academic, community clinical delivery sites that used existing personnel and workflows to deliver either standardized or patient-driven diabetes SMAs to adult patients with type 2 diabetes (Kwan et al., 2020b; Glasgow et al., 2021). RE-AIM was used to structure the evaluation of setting-level Adoption, Implementation and Maintenance of diabetes SMAs and patient-level Reach and Effectiveness (Kwan et al., 2020a). As a hybrid type II implementation-effectiveness study (Landes et al., 2020), there was equal emphasis on studying the comparative effectiveness of the two SMA models as well as testing an implementation strategy based on the Enhanced Replicating Effective Programs (REP) implementation process framework (Kilbourne et al., 2014).

Adoption

We documented the number and characteristics of practices choosing to participate (Kwan et al., 2020b). Practices were recruited through two practice-based research networks (PBRNs). Practice characteristics such as practice type (Federally Qualified Health Centers [FQHCs] serving Medicaid beneficiaries and uninsured patients versus non-FQHCs serving primarily patients with commercial insurance and/or Medicare), size (number of clinicians and health educator staff), patient population (number of patients with diabetes, patient population demographics) were assessed via a baseline survey administered to a key practice representative such as a practice manager. One challenge to reporting Adoption was that the true denominator of eligible practices that offered participation was difficult to track (e.g. availability of personnel to deliver SMAs was not a common practice characteristic known to PBRN coordinating centres).

Implementation

Multiple methods were used to evaluate SMA delivery adaptations, fidelity and cost during the REP implementation phase (Holtrop et al., 2022). Fidelity and adaptations were evaluated using qualitative key informant interviews with practice leadership and staff, observations conducted by practice staff for a semi-random selection of SMA sessions at each practice using a structured fidelity checklist, field notes kept by practice coaches, and a tracking spreadsheet in which practices recorded SMA session dates, topics, facilitators present and patient attendance. Costs for practices to set up and deliver both their first and last SMA session were recorded using a time-driven activity-based costing method (Keel et al., 2017). Results showed that when practices made adaptations to SMAs, they were mostly consistent with fidelity (e.g. changing the time of day); but certain elements of the more complex patient-driven SMA model showed lower fidelity (e.g. integration of diabetes peer mentors as co-facilitators). Initial set-up costs were higher for patient-driven SMAs, but delivery costs were comparable between conditions.

Maintenance

The final practice qualitative interviews included questions about plans for sustaining SMAs, including any anticipated adaptations and reimbursement strategies as well as barriers to sustainability.

Reach

Strategies used to support practices' patient recruitment efforts were summarized (Dailey-Vail et al., 2022) and details of the number and characteristics of patients enrolled in the study (Nederveld et al., 2022) and their reasons for participating were recorded. Data sources included the practice tracking spreadsheet and baseline practice characteristics survey, practice coach field notes, data from EHRs (e.g. patient co-morbidities) and qualitative interviews with a subset of patients who participated in SMAs. Results showed that practices were able to recruit on average 6% of their adult patients with type 2 diabetes to participate in the study. These patients participated in 4 of 6 sessions on average and reported they were motivated to participate because of recommendations from their primary care provider and other practice staff and a desire to improve their education so they could better manage their diabetes. Patient satisfaction with SMAs was high (especially when they had a skilled facilitator), and they reported few if any costs to participate. Patients in FQHCs reported more psychosocial needs (e.g. lower health literacy, higher food insecurity, higher levels of diabetes distress) than patients in non-FQHCs. In addition, patients in FQHCs were more likely to attend virtual SMAs (a COVID-related adaptation), whereas patients in non-FQHCs were more likely to attend SMAs in person.

Effectiveness

Both practice-level and patient-level outcomes were assessed using both quantitative and qualitative methods. Practice-level outcomes included the impact of delivering SMAs on team-based care (using the Relational Coordination Survey) and quality of care (using the Assessment of Chronic Illness Care). These outcomes were assessed using survey methods at baseline, the mid-point and the end of implementation administered to all practice care team members involved in delivering SMAs. The results showed that SMAs had a positive effect on both team-based care and quality of care initially, with no differences between conditions, but that both metrics decreased substantially by the end of the implementation period (mid to late 2021), likely due to the impact of the COVID-19 pandemic on practice morale and staffing challenges. Patient-level outcomes included both patient-centred outcomes (diabetes distress, diabetes self-care behaviours, autonomy support, competence) and clinical outcomes (HbA1c, blood pressure, body mass index). Surveys of patient-reported outcome measures were administered by practice staff as part of the intervention at the first and last SMA sessions. Clinical outcomes were gleaned from EHR data collected in routine care. Results showed that overall, standardized and patient-driven diabetes SMAs showed comparable effectiveness, with some benefits for the standardized model and some benefits for the patient-driven model.

Concluding remarks

Using RE-AIM provided a systematic and rigorous structure to gain insights on the trade-offs and relative benefits of two diabetes SMA delivery models. Reach and Effectiveness were comparable across conditions; the main differences related to slightly increased costs and lower fidelity to the more complex patient-driven SMAs relative to standardized SMAs. Attention to elements of representativeness and diversity in patient populations and practice types (assessed in the context of Reach, Adoption and

Implementation evaluations) yielded key insights into the needs, priorities and preferences of patients receiving diabetes care in FQHCs.

Case 2: Testing a multi-faceted strategy supporting the implementation of adverse childhood experiences screenings in primary care clinics

Adverse childhood experiences (ACEs) are defined as traumatic events occurring before age 18 years, such as maltreatment, a life-threatening accident, harsh migration, exposure to violence and experiences of racism (Perreira and Ornelas, 2013). ACEs can lead to toxic stress and mental health needs and can place children at higher risk for negative life outcomes (Herzog and Schmahl, 2018). The Surgeon General of the state of California sought to address this care gap by issuing a 2020 ACEs Aware healthcare policy. This fee-for-service policy reimburses primary care settings for using the Pediatric ACEs and Related Life-events Screener (PEARLS) to screen children during annual wellness visits to (general) community-based clinics in northern and southern California. This policy was adopted in 2019–2020 and partnered with a multidisciplinary research team to support the implementation with children aged 0–5 years (Office of the California Surgeon General, 2019).

This study used a cluster randomized design, mixed methods, and a co-created participatory approach to identify and refine a multi-faceted implementation strategy being tested in four clinical research sites representing rural, mid-urban and large urban geographic areas. This project capitalized on a rare opportunity to use a natural experiment to leverage implementation research to inform efforts to assess the impact of a state-wide policy in under-resourced settings. A hybrid type II effectiveness-implementation study (Curran et al., 2022) allowed for equal attention to testing the impact of ACEs screening while evaluating the implementation strategy in real-world settings using a pragmatic trial. This study integrated the Exploration, Preparation, Implementation and Sustainment (EPIS) framework (Moullin et al., 2020) to guide the research process; RE-AIM was used to guide evaluation of the impact of both the ACEs screening and the implementation strategy.

EPIS: Exploration and Preparation

During the EPIS Exploration and Preparation phases, clinical partners and a group of Latinx caregivers partnered with the research team to co-create knowledge and the direction of the study (Pérez Jolles et al., 2022b) using implementation mapping (Pérez Jolles et al., 2022a). Partners shared their concerns with researchers that ACEs universal screening may not reach all eligible children due to a lack of capacity within clinics and under-reporting from caregivers. In addition, there was a need to establish clear and efficient workflows for clinics to adopt the ACEs Aware policy and for this intervention to trigger a service referral for children in need of services. This information informed the selection and measurement of the study's outcomes of Reach, Effectiveness, Adoption and Implementation. Due to the negative impact of contextual changes on FQHCs, such as the COVID-19 pandemic and high workforce turnover, Maintenance as an outcome was an area that partners were not able to plan for during the Exploration and Preparation phases.

Reach

The outcome of ACEs screening, Reach, was defined by the team as the percentage of all eligible children attending their wellness visit at the clinic who were invited to or screened for ACEs, as well as the representativeness of those who were screened. Reach data were collected using data gathered in the field using REDCap (Harris et al., 2009) and integrated with the clinic's EHRs every 10 weeks. The representativeness of the children was assessed using sub-group analysis by age, gender, race and ethnicity. A deeper understanding of the experiences of caregivers involved in screening and care team members implementing screening was explored using one-on-one interviews in English and Spanish.

Effectiveness

The intervention's Effectiveness in generating a service referral based on information gathered during screening was reported through REDCap and EHR data. Effectiveness outcomes included reporting on changes in the rate of child referrals to mental health support services before and after the date of the ACEs screening and the implementation of the multi-faceted strategy.

Adoption

Adoption of universal screening within clinics was defined as the number of care teams in a clinic implementing screening and the implementation strategy. Due to extreme turnover of employees in these community-based safety net systems clinics, lack of additional time to add ACEs screening, and concerns about unintended consequences of ACEs screening, Adoption was limited to a single care team, deviating from a planned clinic-wide adoption effort. Interviews with clinic staff were used to generate a better understanding of the impact of outer context challenges, such as the effects of the COVID-19 pandemic on the FQHC system's ability to innovate.

Implementation

Implementation of the ACEs screening and the multi-faceted implementation strategy was measured by the fidelity of the workflow developed for these new screenings and reported through weekly EHR output reports and ongoing coaching calls every 5–6 weeks between the research team and the care team at each clinical site. To address the balance between the Implementation issues of fidelity and adaptation, we used a matrix tool to allow us to track the goals of the strategy set by all partners during the planning phase and informed by the literature (i.e. core functions), the concrete activities tailored to each clinic and designed to accomplish each goal (i.e. forms). We then tracked changes in the relevance of each core function and adaptations to the forms over time (i.e. informed by the FRAME-IS [Framework for Reporting Adaptations and Modifications to Evidence-based Implementation Strategies]) (Miller et al., 2021).

Maintenance

Challenges to the Maintenance of the ACEs Aware policy and of the study's implementation strategy, including unintended consequences, such as further stigmatizing minoritized patient populations, and further traumatizing families and care team members by triggering as a result of ACEs questions, are being explored during coaching calls and one-on-one interviews with clinical care teams and caregivers.

Concluding remarks

The integration of the EPIS framework with RE-AIM outcomes allowed us to account for key inner contextual factors affecting the study outcomes: readiness for change (baseline), and changes in implementation climate and leadership before, during and after the implementation of the multi-faceted implementation strategy. Detailed information on the study's research protocol is provided by Perez Jolles et al. (2021). This framework integration allowed partners to map the dynamic contextual characteristics of clinics and the nature of the ACEs Aware policy during the Exploration and Preparation phases, inform the multi-faceted implementation strategy and identify outcomes that mattered to all partners.

Case 3: Implementation of Unstuck and On Target in elementary schools in Virginia and Colorado

Executive functioning (EF) problems include difficulties with emotion regulation, organization, planning, flexibility, goal-setting and other skills important for participation in school, work and social settings (Sparapani et al., 2016). These difficulties are especially common among children with autism spectrum disorder (ASD) and/or attention deficit hyperactivity disorder (ADHD). Unstuck and On Target (henceforth Unstuck) is an intervention shown to improve EF skills in children with symptoms of ASD and/or ADHD (Kenworthy et al., 2014). The 21-lesson programme can be delivered by any school staff member (e.g. guidance counsellor, special education teacher, regular classroom teacher, paraprofessional) to groups of students in grades 3–5.

This 3-year project was designed to enhance the scalability of Unstuck by replacing the original in-person intervention training with a free, interactive, asynchronous training programme and tele-mentoring of implementers (developed in year 1). The RE-AIM framework was used to plan the project and guide the assessment of multi-level outcomes among schools, implementers and students. A logic model captured the needs (11% of elementary students estimated to have EF challenges); the intervention (Unstuck); implementation strategies (interactive asynchronous online training, intervention curriculum and resources, and remote tele-mentoring); and RE-AIM outcomes to be assessed.

In year 2, the elementary schools enrolled in Colorado ($n = 130$) and Virginia ($n = 99$) each identified one or more implementers to complete the online Unstuck training, have access to tele-mentoring and intervention resources and deliver the intervention to students with EF challenges during the school year. Implementation strategies were delivered in years 2 and 3. RE-AIM outcomes were assessed using a mixed methods approach with measures at multiple time points.

Reach

Reach was operationalized as the number, proportion and representativeness of children who received the Unstuck intervention. Reach was measured using post-implementation implementer surveys at the end of years 2 and 3 by asking how many children participated in groups led by the implementer that year. Semi-structured interviews with implementers and administrators at the end of year 2 explored the characteristics of the children who participated in intervention groups and those who could have benefited but did not receive the intervention, as well as multi-level barriers and facilitators to achieving high and representative Reach.

Effectiveness

Effectiveness was defined as changes in child behaviours related to EF. In year 2, child behaviours were assessed pre- and post-participation in Unstuck in two ways: (a) trained research staff conducted in-classroom behavioural observation ratings of participating children (n = 100) from randomly selected enrolled schools with a focus on EF-related classroom behaviours; (b) parents/caregivers completed surveys including the Behavior Rating Inventory of Executive Funtioning-2 (Gioia et al., 2015) measure of child EF. Perceptions of Effectiveness were also explored using semi-structured interviews with implementers and administrators at the end of year 2.

Adoption

Adoption was operationalized as (a) the number, proportion and representativeness of schools that enrolled in the project of those invited, and (b) the number, proportion and representativeness of implementers in enrolled schools who led at least one Unstuck session. School characteristics (including state, rural versus urban location, size and public versus private) were obtained using publicly available information and pre-implementation survey responses from school administrators, and implementer characteristics (including demographic characteristics, professional role, and knowledge about EF) were assessed with pre- and post-implementation surveys in year 2. Multi-level barriers and facilitators to Adoption were assessed in semi-structured implementer and administrator interviews at the end of year 2.

Implementation

Implementation was conceptualized as having three facets: fidelity, adaptations and cost. The fidelity of intervention delivery was rated by trained research staff who observed and coded randomly selected live or remote Unstuck sessions for adherence to intervention content and process. Implementers also reported the number of intervention lessons delivered in post-implementation surveys as an indicator of fidelity. Adaptations made to the intervention or its delivery were identified during fidelity observations, in semi-structured implementer and administrator interviews at the end of year 2, and in the post-implementation survey completed by implementers at the end of year 3. The costs of intervention delivery were assessed using time-driven activity-based costing (Cidav et al., 2020) for which implementers completed brief time logs during randomly assigned weeks of the school year reporting time spent in specific intervention-related activities that week (e.g. completing training, receiving tele-mentoring, preparing lessons, pulling students from class, delivering lessons, communicating with parents or teachers, documentation). Time log data were supplemented with responses on post-implementation surveys and semi-structured interviews to clarify the amount of time, types of activities and costs of implementing Unstuck. General implementation experiences were assessed with survey measures of implementers' and administrators' perceptions of the acceptability, feasibility and appropriateness (Weiner et al., 2017) of the intervention and the implementation strategies, as well as with semi-structured interviews with implementers and administrators at the end of year 2.

Maintenance

Maintenance of intervention delivery was operationalized as the proportion and representativeness of participating schools and implementers continuing to deliver the intervention in year 3. Surveys administered to implementers and administrators at the end of year 3 assessed whether and when the online training was accessed, whether and how many intervention lessons were delivered, and the number of children who received the intervention. Items from the Program Sustainability Assessment Tool (Calhoun et al., 2014) were adapted for the elementary school setting and included administrators' surveys to assess factors potentially important for Maintenance. Potential barriers and facilitators to the Maintenance of delivery of Unstuck were assessed in semi-structured interviews with implementers and administrators at the end of year 2. Maintenance of the effects of the intervention on child EF was assessed by repeating the observational and parent-report assessments used to assess Effectiveness in year 2 at a 6-month follow-up time point in year 3.

Concluding remarks

In this project aiming to enhance the scalability of the Unstuck intervention to improve EF skills in elementary school students, the RE-AIM framework guided the development of a logic model, selection of implementation strategies, and operationalization of child, implementer and school outcomes. Although frequently used in clinical and public health contexts, this application of RE-AIM highlights its utility and potential impact in educational settings; its relevance for pragmatic evaluation projects; and its natural fit with mixed methods approaches.

Summary of RE-AIM application case examples

Table 20.1 summarizes the different contexts in which RE-AIM was used in the three case examples.

Broader considerations and lessons learned

There is sometimes confusion about and challenges in applying RE-AIM, such as understanding the differences between domains (e.g. Reach versus Adoption); the value of RE-AIM beyond evaluation; or the extent to which RE-AIM can be used in conjunction with other theories, frameworks or models. In planning, RE-AIM aids in informing decisions about target populations (e.g. for whom is Reach most important/likely?) and settings (e.g. what types of organizations and providers have the capacity to adopt and maintain an intervention?) (King et al., 2010, 2020; Glasgow et al., 2019). Recently, RE-AIM has been used more pragmatically as part of an iterative strategy for engaging local implementers of evidence-based practice in a cycle of evaluation, prioritization and refinement over the course of an implementation effort (Glasgow et al., 2020; D'Lima et al., 2022).

The examples described in this chapter demonstrate ways to address several of the common challenges in applying RE-AIM. Here, we enumerate the common challenges

Table 20.1 Characteristics of Reach, Effectiveness, Adoption, Implementation and Maintenance (RE-AIM) application case examples. ACEs, adverse childhood experiences; FQHC, Federally Qualified Health Center.

Case characteristics	Case 1: Invested in Diabetes	Case 2: ACEs screening in primary care	Case 3: Unstuck and On Target
Context (setting, population)	Primary care practices (FQHCs and non-FQHCs); adult patients with type 2 diabetes	Community-based clinics (FQHCs) serving children aged 0–5 years	Elementary schools; children with executive functioning challenges
Intervention	Diabetes shared medical appointments	Psychosocial screening during the child's wellness visit	Unstuck and On Target (group sessions addressing executive functioning skills)
Implementation strategy	Care team training, practice facilitation, learning communities, Enhanced Replicating Effective Programs framework	Remote learning, use a scoring algorithm to triage children to services, ongoing coaching and peer support	Interactive, asynchronous online training; tele-mentoring; curriculum and resources for implementers
Study type	Type II hybrid implementation-effectiveness study	Type II hybrid implementation-effectiveness study	Type III hybrid implementation-effectiveness study
RE-AIM use (planning, evaluation, iteration)	Evaluation, iteration	Planning, evaluation	Planning, evaluation
Qualitative data sources to assess RE-AIM domains	Qualitative interviews with patients and practice clinicians, staff and leadership; observations and field notes	Interviews with clinic personnel and caregivers	Interviews with implementers and administrators
Quantitative data sources to assess RE-AIM domains	Practice and patient-level surveys; electronic health records data; observer ratings; project records and tracking spreadsheets	Electronic health records, surveys from clinic personnel, tracking spreadsheets	Implementer and administrator surveys; parent surveys; observational ratings of child behaviour; observational ratings of intervention fidelity; project records

we have found in practical applications of RE-AIM and suggest solutions to these challenges, and we elaborate on some of the most frequent questions about applying RE-AIM. Table 20.2 summarizes these issues by RE-AIM dimension and then cross-cutting issues.

The frequent question regarding Reach (and other dimensions when addressing representativeness) concerns the lack of good information on the "denominator" of persons approached or who could have participated. When information on non-participants is not available, we suggest two strategies. The first is to use existing administrative data on the target population (or as close as possible). For example, census data for the local community or region, increasingly available geospatial data, or information on all patients with the relevant conditions in the healthcare systems being studied. The second approach is to use sensitivity analyses to provide both conservative and liberal estimates of the denominator population; for example, assuming that almost all persons received an invitation or could have participated, and then a smaller denominator (liberal estimate) using those you are sure had an opportunity to participate.

Differentiating Adoption from Reach and Implementation can be challenging. Adoption refers to the same issues as Reach (the proportion and representativeness of those participating) but Reach is at the individual level (e.g. patient, student, community

Table 20.2 Common challenges and solutions in applying Reach, Effectiveness, Adoption, Implementation and Maintenance (RE-AIM).

RE-AIM dimension	Frequent issues or questions	Example solution
Reach	Do not know denominator or non-participant characteristics	Do high and low denominator estimates for sensitivity analyses. Use existing data (e.g. census, clinic or workplace records)
Effectiveness	Not clear on what to measure for generalization or unintended consequences	Use quality of life or well-being measures; use equity measures
Adoption	Not clear on the denominator, who is invited or their characteristics; differentiating Reach and Implementation; number of levels for adoption	Do sensitivity analyses as above; use summary employee records for comparison; Adoption is initial agreement; usually three or more levels for adoption; include implementing staff and at least the most proximal setting level
Implementation	Not sure how to assess adaptations; insufficient resources for cost assessment	Use interview guides and coding frameworks; just track implementation time if few economic resources
Maintenance	Not sufficient time to assess follow-up; not clear on the time frame; no objective measure	If not enough observation time, can collect intent to sustain; best if there can be 12–24 months of follow-up or longer; use new brief survey measures
All dimensions: cross-cutting issues	Not reporting on representativeness; understanding why these results were obtained	Representativeness/equity should be reported for all dimensions; qualitative and mixed methods are strongly encouraged to understand why/how results obtained

member), whereas Adoption is multi-level, at the staff or implementer level and at one or more larger setting levels as applicable. One or more larger levels are almost always applicable and should include the proximal setting (e.g. clinic, worksite, school) and usually one or more larger units such as a healthcare system, school district, state or region. In differentiating Adoption from Implementation, Adoption refers to the initial decision to participate (e.g. being willing to attend training). Anything after this initial step (e.g. starting to apply an intervention and extent of engagement) is Implementation. That said, some situations are not clear-cut and what is important is to clearly define how each RE-AIM dimension is being defined and assessed, regardless of whether it is called Adoption or Implementation (Glasgow and Estabrooks, 2018).

RE-AIM resources and future directions

Resources are increasingly available to facilitate the application of RE-AIM. Many of these are on the www.re-aim.org and University of Colorado D&I resources website (University of Colorado Anschutz Medical Campus Adult, Child Center for Outcomes Research, Delivery Science, 2023) The *iPRISM and REAIM Guidebook for Planning, Implementation, and Sustainment* includes templates, assessments, and examples to inform the use of PRISM (Practical, Robust Implementation and Sustainability Model) and RE-AIM, including iterative use of RE-AIM during implementation. Current and future directions for practical application of RE-AIM fall into four inter-related areas: (1) making RE-AIM more accessible to non-academic audiences through provision of sample interview guides, exercises, and examples of applications; (2) supporting the application of RE-AIM in low-resource and international settings (Glasgow and Estabrooks, 2018; Kwan et al., 2019) and for health equity and systems issues (Kikuchi et al., 2021; Fort et al., 2023); (3) enhancing iterative use of RE-AIM across different programme phases and helping to assess and guide adaptations (Glasgow et al., 2022); (4) encouraging integrated use of RE-AIM with other frameworks, especially those focused on context such as PRISM, which includes RE-AIM (Chapter 17), and on health equity. In summary, RE-AIM has evolved considerably since its inception and will continue to do so. Work continues to increase its accessibility and applicability across contexts. We hope that this chapter as well as the resources noted above will help others to successfully apply the framework.

References

Calhoun, A., Mainor, A., Moreland-Russell, S., Maier, R.C., Brossart, L., Luke, D.A. (2014) Using the program sustainability assessment tool to assess and plan for sustainability. *Preventing Chronic Disease* 11, 130185. https://doi.org/10.5888/pcd11.130185

Cidav, Z., Mandell, D., Pyne, J., Beidas, R., Curran, G., Marcus, S. (2020) A pragmatic method for costing implementation strategies using time-driven activity-based costing. *Implementation Science* 15, 28. https://doi.org/10.1186/s13012-020-00993-1

Curran, G.M., Landes, S.J., McBain, S.A., Pyne, J.M., Smith, J.D., Fernandez, M.E., et al. (2022) Reflections on 10 years of effectiveness-implementation hybrid studies. *Frontiers in Health Services* 2, 125. https://doi.org/10.3389/frhs.2022.1053496

Dailey-Vail, J., Begum, A., Kwan, B.M., Koren, R., Trujillo, S., Phimphasone-Brady, P., et al. (2022) A value proposition design approach to creating recruitment messages for diabetes shared medical appointments. *ADCES in Practice* 10, 14–20. https://doi.org/10.1177/2633559X211070268

D'Lima, D., SOUKUP, T., HULL, L. (2022) Evaluating the application of the RE-AIM planning and evaluation framework: an updated systematic review and exploration of pragmatic application. Frontiers in Public Health, 9, 2189. https://doi.org/10.3389/fpubh.2021.755738

Estabrooks, P.A., Gaglio, B., Glasgow, R.E., Harden, S.M., Ory, M.G., Rabin, B.A., et al. (2021) Use of the RE-AIM framework: translating research to practice with novel applications and emerging directions. *Frontiers in Public Health* 9, 691526. https://doi.org/10.3389/fpubh.2021.691526

Fort, M.P., Manson, S.M., Glasgow, R.E. (2023) Applying an equity lens to assess context and implementation in public health and health services research and practice using the PRISM Framework. *Frontiers in Health Services* 3, 1139788. https://doi.org/10.3389/frhs.2023.1139788

Gioia, G., Isquith, P., Guy, S., Kenworthy, L. (2015) *Behavior Rating Inventory of Executive Function-Second Edition (BRIEF2)*. Lutz, FL: Psychological Assessment Resources.

Glasgow, R.E., Estabrooks, P.E. (2018) Pragmatic applications of RE-AIM for health care initiatives in community and clinical settings. *Preventing Chronic Disease* 15, E02. https://doi.org/10.5888/pcd15.170271

Glasgow, R.E., Harden, S.M., Gaglio, B., Rabin, B., Smith, M.L., Porter, G.C., et al. (2019) RE-AIM planning and evaluation framework: adapting to new science and practice with a 20-year review. *Frontiers in Public Health* 7, 64. https://doi.org/10.3389/fpubh.2019.00064

Glasgow, R.E., Battaglia, C., McCreight, M., Ayele, R.A., Rabin, B.A. (2020) Making implementation science more rapid: use of the RE-AIM framework for mid-course adaptations across five health services research projects in the Veterans Health Administration. *Frontiers in Public Health* 8, 194. https://doi.org/10.3389/fpubh.2020.00194

Glasgow, R.E., Gurfinkel, D., Waxmonsky, J., Rementer, J., Ritchie, N.D., Dailey-Vail, J., et al. (2021) Protocol refinement for a diabetes pragmatic trial using the PRECIS-2 framework. *BMC Health Services Research* 21, 1039. https://doi.org/10.1186/s12913-021-07084-x

Glasgow, R.E., Battaglia, C., McCreight, M., Ayele, R., Maw, A.M., Fort, M.P., et al. (2022) Use of the reach, effectiveness, adoption, implementation, and maintenance (RE-AIM) framework to guide iterative adaptations: applications, lessons learned, and future directions. *Frontiers in Health Services* 2, 959565. https://doi.org/10.3389/frhs.2022.959565

Hamilton, A.B., Finley, E.P. (2019) Qualitative methods in implementation research: an introduction. *Psychiatry Research* 280, 112516. https://doi.org/10.1016/j.psychres.2019.112516

Harris, P.A., Taylor, R., Thielke, R., Payne, J., Gonzalez, N., Conde, J.G. (2009) Research electronic data capture (REDCap)-a metadata-driven methodology and workflow process for providing translational research informatics support. *Journal of Biomedical Informatics* 42, 377–381. https://doi.org/10.1016/j.jbi.2008.08.010

Herzog, J.I., Schmahl, C. (2018) Adverse childhood experiences and the consequences on neurobiological, psychosocial, and somatic conditions across the lifespan. *Frontiers in Psychiatry* 9, 420. https://doi.org/10.3389/fpsyt.2018.00420

Holtrop, J.S., Rabin, B.A., Glasgow, R.E. (2018) Qualitative approaches to use of the RE-AIM framework: rationale and methods. *BMC Health Services Research* 18, 177. https://doi.org/10.1186/s12913-018-2938-8

Holtrop, J.S., Gurfinkel, D., Nederveld, A., Phimphasone-Brady, P., Hosokawa, P., Rubinson, C., et al. (2022) Methods for capturing and analyzing adaptations: implications for implementation research. *Implementation Science* 17, 1–16. https://doi.org/10.1186/s13012-022-01218-3

Jilcott, S., Ammerman, A., Sommers, J., Glasgow, R.E. (2007) Applying the RE-AIM framework to assess the public health impact of policy change. *Annals of Behavioral Medicine* 34, 105–114. https://doi.org/10.1007/BF02872666

Keel, G., Savage, C., Rafiq, M., Mazzocato, P. (2017) Time-driven activity-based costing in health care: a systematic review of the literature. *Health Policy* 121, 755–763. https://doi.org/10.1016/j.healthpol.2017.04.013

Kenworthy, L., Anthony, L.G., Naiman, D.Q., Cannon, L., Wills, M.C., Luong-Tran, C., et al. (2014) Randomized controlled effectiveness trial of executive function intervention for children on the autism spectrum. *Journal of Child Psychology and Psychiatry* 55, 374–383. https://doi.org/10.1111/jcpp.12161

Kessler, R.S., Purcell, E.P., Glasgow, R.E., Klesges, L.M., Benkeser, R.M., Peek, C. (2013) What does it mean to "employ" the RE-AIM model? *Evaluation & the Health Professions* 36, 44–66. https://doi.org/10.1177/0163278712446066

Kikuchi, K., Gyapong, M., Shibanuma, A., Ansah, E., Okawa, S., Addei, S., et al. (2021) EMBRACE intervention to improve the continuum of care in maternal and newborn health in

Ghana: the RE-AIM framework-based evaluation. *Journal of Global Health* 11, 04017. https://doi.org/10.7189/jogh.11.04017

Kilbourne, A.M., Almirall, D., Eisenberg, D., Waxmonsky, J., Goodrich, D.E., Fortney, J.C., et al. (2014) Protocol: Adaptive Implementation of Effective Programs Trial (ADEPT): cluster randomized SMART trial comparing a standard versus enhanced implementation strategy to improve outcomes of a mood disorders program. *Implementation Science* 9, 132. https://doi.org/10.1186/s13012-014-0132-x

King, D.K., Glasgow, R.E., Leeman-Castillo, B. (2010) Reaiming RE-AIM: using the model to plan, implement, and evaluate the effects of environmental change approaches to enhancing population health. *American Journal of Public Health* 100, 2076–2084. https://doi.org/10.2105/AJPH.2009.190959

King, D.K., Shoup, J.A., Raebel, M.A., Anderson, C.B., Wagner, N.M., Ritzwoller, D.P., et al. (2020) Planning for implementation success using RE-AIM and CFIR frameworks: a qualitative study. *Frontiers in Public Health* 8, 59. https://doi.org/10.3389/fpubh.2020.00059

Kwan, B.M., Jortberg, B., Warman, M.K., Kane, I., Wearner, R., Koren, R., et al. (2017) Stakeholder engagement in diabetes self-management: patient preference for peer support and other insights. *Family Practice* 34, 358–363. https://doi.org/10.1093/fampra/cmw127

Kwan, B.M., McGinnes, H.L., Ory, M.G., Estabrooks, P.A., Waxmonsky, J.A., Glasgow, R.E. (2019) RE-AIM in the real world: use of the RE-AIM framework for program planning and evaluation in clinical and community settings. *Frontiers in Public Health* 7, 345. https://doi.org/10.3389/fpubh.2019.00345

Kwan, B.M., Dickinson, L.M., Glasgow, R.E., Sajatovic, M., Gritz, M., Holtrop, J.S., et al. (2020a) The Invested in Diabetes Study Protocol: a cluster randomized pragmatic trial comparing standardized and patient-driven diabetes shared medical appointments. *Trials* 21, 65. https://doi.org/10.1186/s13063-019-3938-7

Kwan, B.M., Rementer, J., Ritchie, N.D., Nederveld, A.L., Phimphasone-Brady, P., Sajatovic, M., et al. (2020b) Adapting diabetes shared medical appointments to fit context for practice-based research (PBR). *Journal of the American Board of Family Medicine* 33, 716–727. https://doi.org/10.3122/jabfm.2020.05.200049

Landes, S.J., McBain, S.A., Curran, G.M. (2020) Reprint of: an introduction to effectiveness-implementation hybrid designs. *Psychiatry Research* 283, 112630. https://doi.org/10.1016/j.psychres.2019.112630

Miller, C.J., Barnett, M.L., Baumann, A.A., Gutner, C.A., Wiltsey-Stirman, S. (2021) The FRAME-IS: a framework for documenting modifications to implementation strategies in healthcare. *Implementation Science* 16, 36. https://doi.org/10.1186/s13012-021-01105-3

Moullin, J.C., Dickson, K.S., Stadnick, N.A., Becan, J.E., Wiley, T., Phillips, J., et al. (2020) Exploration, Preparation, Implementation, Sustainment (EPIS) framework. In: Nilsen, N., Birken, S.A. (Eds.) *Handbook on Implementation Science*. Cheltenham, UK: Edward Elgar, pp. 32–61. https://doi.org/10.4337/9781788975995.00009

Nederveld, A.L., Gurfinkel, D., Hosokawa, P., Gritz, R.M., Dickinson, L.M., Phimphasone-Brady, P., et al. (2022) The psychosocial needs of patients participating in diabetes shared medical appointments. *Journal of the American Board of Family Medicine* 35, 1103–1114. https://doi.org/10.3122/jabfm.2022.220062R1

Office of the California Surgeon General (2019) ACEs Aware. Retrieved from www.acesaware.org/ (accessed 12 February 2023).

Perez Jolles, M., Mack, W.J., Reaves, C., Saldana, L., Stadnick, N.A., Fernandez, M.E., et al. (2021) Using a participatory method to test a strategy supporting the implementation of a state policy on screening children for adverse childhood experiences (ACEs) in a Federally Qualified Health Center system: a stepped-wedge cluster randomized trial. *Implementation Science Communications* 2, 143. https://doi.org/10.1186/s43058-021-00244-4

Pérez Jolles, M., Fernández, M.E., Jacobs, G., De Leon, J., Myrick, L., Aarons, G.A. (2022a) Using Implementation Mapping to develop protocols supporting the implementation of a state policy on screening children for Adverse Childhood Experiences in a system of health centers in inland Southern California. *Frontiers in Public Health* 10, 876769. https://doi.org/10.3389/fpubh.2022.876769

Pérez Jolles, M., Willging, C.E., Stadnick, N.A., Crable, E.L., Lengnick-Hall, R., Hawkins, J., et al. (2022b) Understanding implementation research collaborations from a co-creation lens: recommendations for a path forward. *Frontiers in Health Services* 2, 942658. https://doi.org/10.3389/frhs.2022.942658

Perreira, K.M., Ornelas, I. (2013) Painful passages: traumatic experiences and post-traumatic stress among US immigrant Latino adolescents and their primary caregivers. *International Migration Review* 47, 976–1005. https://doi.org/10.1111/imre.12050

Sparapani, N., Morgan, L., Reinhardt, V.P., Schatschneider, C., Wetherby, A.M. (2016) Evaluation of classroom active engagement in elementary students with autism spectrum disorder. *Journal of Autism and Developmental Disorders* 46, 782–796. https://doi.org/10.1007/s10803-015-2615-2

Sweet, S.N., Ginis, K.A.M., Estabrooks, P.A., Latimer-Cheung, A.E. (2014) Operationalizing the RE-AIM framework to evaluate the impact of multi-sector partnerships. *Implementation Science* 9, 74. https://doi.org/10.1186/1748-5908-9-74

University of Colorado Anschutz Medical Campus Adult, Child Center for Outcomes Research, Delivery Science. (2023) ACCORDS D&I Program Resources and Services: Interactive Tools. Retrieved from https://medschool.cuanschutz.edu/accords/cores-and-programs/dissemination-implementation-science-program/resources-services#Resources-Services-InteractiveTools (accessed 1 May 2023).

Weiner, B.J., Lewis, C.C., Stanick, C., Powell, B.J., Dorsey, C.N., Clary, A.S., et al. (2017) Psychometric assessment of three newly developed implementation outcome measures. *Implementation Science* 12, 108. https://doi.org/10.1186/s13012-017-0635-3

21 A critique of implementation science

Julia Moore and Sobia Khan

Introduction

Implementation science was established to serve the needs of communities, patients, clients, families and the general public (Eccles and Mittman, 2006). A fundamental concept underlying the field is that implementing evidence-based programmes (the term used in this chapter to generally denote the "implementation object", noting that sometimes the implementation object is not an evidence-based programme but a practice, policy, etc.) can yield better outcomes for end users. The field has traction in diverse domains of human services, such as health, behavioural health, social work, education, mental health, criminal justice and public health, for the very reason that people affected by various challenges stand to benefit from what implementation science brings to the table. Despite the expectation that individuals, organizations, communities and societies, as the beneficiaries of such evidence, could play a central role in implementation research, this is often not the case (Wallerstein and Duran, 2010). Researchers in the field have recently started publishing articles reflecting on and critiquing the existing approaches and the impact of the field (Grimshaw et al., 2019; Wensing et al., 2019; Boulton et al., 2020; Stange, 2020; Wensing et al., 2020; Rapport et al., 2021; Beidas et al., 2022). In this chapter, we build on these critiques, bringing in our perspective as professionals who synthesize and translate implementation science for those doing implementation practice and attempting to bridge the implementation science to practice gap. Our perspective is derived from our role, synthesizing and translating implementation science and providing implementation support to practitioners.

Before we dive in, it is imperative to acknowledge that the field inherently has terminology challenges. The same words are used to describe different concepts and different words are used to describe similar concepts. Even the term "implementation science" is not used in a standard way across fields and countries; alternate terms include "dissemination and implementation" and "knowledge translation". In addition, there are challenges with understanding the existing implementation science roles. We use the term implementation science researchers when referring to people who are studying the science of implementation and using implementation science comprehensively in their studies. This term may be synonymous with implementation researchers, that is, people who do "implementation research" or are "dissemination and implementation researchers". People who do not conduct research but do implementation are broadly referred to as "practitioners" although this is a highly heterogeneous group; for example, implementation teams, implementation supports, leaders, funders, etc. Throughout this chapter, we have clarified the terminology where appropriate.

DOI: 10.4324/9781003318125-23

In this chapter, we reflect on five broad areas where people have identified opportunities for improvement in the field of implementation science. For each theme, we believe a shift in focus could enhance how the field approaches implementation and achieves impact. The five priority shifts are:

- Prioritizing those closest to the problem.
- Prioritizing innovation and usability of theories, models and frameworks.
- Prioritizing feasibility and scalability.
- Prioritizing support of implementation researchers and practitioners.
- Prioritizing implementation generalists.

Prioritizing those closest to the problem

Implementation research questions are often driven by researchers based on topics that are more readily funded and publishable and that tend to align with their interests and expertise. Many of the existing theories, models and frameworks (TMFs) centre primarily on the actions of researchers and assume that they drive implementation by developing and implementing evidence-based programmes. In these TMFs, individuals in the various settings being studied are often not centred in the process, and in some cases, are depicted as passive recipients, particularly when they are considered end users or beneficiaries (i.e. people who are affected by the problem and stand to benefit most from the change).

There is an increasing shift towards greater inclusivity of practitioners and end users (e.g. the individuals, organizations, communities and societies that might benefit from the research), with a focus on fostering more community-academic partnerships (Pellecchia et al., 2018), co-creation, co-design and co-production of evidence-based programmes (Vargas et al., 2022) and embedded research (Damschroder et al., 2021), but these approaches face inherent challenges. Academia is not set up structurally to enable true collaboration in ways that prioritize the needs of practitioners and end users. Often the needs of practitioners and end users are de-prioritized because researchers, as the people bringing funding into a space, hold more power (whether they are conscious of these power dynamics or not). Overall, researchers often mean well but have their hands tied by funding and institutional expectations that lead to job security, such as meeting specific timelines, exploring specific topics and publishing papers. These expectations cause tension when they do not align with the values and needs of practitioners and end users. Collaborating with implementation researchers can be seen as a burden that may cause delays, restrict services to specific groups and impose rigid protocols that do not necessarily benefit those being served.

Moreover, there is an underlying cultural norm within the implementation science community whereby researchers are implicitly assumed to be the primary experts on implementation. There is little discussion of the fact that implementation occurs irrespective of the involvement of implementation science researchers in the process. Implementation and scale-up efforts continue to take place regardless of the state of the science, because organizations, communities and people's lives depend on it (Blitz and Bumbarger, 2022). Social workers, teachers, healthcare providers and community engagement organizations are continuously answering practical questions and have no choice but to respond to these in the best way they know how, which may result in varying quality of implementation but can also lead to great innovation that is not typically recognized by researchers. Thus, lifting the expertise of practitioners and end users not only serves the practice of implementation but can also serve the science of implementation.

Based on our experience of providing implementation support to programme implementers, we have encountered professionals who are eager to improve how they implement. Through their work, they generate numerous questions that could easily be transformed into research inquiries, yet there are limited opportunities to share these questions. Some initiatives, such as the National Council for Mental Health Wellbeing's evidence-based practice implementation science pilot (National Council for Mental Wellbeing, 2023), are emerging to collect and compile practice-based questions, thus fostering a bridge between implementation support and research. Multiple implementation researchers have published on the desire to centre practitioners and end users in research (Danitz et al., 2019; Albers et al., 2020; Chen et al., 2021). A fundamental change in both the structure and culture of implementation science is required from funders, institutions and researchers to turn this vision into a reality.

Prioritizing innovation and usability of theories, models and frameworks

TMFs play a fundamental role in the work of implementation researchers and practitioners because they offer a systematic and rigorous approach to understanding and enhancing the implementation of evidence-based programmes in real-world settings (Nilsen, 2015). The consistent use of the same TMFs facilitates comparisons across diverse research studies, even when they involve different programmes and contexts (Ridde et al., 2020). Moreover, TMFs can serve as the foundation for implementation practitioners to utilize evidence from implementation science to inform their implementation and scale-up efforts (Moullin et al., 2020). However, the field of implementation science faces several challenges concerning TMFs, including an abundance of TMFs, lack of generalizability across programmes and contexts, reinventing the wheel without drawing from established TMFs in other disciplines, insufficient consideration of implementation complexity and researcher-centric TMFs that require significant synthesis and translation to support implementation by practitioners.

One of the most notable challenges is the proliferation of TMFs; scoping reviews have identified hundreds of them (Tabak et al., 2012; Esmail et al., 2020) and new ones are being published regularly. This poses difficulty in identifying and selecting appropriate and relevant TMFs. Although tools are available to assist professionals in navigating TMFs (Birken et al., 2018), they do not address the root causes contributing to this surplus.

Rather than continually producing more TMFs, the field of implementation science would benefit greatly from critically analysing existing TMFs (Glasgow et al., 2019; Kislov et al., 2019; Moullin et al., 2020; Nilsen et al., 2022) and gaining a better understanding of established TMFs used in related fields (such as quality improvement, systems thinking, health equity, design thinking, organizational psychology). This knowledge could then be used to create generalizable TMFs that integrate high-quality existing TMFs into cohesive frameworks. Many existing TMFs have been developed within specific contexts and may lack generalizability. Therefore, there is a need for adaptable and applicable TMFs that can be applied across diverse healthcare settings and populations. However, instead of leveraging existing TMFs from both within and outside the field of implementation science, the tendency is to create new ones (which has the potential benefit of creating a highly cited publication). An important consideration is the complexity of implementation, which is a dynamic process influenced by various factors at multiple levels, including individuals, organizations, communities and the broader society. Developing TMFs that can account for this complexity presents a significant challenge, despite increasing evidence that doing so can improve outcomes (Rowland et al., 2023).

Returning to the original purpose of implementation science, which is to enhance population-level outcomes, it is crucial that the TMFs used by practitioners are practical, user-friendly and relevant to those supporting implementation and scale-up efforts (Moore and Khan, 2023). Currently, most TMFs are not readily applicable to implementers, widening the gap between implementation research and practice (Westerlund et al., 2019). As we have already noted, TMFs also tend to assume that researchers are the drivers of implementation, which makes it difficult for practitioners who drive implementation to see themselves in the existing TMFs. To increase the use of TMFs in implementation practice, there is a need to synthesize and translate TMFs into practical and usable tools, ensuring that implementation efforts are structured and guided by relevant theory and the best available evidence regarding implementation processes and factors that influence outcomes.

Prioritizing feasibility and scalability

Scalability is often the goal of many programmes to enable more widespread access to the programme and have the greatest possible impact. What we know about scalability in implementation science, however, is not entirely applicable to practice contexts. First, the evidence-based programme that is being scaled up is often not designed to be feasible; rather, it is designed for maximum efficacy to achieve statistically significant improvements, resulting in comprehensive and intensive approaches aimed at maximizing outcomes (Strosahl and Robinson, 2018). When programmes cannot be feasibly adopted and implemented (e.g. because they place a significant burden on programme deliverers or recipients; Becker-Haimes and Beidas, 2018), the effectiveness of the programme decreases once it is no longer being implemented with the rigour of a research study. For instance, an evidence-based programme might have been tested using 12 therapy sessions, but if similar results can be achieved in just three sessions, it would increase programme enrolment, retention and scalability. Given the limited time and resources of many professionals and settings, more is not always better. Therefore, programmes must walk the line between evidence and practicality because emphasizing intensive programmes can have detrimental outcomes and ultimately undermine the initial goal of implementation science: improving population-level outcomes.

Second, implementation science had long been trapped in the ideal of "maintaining fidelity" to some gold standard or level of evidence, which proved to be an intense pain point for both researchers and practitioners because absolute fidelity is not compatible with scale-up. Intensive programmes are often not scalable and may fail to accommodate the needs of individuals, organizations and communities, and the complexity of implementation settings, limiting access and population-level impact. There are also equity implications when promoting non-scalable evidence-based programmes; who gains access, and at what cost to those who are excluded? These programmes may not have been designed and evaluated with the same population in mind, leading to challenges when implementing them in different contexts (e.g. implementing programmes tested with middle-class white families in racially diverse neighbourhoods with low socioeconomic status). Implementation in organizations and across different settings requires careful consideration of context and complexity (Nilsen and Bernhardsson, 2019). Introducing evidence-based programmes that do not align well with these factors can lead organizations to believe that implementing evidence is overly burdensome and does not cater to their needs and capacities. Although this may seem like a minor setback, organizations avoiding evidence or being sceptical of the value of research can have long-term and large-scale detrimental outcomes.

Acknowledging that implementation efforts often occur in complex adaptive systems (which can encompass large organizations, communities or broader systems) can help reframe the notion of scaling evidence. These systems involve numerous inter-connected individuals and organizations, with various moving parts and changing contexts that need to be considered. Implementation researchers are now striving to acknowledge and address the inherent complexity of implementation in most settings. In the pursuit of implementing and scaling programmes across systems, there is a shift away from rigid fidelity to "ideal" or gold-standard programmes, and an emphasis that adaptation is required for feasibility, scale-up and sustainability (Chambers, 2023). To better meet local needs, there is also a movement towards creating brief, cost-effective and community-centred programmes and practices that benefit both programme deliverers and recipients (Strosahl and Robinson, 2018).

In addition, there is an opportunity to examine push and pull mechanisms for change when scaling up programmes. The premise of implementation science was historically rooted in "pushing" evidence, as reflected in its definition: promoting the uptake of research evidence into practice (Eccles and Mittman, 2006). Push models make many assumptions: that people value the same things that researchers value or that they will adopt something because they are being asked to and/or can be convinced. Recognizing the challenges associated with the push model, researchers have explored "pull" models, but they have not been as widely embraced as anticipated (Boaden, 2020). Several reasons contribute to the limited success of pull models. For instance, they do not align well with existing funding models, the timeliness of available evidence (Lamont, 2016) and the absorptive capacity of organizations (Currie et al., 2020). Examining scale-up through social networks (i.e. through the formation and strengthening of relationships) and as a mechanism that occurs through self-recognized needs and motivation to adopt and innovate as opposed to something being imposed onto individuals, organizations and communities is vital. As implementation support practitioners, we understand the need for effective implementation support capacities, which are often lacking.

Advancing in this field necessitates focusing on the science of relationships and adaptation. For example, considering the inter-connectedness of barriers and facilitators, and looking for constellations of determinants of change at multiple levels (e.g. individual, organizational and system levels), rather than considering barriers and facilitators as discrete determinants, can help researchers better comprehend drivers of change. This shift entails moving away from deterministic TMFs and embracing the role of relationships as an implementation process, while also exploring how to incorporate and measure adaptability at scale.

Prioritizing support of implementation researchers and practitioners

The challenges faced by implementation science stem from the structures and cultures within which we operate. We have alluded to many of these challenges and want to draw this out as a salient and standalone point to emphasize how crucial it is to think differently about how we approach implementation outside of the status quo. The current academic and practice partnerships are often hindered by structural and cultural issues in academia. Implementation researchers who want to prioritize the impact of their research on communities have expressed that they feel hindered and stifled by the expectations of an academic trajectory. The emphasis on bibliometrics and publications as a measure of performance, promotion, job security and funding entrenches a culture that can discourage deep authentic collaboration and trust building between academics and practitioners. To achieve population-level impacts through the implementation of evidence-based programmes, it is crucial to reimagine a structure and a culture that support both implementation science researchers and practitioners. For example, significant relationship building is required before research projects can begin, a process that is often not accounted for by funders or incentivized within the academic community, leading researchers, particularly early-career researchers, to focus on research topics that require less collaboration. There are ways to restructure grant timelines and planning of programmes to address community needs and sufficiently allow the community to drive research questions.

Beneath these structural issues lie the prevailing academic culture that shapes research practices. A deep reflection on how this culture is informed historically by colonialism and therefore can unintentionally cause individuals and communities to have negative experiences with academic structures and institutions can help pinpoint where structures can be changed and equity can be advanced. For example, academia has traditionally mined communities for data without feeding data back to these communities; although research serves to improve outcomes in the long term, the shorter-term benefits are perceived to service the purpose of meeting academic goals rather than being of immediate use to the people closest to the problem (Boaz, 2021). In addition, knowledge produced by academia is often positioned as superior to other forms of knowledge, such as practice-based knowledge and lived experience, which is built up from experience serving to solve problems that occur in everyday life and work (Nilsen et al., 2012). From a global perspective, a large proportion of research conducted in the global south is spear-headed by the global north, which inhibits local capacity for research and the generation of local solutions (Reidpath and Allotey, 2019).

Power imbalances also manifest in other ways. For example, the existing academic and funding systems create a power dynamic that hinders the formation of meaningful academic-practice partnerships by privileging individuals with PhDs and academic positions. Consequently, individuals with PhDs and academic appointments often wield more influence and are more visible than those with implementation experience and long-standing community relationships. These practices contribute to mistrust, which may make practitioners, implementers, organizations and communities reluctant to collaborate with academics and engage in research projects (Cargo and Mercer, 2008).

Addressing the power dynamics in academic-practice partnerships alongside existing structural and cultural issues (including issues related to equity) (Shelton et al., 2021) requires re-imagining implementation science and, specifically, the partnerships crucial for success between implementation science researchers and practitioners, implementers, organizations and communities. We need to consider the impact of institutions providing support infrastructures to foster collaborative partnerships between academics and practitioners, allocating resources to build capacity in implementation science and practice and supporting innovation in the translation of evidence-based practices. Fundamentally, this shift would place greater value on the unique skills and experiences of individuals outside of academia: the practitioners, implementers, organizations and communities that enact change on a daily basis.

Prioritizing implementation generalists

Recent critiques of implementation science have drawn attention to the widening gap between implementation research and practice, along with the associated tensions (Westerlund et al., 2019). An analogy of a bridge has often been used to understand this gap by illustrating how implementation science can connect research to practice. However, this analogy is often used without delving into the distinct roles of different groups in building this bridge. Implementation researchers play a crucial role in studying and understanding the essential components, such as contextual factors, mechanisms of change and sustainability planning, that form the "bricks, mortar and steel" of a high-quality bridge from research to practice. However, researchers typically do not construct complete bridges because that is not their designated role. Instead, they are encouraged to specialize in specific aspects, which can lead to frustration and confusion among other researchers who may perceive the work of implementation researchers as irrelevant to their own research. Yet, all these pieces are necessary to build a comprehensive bridge that effectively translates research into practice.

What is missing are individuals who can integrate all these components and figure out how to construct bridges based on the TMFs and evidence developed by implementation researchers. Although the implementation system already includes implementation researchers and implementers, there is a need to bridge the gap between these two groups by fostering the development of more implementation generalists rather than specialists. Implementation generalists can support teams throughout the implementation process, identifying and addressing challenges by selecting appropriate and relevant theoretical and methodological frameworks. In contrast, implementation specialists possess in-depth knowledge of specific implementation aspects, such as sustainability, context or feedback strategies. Currently, there is an imbalance between supply and demand; governments, non-profit organizations, healthcare organizations and other service sectors are eager to apply implementation science but face a shortage of implementation generalists to support their efforts. Consequently, organizations are hiring individuals for implementation support roles who do not have adequate training and experience in applying implementation science.

Implementation generalists require two additional systems to enable effective functioning that are presently under-resourced and under-valued: a synthesis and translation system and an implementation support system (Wandersman et al., 2008). The synthesis and translation system aims to unravel the complexities of implementation science and make it practical and accessible for those engaged in implementation practice, essentially providing guidance on how to construct the bridge. Subsequently, an implementation support system is necessary to assist individuals in crossing the bridge, facilitating the integration of research into practice and providing support to implementers in utilizing the science of implementation to inform their efforts.

Concluding remarks

The field of implementation science holds great promise to achieve a more evidence-based practice in various domains for improving health, well-being and societal outcomes. However, several challenges need to be overcome to fully realize its potential. By centring those affected by the work, prioritizing the innovation and usability of TMFs, considering feasibility and scalability across systems, re-imagining systems and structures and building a bridge from research to practice, implementation science can become more effective and impactful. It is essential to foster collaboration, trust and inclusivity between researchers, practitioners, communities and organizations to create a thriving ecosystem that supports the successful implementation of evidence-based programmes. With concerted efforts and a commitment to continuous improvement, implementation science can truly transform the lives of individuals, communities and societies, leading to better health, well-being and societal outcomes.

References

Albers, B., Shlonsky, A., Mildon, R. (Eds.) (2020) *Implementation Science 3.0*. Cham, Switzerland: Springer. https://doi.org/10.1007/978-3-030-03874-8

Becker-Haimes, E.M., Beidas, R.S. (2018) Playing dissemination and implementation limbo—How low can we go? A commentary on Strosahl and Robinson (2018). *Clinical Psychology: Science and Practice* 25, e12255. https://doi.org/10.1111/cpsp.12255

Beidas, R.S., Dorsey, S., Lewis, C.C., Lyon, A.R., Powell, B.J., Purtle, J., et al. (2022) Promises and pitfalls in implementation science from the perspective of US-based researchers: learning from a pre-mortem. *Implementation Science* 17, 55. https://doi.org/10.1186/s13012-022-01226-3

Birken, S.A., Rohweder, C.L., Powell, B.J., Shea, C.M., Scott, J., Leeman, J., et al. (2018). T-CaST: an implementation theory comparison and selection tool. *Implementation Science* 13, 143. https://doi.org/10.1186/s13012-018-0836-4

Blitz, C., Bumbarger, B. (2022). Practitioner Network of Expertise (NoE) Implementation Infrastructure Initiative (I3) Updates. Presented at Society for Implementation Research Collaboration Conference, San Diego, CA.

Boaden, R. (2020) Push, pull or co-produce? *Journal of Health Services Research & Policy* 25, 67–69. https://doi.org/10.1177/1355819620907352

Boaz, A. (2021). Lost in co-production: to enable true collaboration we need to nurture different academic identities. Retrieved from https://blogs.lse.ac.uk/impactofsocialsciences/2021/06/25/lost-in-co-production-to-enable-true-collaboration-we-need-to-nurture-different-academic-identities (accessed 12 August 2023).

Boulton, R., Sandall, J., Sevdalis, N. (2020) The cultural politics of "implementation science". *Journal of Medical Humanities* 41, 379–394. https://doi.org/10.1007/s10912-020-09607-9

Cargo, M., Mercer, S.L. (2008) The value and challenges of participatory research: strengthening its practice. *Annual Review of Public Health* 29, 325–350. https://doi.org/10.1146/annurev.publhealth.29.091307.083824

Chambers, D.A. (2023) Advancing adaptation of evidence-based interventions through implementation science: progress and opportunities. *Frontiers in Health Services* 3, 1204138. https://doi.org/10.3389/frhs.2023.1204138

Chen, E., Neta, G., Roberts, M.C. (2021). Complementary approaches to problem solving in healthcare and public health: implementation science and human-centered design. *Translational Behavioral Medicine* 11, 1115–1121. https://doi.org/10.1093/tbm/ibaa079

Currie, G., Kiefer, T., Spyridonidis, D. (2020) From what we know to what we do: enhancing absorptive capacity in translational health research. *BMJ Leader* 4, 18–20. https://doi.org/10.1136/leader-2019-000166

Damschroder, L.J., Knighton, A.J., Griese, E., Greene, S.M., Lozano, P., Kilbourne, et al. (2021) Recommendations for strengthening the role of embedded researchers to accelerate implementation in health systems: Findings from a state-of-the-art (SOTA) conference workgroup. *Healthcare* 8(Suppl 1), 100455. https://doi.org/10.1016/j.hjdsi.2020.100455

Danitz, S.B., Stirman, S.W., Grillo, A.R., Dichter, M.E., Driscoll, M., Gerber, M.R., et al. (2019) When user-centered design meets implementation science: integrating provider perspectives in the development of an intimate partner violence intervention for women treated in the United States' largest integrated healthcare system. *BMC Women's Health* 19, 145. https://doi.org/10.1186/s12905-019-0837-8

Eccles, M.P., Mittman, B.S. (2006). Welcome to Implementation Science. *Implementation Science* 1, 1. https://doi.org/10.1186/1748-5908-1-1

Esmail, R., Hanson, H.M., Holroyd-Leduc, J., Brown, S., Strifler, L., Straus, S.E., et al. (2020) A scoping review of full-spectrum knowledge translation theories, models, and frameworks. *Implementation Science* 15, 11. https://doi.org/10.1186/s13012-020-0964-5

Glasgow, R.E., Harden, S.M., Gaglio, B., Rabin, B., Smith, M.L., Porter, G.C., et al. (2019) RE-AIM planning and evaluation framework: adapting to new science and practice with a 20-year review. *Frontiers in Public Health* 7, 64. https://doi.org/10.3389/fpubh.2019.00064

Grimshaw, J.M., Ivers, N., Linklater, S., Foy, R., Francis, J.J., Gude, W.T., et al. (2019) Reinvigorating stagnant science: implementation laboratories and a meta-laboratory to efficiently advance the science of audit and feedback. *BMJ Quality & Safety* 28, 416–423. https://doi.org/10.1136/bmjqs-2018-008355

Kislov, R., Pope, C., Martin, G.P., Wilson, P.M. (2019) Harnessing the power of theorising in implementation science. *Implementation Science* 14, 103. https://doi.org/10.1186/s13012-019-0957-4

Lamont, T. (2016). Seize the day or the decision maker-making research count. Retrieved from https://blogs.bmj.com/bmj/2016/12/14/tara-lamont-seize-the-day-or-the-decision-maker-making-research-count (accessed 12 July 2023).

Moore, J.E., Khan, S. (2023) Promises and pitfalls of bridging the implementation science to practice gap from the perspective of implementation practitioners. Retrieved from https://thecenterforimplementation.com/toolbox/white-paper-promises-and-pitfalls (accessed 13 August 2023).

Moullin, J.C., Dickson, K.S., Stadnick, N.A., Albers, B., Nilsen, P., Broder-Fingert, S., et al. (2020) Ten recommendations for using implementation frameworks in research and practice. *Implementation Science Communications* 1, 42. https://doi.org/10.1186/s43058-020-00023-7

National Council for Mental Wellbeing (2023) Evidence-based practice implementation science pilot. Retrieved from www.thenationalcouncil.org/program/ccbhc-e-national-training-and-technical-assistance-center/ccbhc-ebp-implementation-science-pilot/?mc_cid=f9748d40f3&mc_eid=53caf25579 (accessed 17 July 2023).

Nilsen, P. (2015). Making sense of implementation theories, models and frameworks. *Implementation Science* 10, 53. https://doi.org/10.1186/s13012-015-0242-0

Nilsen, P., Bernhardsson, S. (2019) Context matters in implementation science: a scoping review of determinant frameworks that describe contextual determinants for implementation outcomes. *BMC Health Services Research* 19, 189. https://doi.org/10.1186/s12913-019-4015-3

Nilsen, P., Nordström, G., Ellström, P.E. (2012) Integrating research-based and practice-based knowledge through workplace reflection. *Journal of Workplace Learning* 24, 403–415. https://doi.org/10.1108/13665621211250306

Nilsen, P., Thor, J., Bender, M., Leeman, J., Andersson-Gäre, B., Sevdalis, N. (2022) Bridging the silos: a comparative analysis of implementation science and improvement science. *Frontiers in Health Services* 1, 817750. https://doi.org/10.3389/frhs.2021.817750

Pellecchia, M., Mandell, D.S., Nuske, H.J., Azad, G., Benjamin Wolk, C., Maddox, B.B., et al. (2018) Community-academic partnerships in implementation research. *Journal of Community Psychology* 46, 941–952. https://doi.org/10.1002/jcop.21981

Rapport, F., Smith, J., Hutchinson, K., Clay-Williams, R., Churruca, K., Bierbaum, M., et al. (2021) Too much theory and not enough practice? The challenge of implementation science application in healthcare practice. *Journal of Evaluation in Clinical Practice* 28, 991–1002. https://doi.org/10.1111/jep.13600

Reidpath, D.D., Allotey, P. (2019) The problem of 'trickle-down science' from the Global North to the Global South. *BMJ Global Health* 4, e001719. https://doi.org/10.1136/bmjgh-2019-001719

Ridde, V., Pérez, D., Robert, E. (2020) Using implementation science theories and frameworks in global health. *BMJ Global Health* 5, e002269. https://doi.org/10.1136/bmjgh-2019-002269

Rowland, D., Thorley, M., Brauckmann, N. (2023) The most successful approaches to leading organizational change. Retrieved from https://hbr.org/2023/04/the-most-successful-approaches-to-leading-organizational-change (accessed 15 July 2023).

Shelton, R.C., Adsul, P., Oh, A., Moise, N., Griffith, D.M. (2021) Application of an antiracism lens in the field of implementation science (IS): recommendations for reframing implementation research with a focus on justice and racial equity. *Implementation Research and Practice* 2, 26334895211049482. https://doi.org/10.1177/26334895211049482

Stange, K.C. (2020). Commentary: RE-AIM planning and evaluation framework: adapting to new science and practice with a 20-year review. *Frontiers in Public Health* 8, 245. https://doi.org/10.3389/fpubh.2020.00245

Strosahl, K.D., Robinson, P.J. (2018) Adapting empirically supported treatments in the era of integrated care: a roadmap for success. *Clinical Psychology: Science and Practice* 25, e12246. https://doi.org/10.1111/cpsp.12246

Tabak, R.G., Khoong, E.C., Chambers, D.A., Brownson, R.C. (2012) Bridging research and practice: models for dissemination and implementation research. *American Journal of Preventive Medicine* 43, 337–350. https://doi.org/10.1016/j.amepre.2012.05.024

Vargas, C., Whelan, J., Brimblecombe, J., Allender, S. (2022) Co-creation, co-design, co-production for public health – a perspective on definition and distinctions. *Public Health Research & Practice* 32, 3222211. https://doi.org/10.17061/phrp3222211

Wallerstein, N., Duran, B. (2010) Community-based participatory research contributions to intervention research: the intersection of science and practice to improve health equity. *American Journal of Public Health* 100(Suppl 1), S40–S46. https://doi.org/10.2105/AJPH.2009.184036

Wandersman, A., Duffy, J., Flaspohler, P., Noonan, R., Lubell, K., Stillman, L., et al. (2008) Bridging the gap between prevention research and practice: the interactive systems framework for dissemination and implementation. *American Journal of Community Psychology* 41, 171–181. https://doi.org/10.1007/s10464-008-9174-z

Wensing, M., Grol, R. (2019) Knowledge translation in health: how implementation science could contribute more. *BMC Medicine* 17, 88. https://doi.org/10.1186/s12916-019-1322-9

Wensing, M., Sales, A., Armstrong, R., Wilson, P. (2020) Implementation science in times of Covid-19. *Implementation Science* 15, 42. https://doi.org/10.1186/s13012-020-01006-x

Westerlund, A., Sundberg, L., Nilsen, P. (2019) Implementation of implementation science knowledge: the research-practice gap paradox. *Worldviews on Evidence-Based Nursing* 16, 332–334. https://doi.org/10.1111/wvn.12403

Index

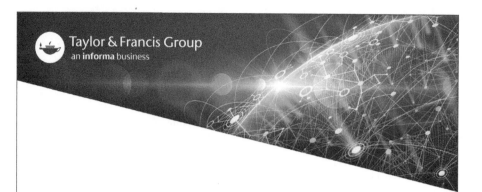

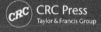